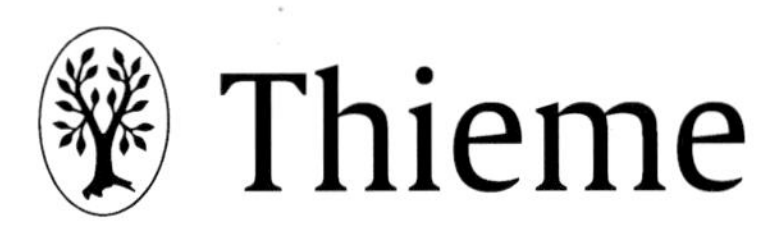
Thieme

Infections in Obstetrics and Gynecology

Textbook and Atlas

Eiko E. Petersen, M.D.
Professor
Gynecologic Clinic
University Hospital
Freiburg, Germany

255 illustrations

Thieme
Stuttgart · New York

Library of Congress Cataloging-in-Publication Data is available from the publisher.

This book is an authorized and revised translation of the 4th German edition published and copyrighted 2003 by Georg Thieme Verlag, Stuttgart, Germany. Title of the German edition: Infektionen in Gynäkologie und Geburtshilfe. Lehrbuch und Atlas

1st German edition 1988
2nd German edition 1994
3rd German edition 1997
4th German edition 2003

Translator: Ursula Vielkind, Ph.D., C.Tran., Dundas, Canada

Illustrators: Christiane and Dr. Michael von Solodkoff, Neckargemünd, Germany

Important note: Medicine is an ever-changing science undergoing continual development. Research and clinical experience are continually expanding our knowledge, in particular our knowledge of proper treatment and drug therapy. Insofar as this book mentions any dosage or application, readers may rest assured that the authors, editors, and publishers have made every effort to ensure that such references are in accordance with **the state of knowledge at the time of production of the book.**

Nevertheless, this does not involve, imply, or express any guarantee or responsibility on the part of the publishers in respect to any dosage instructions and forms of applications stated in the book. **Every user is requested to examine carefully** the manufacturers' leaflets accompanying each drug and to check, if necessary in consultation with a physician or specialist, whether the dosage schedules mentioned therein or the contraindications stated by the manufacturers differ from the statements made in the present book. Such examination is particularly important with drugs that are either rarely used or have been newly released on the market. Every dosage schedule or every form of application used is entirely at the user's own risk and responsibility. The authors and publishers request every user to report to the publishers any discrepancies or inaccuracies noticed. If errors in this work are found after publication, errata will be posted at www.thieme.com on the product description page.

Rüdigerstrasse 14, 70469 Stuttgart, Germany
http://www.thieme.de
Thieme New York, 333 Seventh Avenue,
New York, NY 10001 USA
http://www.thieme.com

Typesetting by primustype Hurler GmbH, Notzingen
Printed in Germany by Karl Grammlich GmbH, Pliezhausen

ISBN 3-13-139811-6 (GTV)
ISBN 1-58890-421-0 (TNY) 1 2 3 4 5 6

Acknowledgment

I would like to take this opportunity to thank my wife, Dagmar, for her sound advice and creative competence, always supporting and encouraging me during all these years, especially while writing this book.

In addition, I would like to thank all of my colleagues who were turning to me with their questions and who trusted me to treat their problem patients. We have been learning a lot together and from each other and, without them, this book would not have become what it is.

Foreword

Since the middle of the 19th century, the fight against infections has been crucial in advancing gynecology and obstetrics. Today, it is hard to imagine the suffering associated with the epidemics of childbed fever in the obstetric hospitals of those days. Ignaz Philipp Semmelweis, a 29-year-old assistant physician at the first maternity hospital in Vienna, Austria, was among the pioneers who—based on observation and with great courage—paved the long and difficult path leading to today's sophisticated diagnostic and therapeutic options. We easily forget that the battle against infections has led us to extraordinary achievements in obstetrics as well as medicine in general. Development of modern surgery would be unthinkable without these successes.

During the course of the 19th century, infectiology in the widest sense developed into a conventional scientific field that gave rise to important findings and impulses for gynecology and obstetrics also. Problems surfaced that were specific for the field, such as in the field of bacteriology of the natural vaginal flora, infections in the genital region with consequences like severe dysfunctions of female reproduction, and obstetric infections with consequences for mother and child.

Even today, infectiology confronts us constantly with new and unexpected problems that are often of vital importance. Such grave viral diseases are still escaping effective therapeutic interventions. Intense scientific attention to infectious diseases is therefore absolutely essential in gynecology and obstetrics, and this includes close cooperation with the appropriate theoretic disciplines, on the one hand, and specialists within the discipline who are most familiar with the specific problems, on the other.

For many years, Eiko E. Petersen has been one of those specialists and has proved himself through systematic, clinical research in gynecologic infectiology. The present monograph originated from his experience as a physician and researcher. In the General Section, the book provides an overview of the current state of infectiology as a whole, with special reference to specific features of the discipline. The extensive Special Section covers the complete range of infection-related questions and problems in gynecology. The book fills a gap in the textbook domain at the right point in time. Not only does it provide information and will thus become an indispensable guide; it will also directly influence the quality of our actions because of its practice-oriented layout. I sincerely hope that this textbook will reach a wide distribution among fellow specialists.

Josef Zander, M.D., M.D. h.c.
Professor Emeritus of Gynecology and Obstetrics
University of Munich
Munich, Germany

Foreword

The diagnosis of specific and, in particular, nonspecific infections in gynecology is, even today, far more difficult than it seems. Cultivation of specific microorganisms from the vulvovaginal region is still difficult and labor- and cost-intensive, and the pathogenesis of many microorganisms is still not clearly understood.

The author's attempt to give gynecologists some insight into this field of diagnosis, but also into the problems of the manifold questions of infectiology and chemotherapy should be applauded in every respect.

Dr. Petersen is one of a few gynecologists who have long-term experience in the fields of microbiology and virology. This is clearly apparent from the General Section. I find this part especially worth reading, not just for the gynecologist but also for every physician in practice.

Current knowledge on the multitude of old and new infections is clearly structured and extremely well illustrated. As a result, the book is no doubt an important reference material for the attending physician. Moreover, the book makes it clear that the field of infectiology is, first, a matter of knowledge.

Hans Knothe, M.D.
Professor Emeritus of Hygiene and Microbiology
Johann Wolfgang Goethe University
Frankfurt am Main, Germany

Preface

Infectiology continues to change. The awareness of infections has noticeably increased in recent years. There is hardly a headline more disturbing than that about a disease that has recently been discovered but is not yet treatable. The incidence and implications of pathogens are changing. The large number of publications and books in this field provides evidence for the increasing interest.

However, it is evident that the perspectives are changing as well, one example being the realization that pathogens sometimes found in the genital region are often overrated. Not every inflammation is always the result of an infection, and many infections of the external genital region cannot be cured in the long term by anti-infectants alone. The infections that bring patients to us today are rarely caused by true pathogens. The majority of infections are caused by microorganisms that do normally not harm us, thanks to our immune system. Many of these microorganisms colonize us for life, or we pick them up temporarily from the environment. Hence, it is not so much the individual pathogen but the host's condition and reaction to the pathogen that lead to infection and inflammation.

Damage to our immune system by wasting diseases like cancer, by chemotherapy, or extensive surgery turn our own flora into a risk factor. However, the individual genetic make-up of a person is also a reason why some people are more susceptible than others. Paying attention to the patient's history is therefore central to good medical care. In addition, resistant pathogens are increasingly spreading in hospitals and seniors' homes. Genetically determined forms of mild, partial immunodeficiencies—which are being increasingly diagnosed—explain some, so far unclear, recurrent infections that are as dangerous as they are annoying.

Clinical assessment has top priority: a patient rarely presents with a known pathogen but rather with complaints and symptoms, and different pathogens may cause very similar clinical pictures. To start with, it is not the detection of the pathogen but the evaluation and assessment of the patient's condition and symptoms that are most important. For this reason, the diseases caused by various pathogens are compared with one another in detail. In particular, the use of photographs helps to illustrate differences between infections, and their similarities, much faster and more permanently than a long text. The original concept of this book—namely, to provide the attending physician with quick information about infections and about the practical aspects arising from them—remains unchanged, even though the range of pathogens and infections has clearly expanded.

In cases of severe, life-threatening infections, particularly those caused by group A streptococci; the recognition of early symptoms is decisive for the prospect of healing. When the clinical presentation is not clear, only the knowledge and identification of the symptoms will lead to the appropriate laboratory tests and to a timely, correct, and therefore sometimes life-saving antibiotic treatment.

Described in greater detail are other causes of complaints in the external genital region, such as skin lesions and dermatoses. Only a few pathogens induce serious infections in the region of the vulva. In this sensitive region, which is richly colonized by bacteria, some infections and many problems result from skin lesions and incorrect skin care. Overrating some bacteria detected in cultures from the vulval region will only burden the patient and cause unnecessary costs.

If it rains into my house, I do not fight the rain but take care of my roof. Applied to the genital region, this means that I need to improve the normal flora (lactobacilli) of the vagina in order to prevent disturbances, and that I take care of the epithelium of the vulval and perianal region. As in previous editions, this book addresses many of my colleagues' questions regarding problems in their daily practice. Such questions still reach me daily, thanks to a trustful and loyal collaboration.

Eiko E. Petersen

Contents

I General

II Infections and Prevention

I General

1 Pathogens

Normal Flora and Virulence

Of the many millions of existing microorganisms, only a few hundreds are capable of causing disease in humans. The number of pathogens relevant for gynecologists is probably far below a hundred.

Many bacteria coexist with humans on good terms. These "friendly" bacteria belong to the normal flora present in the intestinal tract and on the skin and mucosae, where they perform functions that are partly beneficial and essential.

This is different with viruses. If detected, viruses are always pathologically significant. So far, no benefits to humans have been recognized.

Nevertheless, the majority of people are colonized by some viruses throughout life, e. g., with herpesviruses or papillomaviruses.

Whether or not an infection occurs depends, among other things, on the virulence of the individual pathogen. This refers to the degree of pathogenicity (the capacity to cause infections and inflammation). First, the pathogen must be able to invade the organism—or, in the case of viruses, to invade the cells in which to multiply—and, second, it must be able to cause disease. The property of virulence is developed differently in different pathogenic species, even in individual strains (for example, not every *Escherichia coli* strain has the same virulence).

Virulence factors include adhesion properties and the production of certain enzymes (neuraminidases, proteases, mucopolysaccharidases, streptokinases, coagulases, DNases, etc.) that are also called toxins (exotoxins, endotoxins).

The more virulent a pathogen, the less often is it detected as a colonizing germ ("normal flora"), and vice versa.

There are four different types of pathogens:

- viruses
- bacteria
- fungi
- protozoa.

Viruses

These are the smallest pathogens. A virus particle (virion) consists of genetic information (either DNA or RNA) and a protein shell (capsid). Some viruses contain additional enzymes that are required for starting the cycle of viral replication within the infected cell. For example, the herpes simplex virus (HSV) contains thymidine kinase, and the human immunodeficiency virus (HIV) contains reverse transcriptase. It is the presence of these enzymes that provides us with an opportunity for developing and using virus-specific chemotherapeutic agents.

Some viruses also possess an envelope made up of lipoproteins. For the most part, this envelope is derived from the cell in which the virus has multiplied (host cell), and the specific viral antigens have become integrated into it. Because of this envelope, these viruses (HSV, hepatitis B virus, rubella virus, HIV) are very sensitive to environmental influences, such as desiccation, alcohol-containing solvents, etc.

The structures and sizes of individual viruses are shown in Fig. **1.1**.

Viruses do not have a metabolism of their own and thus depend on the enzyme systems of their host cell for replication (obligatory cell parasites).

Certain viruses can only infect cells that express the appropriate receptors (tropism); for example, HIV infects T4 lymphocytes and cells of the central nervous system, while the hepatitis B virus infects liver cells.

The host cell is normally destroyed after viral replication (lytic cycle). With certain viruses, however, the virus may also transform its host and thus gives rise to a neoplastic cell (oncogenic viruses). Certain viruses have the capacity to remain in the cell as episomes that may later result in an endogenous infection (reactivation of the virus). Especially, herpesviruses and papillomaviruses have a tendency to do this.

Viruses are usually identified by immunological methods. Because they are so small, special procedures are required to make the reaction visible (neutralization, complement fixation, hemagglutination, fluorescence test, ELISA, PCR).

Bacteria

Characteristic Features and Staining Properties

Bacteria are the smallest pathogens with a metabolism of their own and thus can multiply on nonliving substrates. Bacteria are superficial parasites with only a few exceptions (e. g., chlamydiae, listeriae, tubercle bacilli).

Bacteria vary considerably in size, shape, and pathogenic properties.

Normally, they can be stained and viewed under a microscope. However, this does not apply, for example, to mycoplasma, which cannot be stained because they lack a solid cell wall and are highly pleomorphic. It applies only partly to chlamydiae, which can multiply only within a host cell.

A common feature of all bacteria is that they possess DNA, RNA, and ribosomes for protein synthesis. Due to their own enzymatic metabolism, all bacteria can be killed by antibiotic and chemotherapeutic agents, or their reproduction can, at least, be inhibited.

In addition to their shape, Gram staining is an important criterion for distinguishing bacteria under the microscope.

Gram-positive Bacteria

They possess a thick, relatively rigid cell wall consisting mainly of murein (peptidoglycan), which is usually covalently bound to teichoic acid. Most gram-positive bacteria are sensitive to penicillins, with the exception of penicillinase-producing staphylococci.

Gram-negative Bacteria

The cell walls of these bacteria are less thick but multilayered. The peptidoglycan portion is less than 10%. Instead, the cell wall also contains lipopolysaccharides and lipoproteins.

The shape of gram-negative bacteria is extremely variable, ranging from very small anaerobic gram-negative cocci (*Veillonella*) and small rods (*Mobiluncus*) to forms of variable length, such as fusobacteria.

Treatment of gram-negative bacteria is rather difficult because they have various mechanisms of resistance (primary resistance, plasmids, β-lactamases).

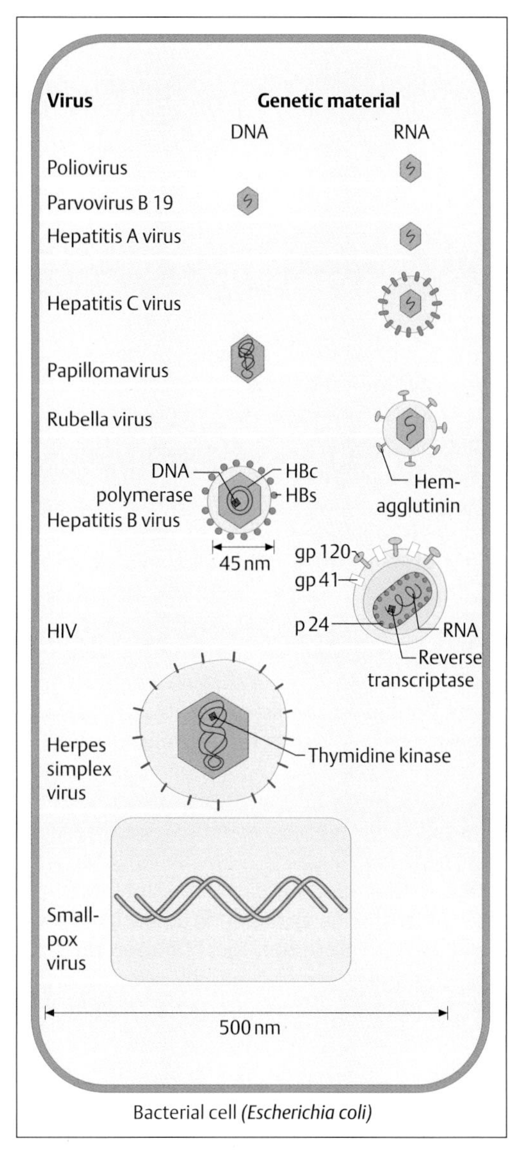

Fig. 1.**1** Schematic illustration of viruses, showing their sizes in comparison with each other and with a bacterium (*Escherichia coli*). In part, structures are pointed out that are important for understanding either the diagnostic procedures (antigens) or the therapeutic approaches (enzymes).

Aerobic Bacteria

Other distinguishing characteristics of bacteria are their growth requirements. We distinguish between aerobic and anaerobic bacteria.

Aerobic bacteria grow well in the presence of molecular oxygen, whereas anaerobic bacteria multiply only in the absence (< 1%) of oxygen. With few exceptions (e. g., pseudomonads) the majority of aerobic bacteria also grow well or, even better, in an anaerobic atmosphere; they are therefore called facultative anaerobes. True anaerobes grow only in an oxygenfree atmosphere and are therefore referred to as obligatory anaerobes. There are also transitional forms.

Aerobic bacteria are the most common pathogens, and they most often cause acute infections.

Anaerobic Bacteria

By contrast, anaerobes rather cause abscess-forming, less rapidly developing infections in soft tissues and in the abdominal region. They originate from the intestine, where synergy plays an important role.

Bacteria are usually identified by their growth requirements (substrates), colony shape on agar, metabolic functions, and microscopy. Other possible methods of distinction include antibiotic sensitivity tests, immunological methods, bacteriophage typing, biochemical analysis of the cell wall, and gas chromatography.

The doubling times of most bacteria lies between 20 and 60 minutes. It is longer for some bacteria (e. g., 24 hours for *Treponema pallidum* and for mycobacteria, and even 48 hours for chlamydiae), which explains why some infections take a slower course and require long-term treatment.

The most important bacteria occurring in the gynecologic region are listed in Table 1.**1** according to their staining properties (Gram stain), their shape, and their growth requirements (aerobic vs. anaerobic).

Fungi

We distinguish yeasts (blastomycetes), mycelial fungi (hyphomycetes), and molds.

Yeasts (blastomycetes):

- *Candida* species (some of them form pseudomycelia) (Tables 1.**2**, 1.**3**)
- *Malassezia furfur* (causing pityriasis versicolor)
- *Saccharomyces.*

Mycelial fungi (hyphomycetes with real ramifications), e. g., dermatophytes:

- *Trichophyton rubrum*
- *Epidermophyton floccosum*
- *Microsporum* species.

Molds:

- *Apergillus* species.

The most relevant fungi for the gynecologist are yeasts and, among them, in particular *Candida albicans. Candida* cells are approximately five to 10 times larger than the average bacterium (Fig. 1.**2**). Reproduction occurs by budding, a feature that makes yeasts easy to recognize under the microscope.

Clinical infections with *Candida* are usually associated with yeast hyphens, i.e., pseudomycelia consisting of single elongated yeast cells. They exhibit enzymatic activities at the growing tip, and this allows them to penetrate into the deeper layers of the tissue (see Fig. 7.**12**, p. 73) where they bring about inflammatory reactions.

In gynecology, we are dealing only with opportunistic fungi, i.e., with pathogens that colonize the intestinal tract of up to half of the human population and cause infections and symptoms only when the body's defenses are weakened, when antibiotics have been administered, or due to other reasons that we do not know in detail.

With the exception of flucytosine, antimycotic agents inhibit cell membrane synthesis in yeasts by disturbing the metabolism of ergosterol, through inhibition of the enzyme cytochrome P450.

Protozoa

Protozoa are unicellular organisms of the animal kingdom. They possess a typical cell nucleus, and are therefore eukaryotes. They cause various infections, such as malaria, sleeping sickness, leishmaniasis, amebic dysentery, toxoplasmosis, pneumocystosis, and giardiasis.

Trichomoniasis plays the most important role in gynecology. However, other diseases caused by protozoa may become a problem during pregnancy, for example, toxoplasmosis.

In the wake of AIDS, pneumonia caused by *Pneumocystis carinii* has increased in frequency.

Normal Flora

Vagina

Lactobacilli

In the vagina, only lactobacilli are regarded as a normal flora with high bacterial counts. Reproduction of lactobacilli and selective colonization of the vagina with these germs depends on estrogen levels. Lactobacilli are therefore found during the first weeks after childbirth and then

Table 1.**1** List of gynecologically relevant bacteria

Gram stain	Bacterial species	Commensal occurrence			Significance in gynecology and obstetrics
		Vagina	Skin	Feces	
○	*Acinetobacter anitratus*	–	–	(+)	Rare in complicated chronic urinary tract infection
●	*Actinomyces*	(+)	–	(+)	Unknown, rare in abscesses
○ A	*Bacteroides fragilis/* **Taxonomy According to** "Dorland's" and "Medizinische Mikrobiologie" (Thieme) **p. 311**, *Porphyromonas asaccharolyticus, Prevotella melaninogenicus/bivius*	+	–	+++	Odor! Involved in bacterial vaginosis, abscesses, endometritis, sepsis
○	*Campylobacter fetus/ jejuni*	–	–	(+)	Rare, sepsis during pregnancy with stillbirth, enteritis
X	*Chlamydia trachomatis*	–	–	–	Sexual transmission, cervicitis, pelvic inflammatory disease
○	*Citrobacter diversus/ freundii*	–	–	+	Rare, urinary tract infection
● A	*Clostridium perfringens/difficile*	– –	– –	++	Pathogen of gas gangrene—pseudomembranous colitis
	Enterobacter cloacae	–	–	++	Problematic pathogen, rare in complicated urinary tract infections
●	Enterococci (streptococci of group D)	+	+	++	Commonly detected pathogen, urinary tract infection
○	*Escherichia coli*	+	(+)	++	Urinary tract infections, soft tissue infections, sepsis, infections of newborns
○	*Eubacterium*	(+)	–	+++	None
○ A	*Fusobacterium nucleatum*	(+)	–	+	Odor! Involved in abscess-forming necrotic infections, bacterial vaginosis
◐	*Gardnerella vaginalis*	++	–	++	Bacterial vaginosis, detected in many infections, significance not clear
○	Gonococci *(Neisseria gonorrhoeae)*	–	–	–	Sexual transmission, definite pathogen, pelvic inflammatory disease
○	*Haemophilus ducreyi*	–	–	–	Sexual transmission, pathogen of soft ulcer (chancroid)
○	*Haemophilus influenzae*	–	–	–	Rare, infection of the child during birth
◐	*Haemophilus vaginalis (Gardnerella vaginalis)*	++	–	++	see above
○	*Klebsiella pneumoniae/ oxytoca*	(+)	–	+	Common after ampicillin therapy, urinary tract infection, soft tissue infection, sepsis
●	Lactobacilli	+++	–	+++	Normal flora of the vagina
●	*Listeria monocytogenes*	–	–	(+)	Listeriosis due to dairy products, especially during pregnancy
○ A	*Mobiluncus*	(+)	–	++	Common in bacterial vaginosis (Fig. 1.**2**)
X	*Mycobacterium tuberculosis*	–	–	–	Rare, genital tuberculosis
X	*Mycoplasma hominis, Ureaplasma urealyticum*	(+)+	––	++	Common pathogen without a firm cell wall, infections are rare

Table 1.**1** (Cont.)

Gram stain	Bacterial species	Commensal occurrence Vagina	Skin	Feces	Significance in gynecology and obstetrics
●	*Neisseria gonorrhoeae* (gonococci)	–	–	–	See gonococci (above)
●	Pneumococci	–	–	–	Rare, sepsis, pneumonia
● A	Peptococci	(+)	–	+++	Involved in bacterial vaginosis, abscesses, endometritis, wound infections
● A	Propionibacteria	(+)	++	(+)	Acne
●	*Proteus mirabilis/vulgaris/rettgeri*	(+)	(+)	++	Common in urinary tract infections, commonly isolated also in soft tissue infections
●	*Pseudomonas aeruginosa/cepacia*	–	–	+	Problematic pathogen, multiresistant, in inpatients, urinary tract infection, sepsis
●	*Salmonella*	–	–	(+)	Rare, typhoid fever, diarrhea
●	*Serratia*	–	–	+	Rare, urinary tract infection, multiresistant
●	*Shigella*	–	–	(+)	Rare, diarrhea, risk of infection during childbirth
●	Streptococci of Lancefield group A (β-hemolysis)	–	–	(+)	Rare, most dangerous pathogen in the genitals, puerperal sepsis, postoperative sepsis, scarlet fever, phlegmon, not uncommon in the nasopharyngeal cavity
●	Streptococci of group B (*S. agalactiae*) (β-hemolysis)	+	(+)	++	Feared during delivery because of risk of infecting the newborn
●	Streptococci of group D *(S. enterococcus)*	+	+	++	Urinary tract infection, often found as an easily detectable germ, minor pathogenicity
●	Other streptococci	(+)	–	+	Soft tissue infections
●	*Staphylococcus aureus*	(+)	+	+	Common pathogen of infections, wound infection, sepsis, mastitis, abscess, toxic shock syndrome
●	*Staphylococcus epidermidis*	(+)	+	+	Urinary tract infection, wound infection, often only a contaminating germ
●	*Staphylococcus saprophyticus*	(+)	+	+	Cystitis
● A	*Mobiluncus*	+	–	++	Common in bacterial vaginosis
● A	*Veillonella parvula*	+	–	++	Common in bacterial vaginosis

● Gram-negative (red); ● gram-positive (blue); A, anaerobe; X, cannot be stained with Gram method

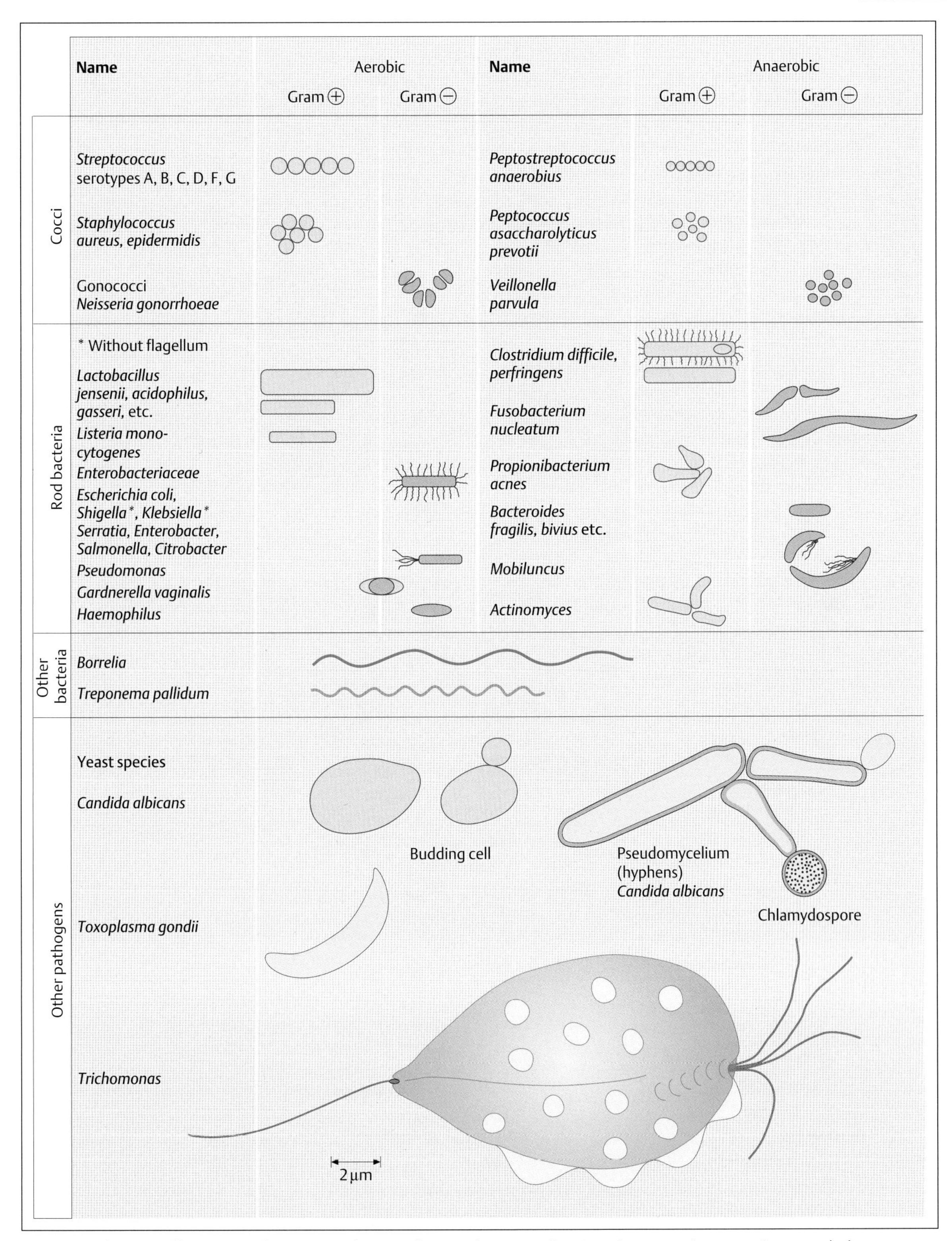

Fig. 1.2 Schematic illustration of various pathogens (bacterial species, fungi, and protozoa), comparing morphology and size. Even within some bacterial species, there may be considerable variation in morphology and size.

Table 1.**2** Occurrence and clinical significance of various yeast species

Candida species	Clinical significance	Morphology	Occurrence
Candida albicans	Most important and common (85 %) pathogen of genital fungal infections	Budding cells (large), form pseudomycelium and chlamydospores on rice agar	Humans, soil, vegetables, water, etc.
Candida glabrata (Torulopsis glabrata)	Second most common genital fungus (10–15 %) isolated, but rather harmless	Only budding, no ability to adhere	Symptoms questionable, therapeutically difficult to eliminate
Candida parapsilosis	Widespread in hospitals, also on skin, nails, genitals, heart	Budding cells (large, elongated), abundant pseudomycelium with clustered blastospores (rice agar)	Humans, environmental pathogen
Candida tropicalis	Widespread, virulence similar to that of *C. albicans*	Budding cells (large, oval), treelike pseudomycelium on rice agar	Humans, water, soil, fish, fruits, etc.
Candida pseudotropicalis (synonym: *C. kefyr*)	Can be isolated from clinical material, rather harmless	Budding cells (large, elongated), treelike pseudomycelium on rice agar	Dairy products, water, air
Candida krusei	Occasionally isolated from genitals, bronchi, nails, skin, intestinal tract	Budding cells (large, elongated), pseudomycelium with coronary blastospores on rice agar, resistant to fluconazole (Diflucan)	
Candida guilliermondii	Environmental germ (water, air, flowers, foods), occasionally important as a pathogen	Budding cells, thick pseudomycelium on rice agar	
Candida lusitaniae	Environmental germ, rarely causing systemic mycotic infections	Ascospores, pseudomycelium	
Candida famata	Similar to *Candida guilliermondii*		

Table 1.**3** Other fungal species, also for purposes of differential diagnosis

Fungal species	Characteristics
Trichophyton rubrum	The most common dermatophyte, a hyphomycete, pathogen of infections on dry skin
Saccharomyces cerevisiae	Brewer/baker yeast, nonpathogenic, only large, elongated budding cells
Geotrichum candidum	Mold fungus, harmless, occurs in feces due to dairy products etc., forms true septate, large mycelium with arthrospores (hockey sticks)
Rhodotorula rubra	Widespread in the environment, harmless, pink-red colonies, homogeneous budding cells, poorly developed pseudomycelium
Trichosporon cutaneum	Hyphomycete, considered opportunistic, infests hairs
Cryptococcus neoformans	Occurs in the soil, in AIDS patients: meningitis, lungs, abscesses
Aspergillus fumigatus	Mold fungus, common air contaminant, aspergilloma in case of immunosuppression (Fig. 7.**166**, p. 167)

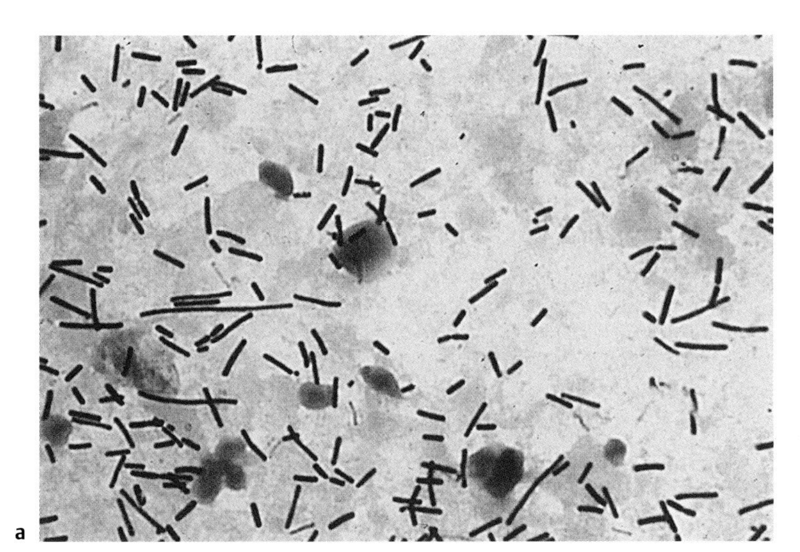

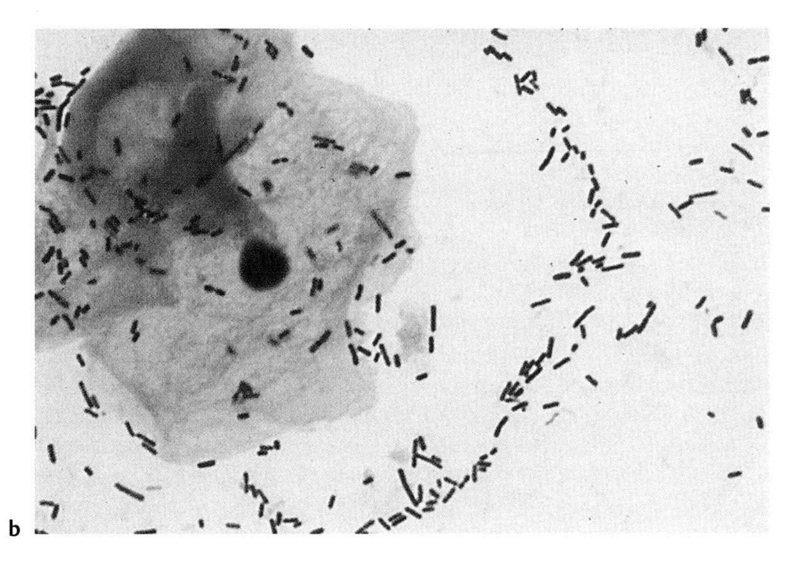

Fig. 1.**3** Normal vaginal flora stained using Gram method, showing (**a**) large lactobacilli (*Lactobacillus jensenii*) and (**b**) small lactobacilli (*Lactobacillus casei*).

again, when the ovaries regain activity, until menopause sets in. Even in old age, high concentrations of lactobacilli in the vagina can still be found in some women, e. g., in obese women who receive medications that have a certain estrogen effect.

During childhood, various skin pathogens—including those derived from the perianal region—are found in the vagina, with no specific pathogen dominating. With the onset of estrogen production, selective multiplication of lactobacilli takes place. These are then found at concentrations between 10^5 and 10^8 bacteria per mL.

The number of germs also depends on the menstrual cycle. Lower concentrations are found during menstruation and immediately thereafter, and the numbers rapidly increase again under the influence of estrogen. In addition, during pregnancy, the effect of estrogens can be easily observed: some women who have a disturbed vaginal flora at the beginning of the pregnancy develop a normal lactobacilli flora during the course of the first months.

Lactobacilli are a heterogenous group of large, gram-positive bacteria without a flagellum, and they produce lactic acid (Fig. 1.**3**). Over 50 different varieties are known. Lactobacilli are difficult to deal with in culture and in terms of identification. In addition, they are not pathogenic but belong to the normal flora. Because of this, they have not been studied extensively and are therefore not well understood.

About five to seven varieties predominate in humans. The most common form is *Lactobacillus jensenii*, followed by *Lactobacillus acidophilus*, *Lactobacillus gasseri*, *Lactobacillus fermenti*, and others. Frequently the vagina is colonized by two or more types simultaneously.

Tabelle 1.4 *Lactobacillus* species and hydrogen peroxide (H_2O_2) formation in women with normal flora and bacterial vaginosis (from Wenz, M.: Dissertation, Freiburg, Germany, 1993)

Number of women	Normal flora 59		Bacterial vaginosis Prior to therapy: 45		After therapy: 45	
	L. type	H_2O_2-positive	L. type	H_2O_2-positive	L. type	H_2O_2-positive
Lactobacillus acidophilus	6	6	3	2	17	15
Lactobacillus jensenii	40	35	3	3	5	5
Lactobacillus gasseri	10	10	1	1	0	–
Lactobacillus delbrueckii	2	1	1	1	1	1
Lactobacillus fermenti	1	1	0	–	4	4
Lactobacillus crispatus	0	–	2	1	1	0
Lactobacillus casei	0	–	0	–	2	1
Nontyped lactobacilli	3	2	0	–	4	4
Atypical lactobacilli	0	–	4	0	16	0
Number of *Lactobacillus* strains	62	55	14	8	50	30

Lactobacilli are largely responsible for the acidity of the vagina. They still grow in relatively acidic milieu, which they create for themselves by lactic acid production. In addition, many strains produce hydrogen peroxide, which is bactericidal especially for anaerobes and thus inhibits those pathogens.

It is not known to what extent colonization of the vagina with a specific strain remains stable in individual women and what effect individual strains have on the resistance of the vaginal flora against other intruding germs.

Preliminary studies have shown that colonization with certain lactobacilli strains, particularly with *Lactobacillus jensenii*, is more stable in women with a normal flora. By contrast, women with recurrent bacterial vaginosis (nonspecific vaginitis) seem to be colonized more by atypical lactobacilli strains, which are often identified only after treatment and which are unable to produce hydrogen peroxide (Table 1.4).

The different species of lactobacilli differ in their morphology:

- large lactobacilli: *Lactobacillus acidophilus, L. fermenti, L. delbrueckii*
- medium-sized lactobacilli: *Lactobacillus jensenii*
- small lactobacilli: *Lactobacillus brevis, L. casei, L. plantarum*
- curved lactobacilli: *Lactobacillus crispatus.*

In addition, lactobacilli can change their shape in culture. Therefore, the microscopic distinction between small lactobacilli and *Escherichia coli, Gardnerella vaginalis*, or even clostridia is often impossible, especially in methylene blue mounts. A normal flora can only be assumed present if the pH is below 4.5 and the microscopic appearance is normal.

Lactobacilli are sensitive to most broad-spectrum antibiotic agents, especially to those affecting gram-positive bacteria (e. g., penicillins, cephalosporins, tetracyclines, erythromycin, cotrimoxazole, etc.). No destruction of the lactobacilli flora is caused by 5-nitroimidazoles (metronidazole, ornidazole, tinidazole) and fluorquinolones.

Significance. Responsible for the acidic pH of the vagina and thus for the inhibition of facultative pathogens introduced into the vagina.

Stimulation. Estrogens, acidification of the vaginal milieu.

Inhibition. Antibiotics (see above), menstrual bleeding, antiseptic agents.

Lactobacillus preparations for treating vaginitis or bacterial vaginosis and restoring a normal vaginal flora are available on the market.

Lactobacillus preparations (such as Lactobacillus GG) are currently also used for treating diarrhea in children. It has been surmised that there is a connection between atopy in children and abnormal lactobacillus colonization during and after birth.

Tabelle 1.**5** Bacterial species often found in the vagina in addition to lactobacilli

Bacterial species	Incidence	Concentration
Gardnerella vaginalis	30–50 %	10^4–10^6/mL
Streptococci of group B	10–30 %	10^4–10^6/mL
Ureaplasma urealyticum	approx. 40 %	10^3–10^4/mL
Enterococci (streptococci of group D)	10–20 %	10^4–10^6/mL

Other Pathogens

Due to its position and function, the vagina is regularly contaminated with various pathogens derived from the skin, the perianal region, and the sexual partner (Table 1.**5**).

Normally, these pathogens remain at low concentrations (up to 10^4–10^5 germs/mL).

There are plenty of studies showing that between three and eight different germs can be detected even in the vagina of a healthy woman. The transition from a normal to a disturbed vaginal flora is blurred, and it is a question of definition as to what constitutes a normal flora.

Only the presence of high numbers of lactobacilli should be regarded as indicative of a normal vaginal flora. The detection of germs in the vagina without any indication of quantity is therefore useless for an evaluation. The only exceptions are definite pathogens, such as gonococci, streptococci of group A, and possibly *Staphylococcus aureus.*

Cervix

As a rule, germs that are found in the vagina can also be detected in the endocervix, though in lower numbers. There is no such thing as a normal flora of the cervix, and there is no easy answer to the question of whether pathogens detected in the cervix represent just contamination or a true colonization of the cervix.

The cervix represents an important barrier to the inner genitals. The stratified squamous epithelium of the ectocervix and the cervical secretion prevent or hamper the intrusion of pathogens.

By contrast, a large ectopia—the evagination of the single-layered columnar epithelium of the endocervix (Figs. 1.**4 a, b,** 1.**5 a–c**)—poses an increased risk of infection with certain sexually transmitted pathogens, e. g., chlamydiae, gonococci, hepatitis B viruses.

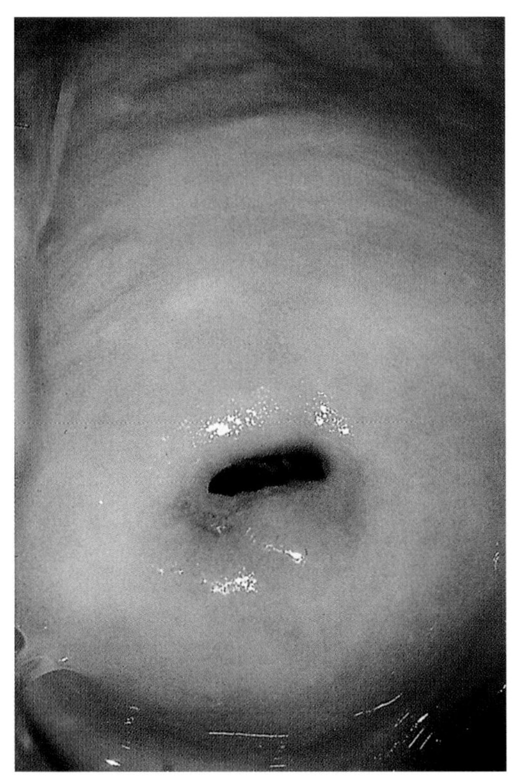

Fig. 1.**4 a** Portio without ectopia in a 28-year-old woman.

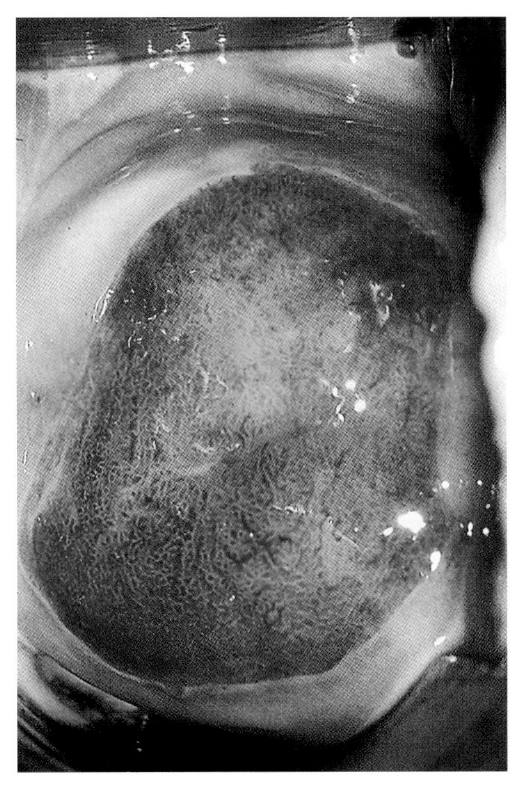

Fig. 1.**4 b** Portio with a large ectopia in an 18-year-old woman.

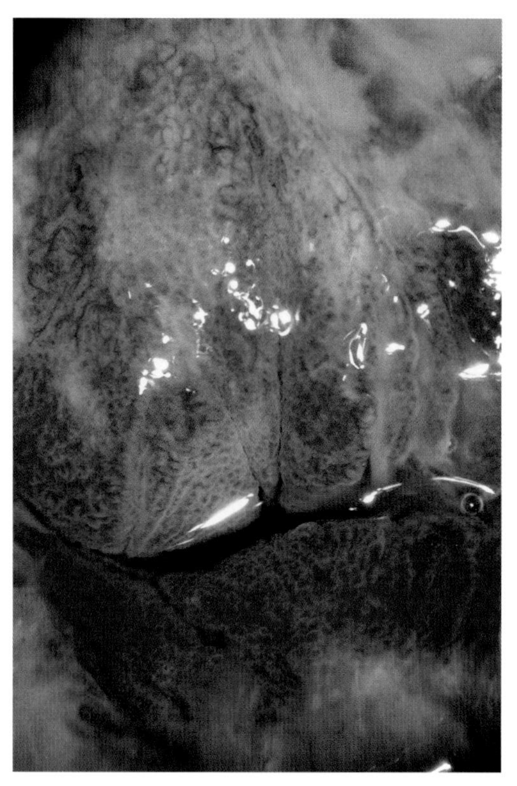

Fig. 1.**5 a** Large ectopia in a 24-year-old patient, mid-cycle.

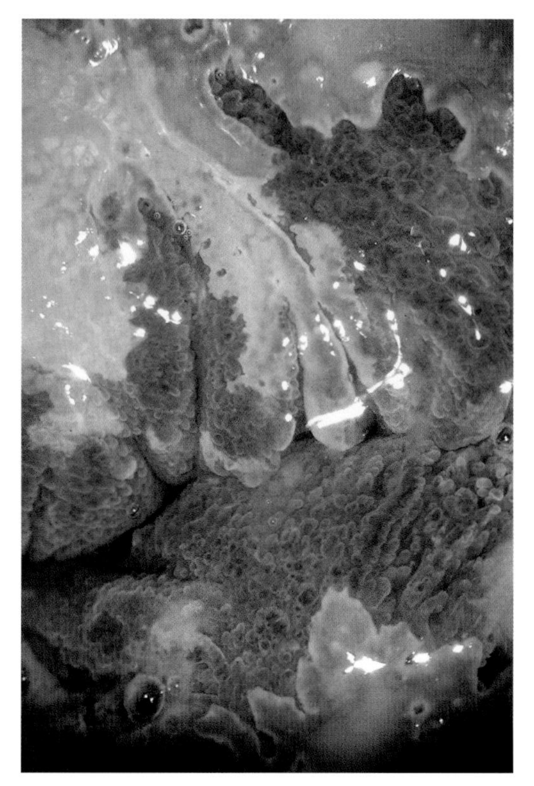

Fig. 1.**5 b** The same portio after treatment with 3% acetic acid.

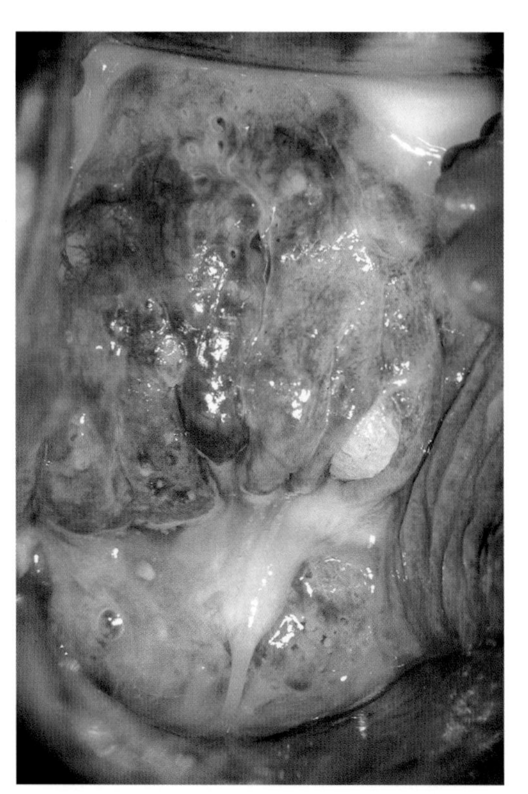

Fig. 1.**5 c** The same portio two years later during the 35th week of pregnancy.

Skin

Normally the skin is colonized by many different germs. The total number of bacteria on the entire skin is estimated to be at least 10^{12}.

A typical skin pathogen is *Staphylococcus epidermidis*. It is, therefore, often found as a contaminant in connection with punctures and swabs, and also in blood cultures. It can cause infections in some patients. Frequently, it is a pathogen of urinary tract infections, as is *Staphylococcus saprophyticus*.

Staphylococcus aureus, which may lead to wound infection or sepsis, is found in up to 30% of the human population on the skin and mucosal regions.

Other typical skin pathogens are propionibacteria, which play a role in acne.

Intestinal Tract

The concentration of bacteria colonizing the gastrointestinal tract increases from stomach to rectum, with the total number of germs reaching more than 10^{14} (Table 1.**6**).

Bacterial colonization of the gastrointestinal tract starts at birth. The first uptake of bacteria

Tabelle 1.**6** Bacteria in the gastrointestinal tract

Bacteria	Concentration
Stomach	$0–10^3$/mL
Jejunum	$0–10^5$/mL
Ileum	$10^3–10^9$/mL
Feces	$10^{10}–10^{12}$/mL

takes place from the flora of the mother's birth canal. Depending on the food uptake during the first weeks and months, different compositions of the intestinal flora will develop. Bifidobacteria predominate in breast-fed children. By the age of two, the intestinal flora of the child has changed to that of adults. Lactobacilli and other facultative anaerobes predominate in the small intestine, whereas anaerobic bacteria dominate in the rectum.

Bacteria perform multiple functions in the intestinal tract. For example, they synthesize vitamins in the colon, ferment food remnants, form a barrier against colonizing pathogens, and represent an important stimulus for the intestine-associated lymphatic tissue.

Early abnormal colonization of the intestinal tract is increasingly considered in connection with atopy and food allergies. An interesting question is whether an improvement in the vaginal flora of the mother during pregnancy would make atopy, and other consequences, less common in the child.

Over 500 different microorganisms are found in the intestinal tract. The germs predominating here are anaerobes (*Bacteroides* species, eubacteria, peptococci, peptostreptococci, clostridia, bifidobacteria).

Enterobacteriaceae (*Escherichia coli, Proteus, Klebsiella, Citrobacter*, and others) are also typical intestinal pathogens, although they represent only 3–10% of the intestinal flora.

Other aerobes are lactobacilli that colonize the vaginal flora, various species of *Streptococcus*, and various staphylococci.

Yeasts can be detected in the feces in approximately 30% of the population. They certainly represent the most common source of yeast colonization and infection in the genital region.

Of course, all these pathogens are also found at relatively high concentrations in the perianal region, from where they can get into the vagina. This is promoted through sexual contacts, wet bathing suits, and frequent soaking in warm water (thermal baths), a gaping vaginal entrance, and absence of a lactobacilli flora.

Also cleansing habits and skin care of the perianal region and vulva play a role that has not yet been sufficiently addressed. Excessive washing, use of unsuitable cleansing agents, and the lack of skin care by means of fatty creams result in desiccation and injury to the skin. Here, intestinal pathogens find favorable conditions and multiply extensively.

Oral Cavity

The oral cavity is colonized by large numbers of microorganisms of a mixed flora. A multitude of different pathogens can be detected here (streptococci, actinomycetes, various anaerobes, etc.). In the dental pockets, especially in cases of periodontitis, synergistic mixtures of bacteria are found that are similar to those of bacterial vaginosis.

In almost half of all adults, *Candida* is detected in the oral cavity and in the intestinal tract. The pathogens are taken up partly with food. From here they reach the intestinal tract. The stomach does not act as a barrier because yeasts are very acid stable. They can infect the genitals through the intestinal tract and anal region or by means of direct contact.

Due to the lower sensitivity of the oral cavity as compared with the vaginal entrance, some infections and abnormal colonization are more easily overlooked here than in the genital region. There are reports describing a connection between the intense bacterial colonization of the oral cavity in pregnant women, their intestinal bacteria, and an increased incidence of premature births.

The Importance of Individual Bacterial Species and Strains

Streptococci

Streptococci are chain-forming cocci and show a wide range of pathogenicity. They include aerobes, which are more important, and anaerobes, such as streptopeptococci.

Aerobic streptococci are classified according to serotype. There are streptococci of groups A, B, C, D, E, F, and G, and those belonging to the *milleri* group. Identification of these streptococci is quick and easy. Following cultivation, the serotype is immediately determined by a serological reaction.

The capacity for β-hemolysis is no indication of pathogenicity, but this property is of diagnostic value. For example, the streptococci of group A and group B are very different pathogens, but both are β-hemolytic.

Streptococci of group A (*Streptococcus pyogenes*) are the most dangerous bacteria in the genital region because they can cause rapidly developing, severe, life-threatening infections. They are the pathogens of puerperal sepsis. They are found in the naso-pharyngeal region in up to 5% of children and also in many adults. If detected in the genital region, the infection should always be treated. Penicillins and cephalosporins are especially effective.

Microbiology of Streptococci of Group A

These gram-positive bacteria are of spherical to ovoid shape and have a diameter of less than 2 µm. They form twisted chains of various lengths, hence their name.

In 1933, Lancefield subdivided the streptococci into 22 groups that differed from each other by a polysaccharide in their cell wall. They have been designated all the way through, from A to V.

The pus-forming *Streptococcus pyogenes* was first described by Rosenbach in 1884. It belongs to the group A streptococci. Because erythrocytes on agar plates containing sheep blood are completely hemolyzed by this bacterium, it belongs to the β-hemolytic streptococci—like the streptococci of group B. The bacteria possess borders (fimbriae) containing the M protein, one of the germ's over 80 different antigens that have been detected so far.

The M protein represents an important marker for typing the individual strains of *Streptococcus pyogenes*. It is a virulence factor because it inhibits phagocytosis. The fimbriae also contain lipoteichoic acid, which is responsible for the adherence of these streptococci to the human mucosa.

Strains of *Streptococcus pyogenes* that are involved in severe infections produce various exotoxins. Of these, exotoxins A and B are of special importance because they stimulate the production of tumor necrosis factors in human monocytes.

Other virulence factors are streptolysin O, streptolysin S, and hyaluronidase. It has been shown in experiments that streptolysin O is cardiotoxic and lethal. Hyaluronidase depolymerizes the extracellular substance hyaluronic acid and thus facilitates the invasion of germs into the tissue.

The virulence of the strains depends on their ability to produce various virulence factors in large quantities.

Thus, strains that are able to produce M protein and hyaluronidase show the highest virulence. Strains that cannot produce M protein are far less virulent. If neither M protein nor hyaluronidase is produced, virulence is very low; as a result these strains require extremely high counts in order to get an infection going.

Streptococci of group B (*Streptococcus agalactiae*) are present in the intestine—and thus also occur in the vagina—in approximately 20–30% of the human population. In isolated cases (1–3% of the newborns are infected, approximately 3% of which may have a lethal outcome), they induce severe neonatal infections (pneumonia, meningitis, sepsis). They are among the main pathogens causing severe neonatal infections.

Streptococci of group D (enterococci, *Enterococcus faecalis*) are part of the intestinal flora. These are relatively stable bacteria; they can often still be cultured when other bacteria have already died during transport. They are frequently detected in the genital region, although they are less important as pathogens and rather represent just colonizing germs. They are resistant to cephalosporins and are therefore found in increased numbers after cephalosporin therapy. The medication of choice for treating infections is amoxicillin.

Enterococcus faecium is occasionally found in the vaginal region and has been isolated from premature infants. Its pathogenic significance is unclear. Infections are difficult to treat because this pathogen—in contrast to *Enterococcus faecalis*—is resistant to most antibiotics, except for vancomycin.

Streptococci of group G are being increasingly identified. They are pathogenic, though not as dangerous as streptococci of group A, and should always regarded seriously if found in the genital region.

Streptococci of the milleri group (*Streptococcus intermedius*, *Streptococcus constellatus*, *Streptococcus anginosus*) are also part of the intestinal flora. They are found occasionally in abscesses. *Streptococcus anginosus* is also known as a pus-forming streptococcus. It is rare and only relevant in pure culture.

Streptococcus pneumoniae is ubiquitous; almost every second person carries pneumococci in the naso-pharyngeal region without showing symptoms. Pneumococci infections endanger splenectomized patients, the elderly, or other persons with a weakened immune system. The overall lethality of pneumococcal bacteremia is 30%, and 50% in persons over 60. Pneumococci now belong to the most common pathogens of severe pneumonia. People with an increased risk are the ones who profit most from vaccination.

In recent years, isolated deaths during pregnancy and after cesarean section (sepsis originating from the genitals) have been reported.

Staphylococci

Staphylococci are relatively large, cluster-forming cocci. However, this is just a morphological criterion. There are aerobic staphylococci as well as obligatory anaerobic ones, e. g., *Peptococcus.* The most important *Staphylococcus* species are the aerobic *S. aureus* and *S. epidermidis.* They, in turn, consist of subgroups and various strains with different properties. The main reservoir are humans, where these germs occur on the skin and hair, and particularly in the nose.

Staphylococcus aureus is one of the most important pathogens in humans. It causes a number of diseases. The various subspecies and strains are ubiquitous and can be detected on the skin and mucosae of many people, even in the absence of any signs of inflammation. Normally the inflammatory process is limited, because these bacteria produce **coagulase**, an important pathogenicity factor that restricts the formation of abscesses. Other typical inflammatory responses include folliculitis, wound infection, mastitis puerperalis, and conjunctivitis (also in newborns). Once the pathogen is present in the blood (bacteremia, sepsis), it spreads throughout the body and can infect various organs (even the brain or poorly vascularized regions), where it causes abscesses.

Individual strains (approximately 5 %) produce special toxins, e. g., TSST 1 and several other enterotoxins, and can induce toxic shock syndrome (TSS) (see p. 159).

About 30–50 % of *Staphylococcus aureus* strains isolated from outpatients, and 50–80 % of those isolated from hospitalized patients, produce β-lactamase and are therefore resistant to penicillins. This is why physicians should preferably prescribe cephalosporins if there is no antibiogram available.

A particular disease due to *Staphylococcus aureus* is food poisoning associated with fever, nausea, vomiting, and diarrhea. It is caused by heat-stable enterotoxins (primarily enterotoxins B and C). A prerequisite for food poisoning is a massive multiplication of pathogens in the food. Cooking does kill the pathogens, but it does not destroy the toxins. Antibiotics are ineffective in such cases.

MRSA strains (methicillin-resistant *Staphylococcus aureus* strains): Their pathogenicity does not differ from that of other *Staphylococcus aureus* strains, but they are responsive to treatment. They occur largely in intensive-care stations and increasingly in old people's homes, where they may also colonize the nursing staff.

They can be treated with teicoplanin (a glycopeptide), vancomycin, and the new antibiotic agent quinupristin–dalfopristin. Immunocompetence is essential for treatment.

Staphylococcus epidermidis (coagulase-negative staphylococcus) belongs to the normal flora of the skin, and this is why it is often detected in the genital region. Only in isolated cases are these cocci regarded as pathogens. Occasionally, they can be cultivated in blood cultures. They are not considered a colonizing germ of the skin, unless they are detected in two different blood cultures. (Blood samples should therefore always be taken from both arms or two different body regions.)

Enterobacteriaceae

This is a large group of gram-negative bacteria occurring in the intestinal tract. There are great differences with respect to pathogenicity and sensitivity to antibiotics not only between the various genera but also within a single genus or even species, such as *Escherichia coli.*

Escherichia coli (E. coli) is one of the most commonly detected bacteria in the genito-urinary region. However, this species consists of very different pathogenic strains. Because of their flagellum, these bacteria adhere especially well to the genitourinary epithelium, and are therefore the most common bacteria associated with cystitis. They are also frequently detected in the vagina, but rather as a colonizing germ derived from the anal region. They do not induce inflammatory reactions in the vagina. However, they may contribute to premature births and neonatal infections—this is why they should be reduced, as much as is possible, during pregnancy. *E. coli* may cause severe infections, or even sepsis, especially in cases of intestinal injuries or complicated urinary tract infections. Together with *Staphylococcus aureus*, *E. coli* belongs to the most common pathogens that can be detected in blood cultures. In the past, endotoxic shock, resulting from sepsis due to gram-negative bacteria, was much feared and probably also frequently observed. It is caused by the lipopolysaccharide of certain strains of *E. coli.*

The more normally found *E. coli* bacterium contributes especially to urinary tract infections, whereas special *E. coli* strains (serotypes) contribute to intestinal tract infections:

- ETEC stains (enterotoxinogenic *E. coli*) cause traveler's diarrhea, also known as Montezuma's revenge.
  Fluorquinolones are therefore much appreciated in cases of diarrhea when traveling in tropical countries.
- EHEC strains (enterohemorrhagic *E. coli*) are feared because of their association with acute bloody diarrhea and kidney damage; they may cause hemolytic uremic syndrome.

Klebsiella. Like *E. coli*, bacteria of the genus *Klebsiella* colonize the human gastrointestinal tract. Together with the genera ***Enterobacter*** and ***Serratia***, they form a special group (KES group) within the *Enterobacteriaceae*. In approx. 10% of healthy people, *Klebsiella* species (*K. pneumoniae* and the indole-positive *K. oxytoca*) are found in the intestinal tract and in the upper respiratory tract, but less often in the vagina. In addition, *Klebsiella* species also occur in the soil, in water, and on plants. Hence, they can colonize a person repeatedly (e. g., through person-to-person contact, but also through food, humidifiers in air conditioners, etc.). In immunocompetent individuals, *Klebsiella* causes predominantly respiratory tract infections and urinary tract infections. In people with a weakened immune system (immunosuppressed cancer patients), they may cause sepsis, meningitis, pneumonia, and urinary tract infections. They usually produce simple β-lactamases—this is why they are often found after penicillin treatment as the result of selection. Normally, they can be adequately treated with cephalosporins. If the selection pressure is high (inadequate antibiotic therapy), strains with extended β-lactamase activity and multiple resistances will be detected, as has been observed with pseudomonads.

Pseudomonas aeruginosa is ubiquitous, even in humans. It is found at 0–2% on the skin, 0–6% in the throat, and 2.6–24% in the feces of healthy people. Detection and colonization increase to 50% after long hospital stays. This pathogen also occurs in the food, on vegetables, in air conditioners and respiratory devices, etc. It produces extracellular polysaccharides (adherence mechanism), exotoxins, and proteases. It exhibits a natural, broad resistance to many antibiotics (e. g., many penicillins, cephalosporins, tetracyclines, and sulfonamides). In the presence of antibiotic treatment, it rapidly develops new types of resistance that are in part genetically stable. Hence, it is one of the most common pathogens originating in hospitals and responsible for approximately 20% of nosocomial infections. It is especially feared among immunosuppressed patients.

Effectiveness of the following antibiotics is limited: acylureidopenicillins (piperacillin), carbapenems (meropenem, imipenem), cephalosporins (among them, most likely ceftazidime), fluorquinolones (e. g., ciprofloxacin, levofloxacin, moxifloxacin), and aminoglycosides (gentamycin, amikacin, tobramycin). Combination therapy can slow down the rapid and intense development of resistances.

Salmonella. Bacteria of the genus *Salmonella* form a huge group with over 1000 varieties. They are the main pathogens of food poisoning, especially via eggs and chicken. Their pathogenicity is only moderate—with the exception of *S. typhi*, the pathogen of typhoid fever, and *S. paratyphi*, which has become extremely rare—so that large quantities of the pathogen must be taken up in order to cause an infection. As with all moderately pathogenic germs, the very young and old are at increased risk. Chronic carriers also pose a problem. The most effective antibiotics are fluorquinolones.

There is no satisfactory answer to the occasional question regarding the risk for newborns during childbirth if the mother has a salmonella infection or is a carrier. The commonly recommended hygienic measures are far easier to adhere to during childbed than during a vaginal birth. Close monitoring and early treatment of the newborn are probably sufficient. A cesarean section seems justified only in cases of a high risk.

Yersinia. Bacteria of the genus *Yersinia* cause, for the most part, intestinal tract infections associated with diarrhea, vomiting, and sometimes high fever. When spreading systemically, *Y. enterocolitica* may cause arthritis or also erythema nodosum. Cephalosporins of the third generation and carbapenems are very effective, also fluorquinolones.

Other species are *Y. pseudotuberculosis* and *Y. pestis.*

Campylobacter. Bacteria of the genus *Campylobacter* are transmitted by animals through food and primarily cause intestinal tract infections. Complications include sepsis (e. g., *C. fetus*), arthritis (e. g., *C. jejuni*), infectious abortion, and possibly Barré–Guillain syndrome. Amoxicillin and metronidazole are effective, and fluorquinolones and others are moderately effective.

Actinomycetes

Actinomycosis is a chronic granulomatous inflammation that is rarely found in the small pelvis, causing pelvic inflammatory disease (PID).

1 2 3 4 5 6 7 8 9 10 11 12 13 14 15

Much more frequent is the cytological diagnosis of an *Actinomyces* infection caused by a removed intrauterine device (IUD). This often causes anxiety and insecurity with respect to the consequences. In many patients, the cytologic suspicion cannot be confirmed by microbiological tests. Even if the difficult detection, involving special cultures and long observation times, is successful, this germ does not seem to pose a risk. *Actinomyces israeli* occurs as a colonizing germ in the feces and, hence, also occasionally in the vagina.

2 Defense Systems

Functions and Disturbances of the Immune System

Our immune system plays the major role in preventing and overcoming infections. In the absence of a functioning immune system, not even the most effective antibiotics can fight infections. The defense system can be affected by various disorders, such as congenital immunoglobulin deficiency, partial weakness of the immune system (cellular as well as humoral), iatrogenic immunosuppression, or acquired immunodeficiency syndrome (AIDS). Other influences that reduce the activity of the immune system include malnutrition, stress, and aging.

The human body can coexist quite well with a multitude of different microorganisms. Skin and intestinal tract are colonized with 10^{12}–10^{16} bacteria. An infection can only occur when the equilibrium between the defense system and microorganisms is disturbed, for example, by the invasion of pathogens into otherwise sterile regions, by the uptake of especially pathogenic germs from the outside, or by weakening of the defense systems.

The number of invading pathogens and their virulence also play a major role in initiating an infection.

Table 2.**1** Defense systems

1. In general:
   - skin
   - mucosa
   - secretions
   - normal flora
2. Immune system:

a) nonspecific:
   - complement system
   - interferons
   - lysozymes, etc.
   - leukocytes (microphages)
   - lymphocytes (macrophages)
   - natural killer cells (T lymphocytes)

b) specific:
   - immunoglobulins (antibodies) IgM, IgA, IgG
   - specific macrophages (T cells)

General Defense Mechanisms

Intact skin and mucosae normally represent an effective mechanical barrier against invading pathogens (Table 2.**1**).

The cornified skin is much more resistant against microorganisms than the stratified or single-layered mucosae. Hence, mucosae represent the main site of entrance for most microorganisms.

However, mucosae have their own protection through the secretion of mucus (e.g., the cervical mucosa) and through various specific defense mechanisms (IgA antibodies) or nonspecific defense mechanisms (e.g., lysozymes).

Another protective mechanism is the colonization of the vagina with lactic acid-producing lactobacilli.

Nonspecific Humoral Defense Systems

Complement system. This complex enzyme system is able to dissolve invading pathogens through a series of cascading reactions of individual components. Many interactions take place between the individual defense systems.

Activation of the complement system is promoted by specific antibodies binding to the invading microorganism. Phagocytosis by macrophages is also increased.

Other nonspecific humoral defense systems include:

- the *properdin system,* which activates the alternative pathway of the complement system
- *lysozymes,* which dissolve certain bacterial cell walls
- the various *interferons*, which exhibit antiviral and antiproliferative activities and also have immunoregulatory functions (cell membrane effects, cell differentiation, increased cytotoxicity).

Apart from these systems, there are also numerous substances (mediators) that are released by macrophages or T lymphocytes upon stimulation.

Nonspecific Cellular Defense System

This includes polymorphonuclear leukocytes (neutrophil and eosinophil granulocytes, also called **microphages**) and mononuclear phagocytes (**macrophages**).

Polymorphonuclear leukocytes are the first cells to reach the site of infection. They have limited resistance, die early, and cause pus formation.

Next in line comes the attack by macrophages. These are monocytes derived from the bone marrow; they differentiate within the tissues to become macrophages. Under the microscope, they can be seen in the cervical secretion together with granulocytes. They are especially numerous in chronic infections, such as chlamydial cervicitis.

Phagocytes migrate by means of chemotaxis toward the invading microorganisms and ingest them so that they are degraded by lysosomal enzymes.

Apart from stimulating the nonspecific defense systems, phagocytes also have a positive effect on specific immune reactions. They produce a multitude of mediators, e.g., interferon, leukotrienes, complement factors, monokines, and prostaglandins.

In addition, there are **natural killer cells**, which are cytotoxic T lymphocytes.

Phagocytosis is stimulated by specific immunoglobulins that have bound to the surface of the pathogens (**opsonization**). The microorganisms thus become, so to speak, more palatable for the macrophages. Some bacteria are adequately phagocytosed only after such opsonization, e.g., listeriae, some staphylococci, mycobacteria, pneumococci, and *Haemophilus influenzae*.

Specific Humoral Defense System

Activation of the specific immune system results in measurable amounts of humoral antibodies (immunoglobulins) and cell-bound antibodies (on T lymphocytes), thus creating a permanent specific defense system.

Cell-bound Antibodies

In response to various mediators, the two mature lymphocyte populations of the blood—**B lymphocytes** and **T lymphocytes**—develop via different intermediates from stem cells in the bone marrow. Many interactions take place between these two cell populations. Programming of the lymphocytes released from the bone marrow takes place once they reach the periphery where they develop into immunologically competent cells.

Upon contact with an antigen (e.g., a microorganism) and with the participation of normal macrophages, clonal proliferation is stimulated in all B lymphocytes that carry the corresponding specific receptor. This creates memory cells, which are long-lived and can store the information for years. Renewed contact with the same antigen triggers a rapid immune response. At the same time, the antigen stimulus causes B lymphocytes to differentiate into immunoglobulin-secreting **plasma cells.**

Immunoglobulins

These are glycoproteins that react specifically with certain immunogenic determinants on the microorganism. Depending on its size, the organism exhibits a multitude of different receptors. Antibodies are generally found only in the extracellular space (IgA and IgG can pass into the mother's milk).

Five different immunoglobulins are known (Table 2.**2**):

IgM Antibodies

They are the initial response to an antigenic stimulus. Each IgM molecule is composed of five basic units. Its molecular weight of 900 000 daltons is the highest among immunoglobulins, and they are not transferred across the placenta. They are produced whenever an antigen is present, and florid infections—including reactivated ones—are recognized through the detection of specific IgM antibodies. They have a half-life of one to three days, which is the shortest among immunoglobulins.

IgA Antibodies

These are secretory antibodies; they are found in the serum as well as on mucosae and in secretions. Normally, IgA molecules occur as monomers (the common antibody structure); however, they may also occur as dimers. IgA antibodies pass into the mother's milk.

Table 2.2 Characteristics and concentration of immunoglobulins in the plasma

Class	Number of units	Heavy chains	Light chains	Subclasses	Molecular weight	Half-life (days)	mg/dL
IgG	1	γ	χ, λ	IgG_1 IgG_2 IgG_3 IgG_4	150 000	22	1250 (750–1500)
IgM	5	μ	χ, λ	IgM_1 IgM_2	900 000	1–3	150 (50–200)
IgA	1–3	α	χ, λ	IgA_1 IgA_2	170 000	6	210 (90–320)
IgD	1	δ	χ, λ		180 000	3	3
IgE	1	ε	χ, λ		200 000	2	0.03

IgG Antibodies

They form the largest subclass of antibodies and represent approximately 75 % of all antibodies in the plasma. They bring about permanent immunity and persist even in the absence of the antigen. Their half-life is approximately three weeks. They are continuously produced; as a result, they usually decrease only slowly over years and decades. With a molecular weight of 150 000 daltons, they do cross the placenta.

IgD Antibodies

They are found only in small quantities in the plasma and are probably involved in the differentiation of B cells.

IgE Antibodies

They occur only at very low concentrations in the plasma. These antibodies are found especially on mast cells present in cutaneous and mucosal regions, where they induce immediate hypersensitivity reactions. They do not cross the placenta.

Antibody Function

The Fab end of the antibody forms a reversible bond with the corresponding receptor on the microorganism. This causes a configurational change on the other end of the immunoglobulin (Fc fragment). This, in turn, triggers various reactions:

- complement activation resulting in enzymatic activity and, as a result, lysis of the microorganism
- neutralization of the pathogen and, as a result, termination of the ability to penetrate into the cell (e.g., in the case of viruses)
- agglutination or precipitation of the pathogen by forming large immunocomplexes
- improved phagocytosis (opsonization effect).

Specific Cellular Defense System

This is based on T lymphocytes that become immunologically programmed in the thymus. These cells express various receptors on their surface that can react with certain antigens. They continuously migrate back and fourth between the lymph nodes, spleen, vascular system, and tissues.

Upon immunological contact, they are activated to differentiate further into T effector cells, which are divided into T helper cells, T suppressor cells, and T killer cells depending on their surface markers and their function. The T helper cells are responsible for antigen recognition, B cell activation, T cell induction, and lymphokine synthesis, whereas the T suppressor cells lead to suppression of the immune response, destruction of tumor cells, destruction of virus-infected cells, and rejection of transplants. Excessive immune reactions are prevented as long as these cell populations are in equilibrium with each other.

By means of various mediators, T lymphocytes have a regulatory effect also on other cell types, such as granulocytes and macrophages.

1 2 3 4 5 6 7 8 9 10 11 12 13 14 15

HIV infections preferably attack T4 lymphocytes, which are destroyed during the course of the disease.

Disorders of the Immune System

There are primary (congenital) and secondary (acquired) forms of immunodeficiency.

Only mild forms exist in case of congenital immune defects because children with severe defects are not able to survive. Many of such mild defects are known to us. The defect may have nonspecific causes, e.g., complement system, phagocytotic function (granulocytic defect), or specific ones, either affecting B cells (immunoglobulin deficiency) or T cells (Table 2.**3**).

Such defects can be uncovered by modern immunological methods. Sometimes, in the case of individual infections taking a serious course, this may be important from a forensic point of view as well.

Acquired immunodeficiency may develop through metabolic disorders, e.g., hypoproteinemia, diabetes mellitus, liver cirrhosis, and uremia. Even disorders of the immune system itself, the cause of which is often still unknown, may lead to immunodeficiency. Cytostatic and immunosuppressive agents as well as radiotherapy cause iatrogenic immunodeficiency.

Table 2.**3** Development of the immune status of the child

6th week of pregnancy	Thymus primordium
12th week of pregnancy	Thymus function begins, surface markers (IgM, IgG, IgA) on lymphocytes, T cells
20th week of pregnancy	Production of IgG and IgM antibodies by plasma cells
30th week of pregnancy	IgA antibody production, start of transmission of maternal IgG antibodies (premature babies thus have an antibody deficit)
3rd to 6th month of life	Lowest antibody levels
1st year	IgM levels are similar to those of adults
8th year	IgG levels are similar to those of adults
11th year	IgA levels are similar to those of adults

Various infections may also cause a disturbed immune system. This has been demonstrated, in particular, by the new disorder caused by HIV infection. However, other infectious diseases also result in altered immune situations, as is the case with tuberculosis.

3 Detection of Pathogens

General Remarks

Direct Detection

Colposcopy: pubic lice, worms.

Microscopy:
- native wet mount: trichomonads, fungi, possibly bacteria
- stained with methylene blue (also as a wet mount) or Gram method: fungi, bacteria
- labeled with immunofluorescent markers: chlamydiae, herpes simplex viruses, *Treponema pallidum*
- special staining methods: malaria, trichomonads
- phase contrast: trichomonads, fungi
- possibly electron microscopy: herpesviruses, HIV, poxviruses, rotaviruses.

Culture and Identification of Pathogens

Culture is the method of choice for almost all bacterial infections. Viruses that can be identified in this way include particularly enteroviruses but also herpes simplex viruses and cytomegaloviruses. Culture is also the method of choice for fungi.

Serological Detection (Antibodies)

This is the most important procedure for detecting viral infections, because viruses are effective antibody inducers and also because their detection through culture methods is expensive and time-consuming. In the case of bacterial infections, serology plays only a minor role because the cross-reactivity between bacterial antibodies is high and the immune response is often negligible. Exceptions include syphilis, which is now exclusively detected by serological means. More recently, serology is also used for detecting *Chlamydia* infections and borreliosis and, among the infections with protozoa, also toxoplasmosis.

In addition, serological procedures are used for the detection of antigens (e.g., the enzyme-linked immunosorbent assay, ELISA).

Detection by Means of Molecular Biology

Up to now, hybridization has been the only procedure for detecting papillomavirus infections. With the invention of polymerase chain reaction (PCR), a new era of pathogen identification has begun.

Detection of Bacteria

Special emphasis is given to the isolation and identification of the pathogen.

Collecting Specimens with a Swab (Soft Tissue Infection)

Specimens should always be collected from a deep area of the wound because the surface usually contains only necrotic material. When collecting material from the cervix, one should reach as deep as possible into the cervix. Prior to that, the external area must be cleaned to ensure that as few contaminating germs as possible will be picked up from the vaginal region. The more contaminating germs are found together with the pathogen, the less convincing are the microbiological findings.

The more careful the collection of material and the more selective the swabbing of the infected site, the greater is the chance that the germ responsible for the infection will be identified.

When swabbing sensitive external regions (e.g., the genitals of a young girl, or the eye lids) it is recommended that one uses a moistened swab (soaked in physiological saline or transport medium—or even tap water, if absolutely necessary). By doing so, more material is picked up and the sampling is less painful.

Urine Analysis (Urinary Tract Infection)

Spontaneously voided urine is regularly contaminated with germs from the external region of the urethra and partly also from the vulvar region. For this reason, only germ counts of 10^5 and more are regarded as an indication of urinary tract infection. Whether or not the results can be used depends therefore on the proper collection of the urine and, hence, on proper instructions for urine collection given to the patient.

The patient is instructed to spread apart the pudendal lips, clean the opening of the urethra, and discard the first part of the urine; only then may she use the container provided for urine collection. Contamination is always suspected when several types of germs are detected in high concentrations.

Another problem is that urine is an excellent culture medium for bacteria. During shipment of urine samples—with transportation times lasting up to several hours—bacteria rapidly multiply and thus simulate high germ counts. For this reason, immersion procedures have been developed (e. g., Urotube, Roche) in which a prefabricated special agar is dipped into the freshly voided urine; after incubation, the actual germ count is indicated fairly accurately.

One disadvantage is the fact that not all bacteria grow equally well, if at all, on these prefabricated culture media. If a urinary tract infection is suspected and the test culture is negative for bacteria (e. g., during pregnancy), the freshly voided urine must reach the laboratory as quickly as possible and be kept at 4 °C during transport. Even relatively low germ counts ($< 10^5$/mL) may indicate a urinary tract infection, especially when the urine has been collected by means of suprapubic bladder puncture or catheter.

The first 10 mL of the spontaneously voided urine (first-stream urine) are used for the **detection of chlamydiae** in the urethra.

Blood Culture (Sepsis)

In cases of severe infections (even without fever, e. g., in the case of septic shock) and/or fever (> 38.5 °C), blood cultures should be collected because there is the possibility of sepsis. For this purpose, ready-to-use culture flasks are available into which 5–10 mL of venous blood are transferred—by means of a direct tube system, if possible. Thorough and repeated disinfection of the collection site is particularly important, otherwise only contaminating germs will be detected (e. g., *Staphylococcus epidermidis*). In addition, one should always prepare an aerobic culture, which is supplied with air, and an anaerobic culture, into which only blood is transferred. It is best to collect one aerobic and one anaerobic culture from each arm (minimum: three cultures, optimal: four cultures). The more often blood cultures are collected, the greater the chance that a pathogen is detected. If at all possible, blood samples should be collected while the fever is still rising. Large statistical studies have shown that pathogens will only grow in approximately 20% of the blood cultures. The results of the blood culture are expected to be available not before 20 hours, because the culture flask has to be incubated for eight hours and the content then transferred to an agar plate.

If, for example, the blood culture yields *Staphylococcus epidermidis* in only one culture, this indicates that one is dealing with a contaminating germ from the skin and not with the pathogen causing the sepsis.

Gardnerella vaginalis cannot be detected with the usual blood culture media, because the presence of heparin inhibits the growth of this pathogen.

Special Procedures

For culturing chlamydiae, epithelial cells from the site of infection (cervix, urethra, infundibulum of uterine tube) are picked up with a swab—or, even better, with a brush or sponge—and transferred to an appropriate transport medium.

Transport Medium

Without the use of a transport medium, only extremely resistant bacteria (e. g., enterococci) can still be cultured after a long period of transport (several hours, one to three days). After 24 hours in a moist swab without transport medium, staphylococci can still be cultured in the original numbers, whereas certain *Bacteroides* species will have declined (by a magnitude of) 10^3–10^5 (in steps of $\log_{10}$) cfu (colony forming units) within hours and can no longer be cultured.

Since the introduction of transport media and the improvement of culture procedures, fastidious bacteria have been detected far more frequently. Gonococci are relatively sensitive as well; they can be cultured after 24 or 48 hours only if shipped in a transport medium.

Transport media are particularly important for anaerobic bacteria, some of which are extremely sensitive to oxygen and can only survive in appropriate media. A multitude of different transport media are commercially available (e. g., Port-A-Cult, Transystem).

Culturing chlamydiae requires transport media other than those used for the usual bacteriological diagnostic procedures. Like viruses, these bacteria require buffered solutions to which the infected cells can be transferred.

Culture Methods

Common Culture Methods

Bacteria are normally cultured on solid agar media containing the essential nutrients. Each bacterium that is able to multiply produces one colony. By smearing the swab onto the culture plate in a fractional way, a first impression can be gained of the amount of bacteria present. Accurate germ counts are obtained by first setting up dilution series of the starting material.

From each swab different culture plates are prepared because different species of bacteria have different nutritional needs, and also because one might want to check simultaneously for certain growth properties, such as hemolysis.

The use of selective culture media, which contain inhibitors (e. g., antibiotics) suppressing the growth of other contaminating germs, allows for easier recognition of certain pathogens. Ever since selective culture media for streptococci of group B have been introduced, there has been a sharp rise in the detection rate in smears from the vagina and cervix. Selective culture media are also required for pathogens occurring only at low germ counts, such as gonococci.

Culture plates for the detection of aerobic bacteria can be incubated in a normal incubator. Culture plates for the detection of anaerobic bacteria, which do not grow in the presence of oxygen, must be incubated in an anaerobic culture container from which the oxygen is removed by physical or chemical means after the plates have been placed.

Normally, agar plates can be inspected after 24 hours. However, incubation may take several days in the case of slow-growing bacteria (e. g., many anaerobes). This is the case when the initial microbiological report mentions only a "physiological flora" or "no growth of pathogens" and, several days later, a subsequent report mentions anaerobes or other bacteria that are difficult to culture.

Tubercle bacteria grow particularly slowly, with a doubling time of 24 hours. Culture results are therefore available only after four to six weeks.

Further identification of the bacteria is based on the microscopic evaluation of gram-stained samples, testing for metabolic activities (e. g., by means of color strip tests), and—in the case of gonococci—the additional detection of peroxidase.

Other methods of determination include gas chromatography for identifying specific metabolites and the determination of the GC content (base composition of the DNA). Serological methods may be used as well for individual pathogens.

Subsequently, agar plates are inoculated with bacteria from the pure culture. By placing small paper discs impregnated with antibiotics onto these cultures, the sensitivity of the pathogen against various antibiotics can be checked; this test is carried out by following a predetermined, standardized procedure. As the antibiotic from each test disc diffuses into the agar and creates a concentration gradient, a more or less extensive zone of inhibition is formed around the test disc, depending on the sensitivity of the pathogen.

Special Culture Methods

They are required for the following bacteria:

- *Chlamydia*: cell culture (e. g., McCoy cells)
- *Mycoplasma*: selective culture media with the addition of penicillin, slow growth even in a CO_2 atmosphere; can be isolated from the usual swabs
- *Mycobacterium*: special culture media, very slow growth (four to eight weeks).

Many other bacteria can only be isolated when appropriate culture media are used, for example, actinomycetes. Also, *Gardnerella vaginalis* requires a special culture medium (a double-layered agar medium with different additives and inhibitors).

Experimental animals are rarely used for the isolation of bacteria today. In the past, they played a role in diagnosing tuberculosis. However, animals (rabbits) are still required for culturing *Treponema pallidum* (the pathogen of syphilis) in their testes, although the only use of this method is for manufacturing material used in diagnostic procedures.

Detection of Viruses

The isolation of viruses is an expensive method because it requires cell cultures. It should only be ordered in special cases where other methods do not yield results, or when the task is to detect and identify the pathogen directly.

Materials and Methods of Specimen Collection

The following materials are suitable for the detection of viruses:

- throat swabs: rubella virus, influenza virus, and herpes simplex virus (HSV)
- cervical swabs: HSV
- swabs from vesicles, lesions, ulcers: HSV, varicella–zoster virus
- urine: cytomegalovirus (CMV)
- feces: enteroviruses (poliovirus, Coxsackie virus, echovirus), hepatitis A virus (HAV), rotaviruses
- blood: HIV, Epstein-Barr virus (EBV), hepatitis B virus (HBV), hepatitis C virus (HCV), CMV
- biopsies: HSV, papillomaviruses, and others
- amniotic fluid: CMV, rubella virus.

In cases of lesions (erosions, ulcers) and small vesicles (e. g., genital herpes), a small sterile swab is vigorously rubbed through the ulcer or the fundus of the vesicle (better still, through several lesions). Unfortunately, this procedure is painful. It is recommended that the swab be moistened with transport medium prior to use because this increases absorbency. The swab is then rinsed out in the transport medium, squeezed, and discarded.

Puncture of a vesicle is only meaningful if it is relatively large; the vesicle content is then aspirated using a small syringe with a thin needle.

Transport Medium

With the exception of papillomaviruses or enteroviruses, viruses are sensitive to desiccation; the swab material must therefore be transferred to a transport medium (e. g., cell culture medium). If this is not available, physiological saline may be used for a brief transport. This applies to all swab material and vesicle contents.

Culture Methods

The isolation of viruses requires cell cultures. Depending on the virus, different cell types are needed because not every virus grows on every cell type. There are permanent cell lines and primary cell cultures, with the permanent cell lines now having gained acceptance. In the majority of cases, multiplication of a virus is recognized by its cytopathic effect (destruction of the monolayer of cells). This may become visible already after 24–48 hours, if one is dealing with a fast-growing virus or if viral numbers were already high at the time of seeding (e. g., herpes simplex virus). With other viruses, it may take up to eight days (e. g., CMV). Sometimes subcultures are required. Some viruses do not destroy the monolayer of cells (e. g., rubella virus). In that case, virus multiplication is demonstrated by detection of the virus-specific hemagglutinin, which is able to bind erythrocytes to the surface of the virus.

Further identification of the virus is carried out by immunological means, i. e., by blocking the cytopathic effects in the next round of cell culture or, more rapidly, by means of immunofluorescence tests using monoclonal antibodies (e. g., HSV).

Polymerase Chain Reaction

Meanwhile the PCR can be used for the detection of many viruses. It is the method of the future for many pathogens (see p. 35–36).

Detection of Fungi (Table 3.1)

Microscopy and Indication for Culture Methods

Due to their size and characteristic morphology, most yeasts can be recognized already under the microscope in the wet mount or, even better, in the stained swab preparation (Fig. 3.**1**).

There are three typical morphologies: budding cells, pseudomycelia, and—on rice agar plates—chlamydospores (Fig. 1.**2** [p. 7] and Figs. 3.**2**, 3.**3**).

Not all *Candida* yeasts express these three morphologies, which otherwise can be used for differentiation. In addition, the pseudomycelia may differ, but only the experienced eye is able to distinguish between them.

A culture is always required for the detection and identification of fungi when a clear microscopic diagnosis is impossible, namely, when only a few fungal cells are present or the fungal elements cannot be recognized due to the presence of other germs and materials (e. g., in oral swabs or stool samples). This also applies when only budding cells can be seen, which may include many different yeast species.

Table 3.1 Procedures for diagnosing yeast fungi

Method	Assessment
1. Native state microscopy (mix the flakes with methylene blue solution)	Budding cells: no evaluation of pathogenicity Pseudomycelia: usually *C. albicans*
2. Sabouraud culture (the addition of antibiotics suppresses bacteria, thus facilitating assessment and identification)	Used for culturing pathogens as budding cells 50–70 % more yeasts detected than by native state microscopy; Sabouraud broth is 20 % more sensitive than Sabouraud agar plate; differentiation between yeast species is not possible (the presence of small budding cells suggests *C. glabrata*) **Caution:** staphylococci (even smaller cells)
3. Rice agar plate (starvation medium)	Pseudomycelia: important as a pathogen; if associated with chlamydospores: *C. albicans,* otherwise differentiation by means of biochemistry is required Budding cells: nonpathogenic, e. g., *Candida (Torulopsis) glabrata,* brewer yeast (*Saccharomyces cerevisiae*) True ramifications: hyphomycetes, e. g., *Geotrichum candidum* (nonpathogenic) or contamination of the plate with airborne germs (older plates)
4. Chrome agar plates	Identification of yeast species by means of a specific color reaction of the colonies (relatively expensive)
5. Biochemistry	Identification of different yeast species based on their biochemical activity (color reaction) during growth on prefabricated carriers
6. Serology	Plays a minor role in genital infections Exception: chronic, frequently recurrent candidiasis. There is evidence that, in the absence of IgA antibodies against *Candida albicans* in the serum, symptoms can be alleviated by immunostimulation—which may be helpful in severely ill and immunosuppressed patients
7. Antimycogram	Normally not required for genital infections, but appropriate in AIDS patients; resistances are very rare and directed only against certain substances, never against nystatin

Collection of Material

Swabs from the vaginal region should be collected, if possible, by vigorous rubbing on the vaginal wall; especially in the case of an infection, fungi adhere with their cell walls and penetrate into the tissue.

As the distribution of fungi is usually not homogenous in the regions of vulva and vagina, it is essential for the detection of the pathogen that the swab material is collected at the proper location. Areas with reddening, and particularly those with floccular and often firmly adherent vaginal discharge, are especially suited. If the flakes for microscopic preparation are selectively picked up with the wooden handle of a swab and rubbed carefully into the methylene blue solution on the microscopic slide, chances for a direct detection are very high.

Transport Medium

This is not essential because fungi are very stable. However, the sample must not be allowed to dry out.

Culture Methods and Differentiation

Fungi are very modest in their growth requirements and thus grow on many media (e.g., Sabouraud 2% glucose agar; Kimmig agar, Merck).

Microscopic-morphological Differentiation

Detection of pseudomycelia, which are characteristic of the filamentous phase of *Candida* yeasts on rice agar subcultures, is used for the morphological differentiation of yeasts (Table 3.2). A pseudomycelium is formed on nutritionally poor or exhausted media, like those also found in the infected host tissue. The simplest culture media for inducing pseudomycelia are rice agar and corn meal agar. Agar plates are inoculated with cells from the isolated culture, and the inoculated surface is covered with a glass cover slip. After 24–48 hours of incubation at room temperature (up to a maximum of 28 °C), the cultures are directly inspected using a microscope with 10× or 40× objectives.

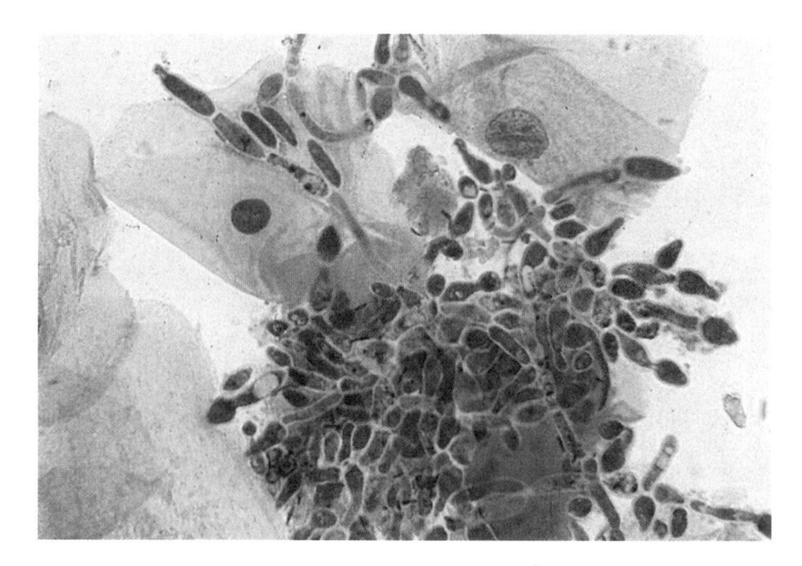

Fig. 3.**1** Microscopic wet mount in 0.1 % methylene blue solution: *Candida* infection. Tangle of fungal elements (*Candida* pseudomycelium) and vaginal epithelial cells; leukocytes are not visible here, though always present with inflammation. Magnification 400×.

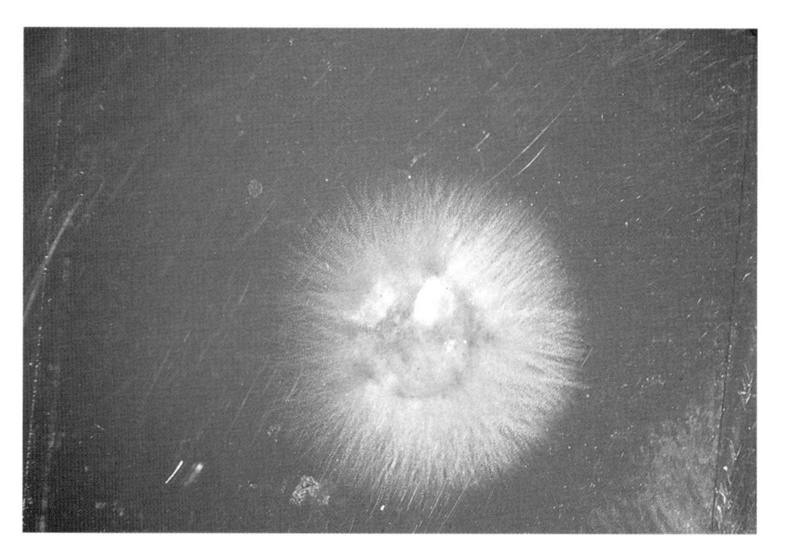

Fig. 3.**2** *Candida albicans* colony on rice agar: macroscopically visible corona of pseudomycelium. Magnification 10×.

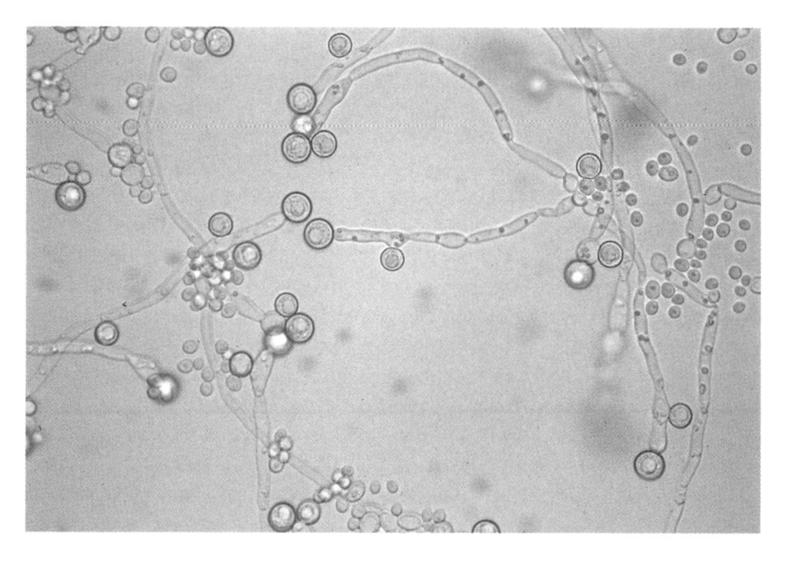

Fig. 3.**3** *Candida albicans* on rice agar: typical chlamydospores. Magnification 400×.

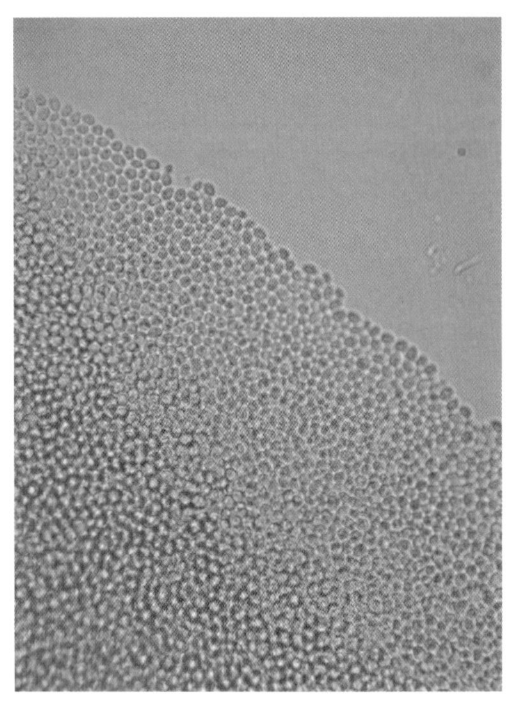

Fig. 3.**4** *Candida glabrata* on rice agar: only small budding cells are visible under the microscope. Magnification 400×.

Table 3.**2** Yeast species that form pseudomycelia

Candida albicans	Pseudomycelium and chlamydospores
Candida stellatoidea	Pseudomycelium and chlamydospores, but no assimilation of sucrose
Candida tropicalis	Extensive pseudomycelium, but no chlamydospores
Candida parapsilosis	Pseudomycelium and blastospores
Candida kefyr (*C. pseudotropicalis*)	
Candida krusei	± Pseudomycelium
Candida guilliermondii	
Candida ceylanoides	

Species of the genus *Trichosporon* (*T. cutaneum*, *T. beigelii*), which are occasionally isolated from vaginal swabs, also develop a mycelium in addition to the budding yeast morphology, and the hyphens of this mycelium form terminal arthrospores by hyphal segmentation (hingelike, kinked single cells).

Candida glabrata and other species of the former genus *Torulopsis* are characterized by a small cell diameter. They grow only as small budding cells even on agar plates (Fig. 3.**4**) and do not develop a pseudomycelium.

Biochemical Differentiation

Because of the sparse expression of different morphological markers, a laboratory diagnosis of yeasts is mostly impossible without determining their biochemical activity. Systematic criteria are based on their capacities to utilize carbohydrates for fermentation and assimilation or to utilize nitrogen compounds for assimilation, and—less often—on tests for vitamin requirements. Industrial ready-made systems for biochemical differentiation have been commercially available for several years now. They are usually adapted to the practical needs of medical mycology and considerably ease the routine work of diagnostic laboratories. When used discriminatingly, at least 95% of all medically relevant yeast fungi can be diagnosed with such systems.

Serological Differentiation

In analogy to the diagnosis of salmonellae in bacteriology, the antigen patterns expressed on the surface of the cell wall can also be used for the diagnosis of yeasts. The medically relevant yeast species can be identified by means of typical antigen patterns. The value of serological differentiation lies in the quickness of this method of determination. In addition, it is possible to distinguish between serotype A and serotype B within the species *Candida albicans*, and this is of interest epidemiologically and also with respect to some therapeutic problems.

Serology

Serology plays only a certain role in diagnosis when a systemic infection with *Candida* is suspected. The detection of antibodies does not say anything about the status of immunity.

Antibody production. Antibodies against *Candida* antigens are produced in humans only when immunocompetent host cells get into contact with the fungal antigens. This is the case when the fungal antigens enter the circulation of the host. In cases of candidiasis of the vaginal epithelium, fungal colonization remains superficial; an invasion of antigens and a subsequent antibody response by the host hardly take place, or not at all. In cases of clinically relevant vulvitis, however, fungal antigens frequently enter into the blood stream and thus induce a humoral immune response.

The following methods for the detection of antibodies are commercially available:

- **Indirect *Candida* hemagglutination test** (*Candida* HA test). It employs formalin-treated sheep erythrocytes that are loaded with *Candida* polysaccharides; these are several serologically active components isolated from serotype A of *Candida albicans*. The test recognizes antibodies of classes IgM, IgG, and IgA directed against cell wall antigens and manna antigens. In part, antigen–antibody complexes are also bound. This explains the high sensitivity of the test. The *Candida HA* test also recognizes antibodies against *Candida tropicalis*, *C. parapsilosis*, and *C. (Torulopsis) glabrata* because of the shared antigens. Titers of 1 : > 160 are considered pathognomonic.
- **Indirect *Candida* immunofluorescence test** (*Candida* IF test). It employs native *Candida albicans* cells. A cell suspension is transferred to subdivided microscopic slides and then dried and fixed. The antigen-coated fields are then overlaid with serial dilutions of the patient's serum to allow specific *Candida* antibodies to bind to the yeast cells. In a second incubation step, the specifically bound antibodies are linked to fluorescein isothiocyanate-labeled (FITC-labeled) antihuman globulin to make them visible in the fluorescence microscope. Because of the reaction kinetics, the test recognizes only IgG antibodies. The immunofluorescence titers therefore take longer to become positive than the hemagglutination titers, but they remain high for a longer period. Titers of 1 : > 160 are considered pathognomonic.

Detection of Protozoa

In the case of trichomonad infections, special emphasis is given to direct microscopic detection of the pathogen, while in the case of toxoplasmosis the focus of attention is on serological detection. There are hardly any routine culture methods available. Both *Trichomonas* and *Toxoplasma* can be cultured in special laboratories. Culture of *Toxoplasma gondii* in the mouse requires at least two weeks. Recently, DNA detection methods have become increasingly available (PCR), and are finding their way into the daily routine of laboratories.

Trichomonas vaginalis:

- microscopy of wet mounts (Fig. 3.**5**) (sensitivity approximately 50 %)
- microscopy of cytological preparations (Fig. 7.**107 a**, p. 119)
- microscopy after Giemsa staining (Fig. 3.**6**)
- concentration through culture, e. g., incubation in Diamond medium at 35 °C and microscopic observation of the sediment after two to three days, and then again after six to seven days (sensitivity 60–80 %)
- DNA sample test (Affirm VP III, BD Diagnostic Systems) (sensitivity 85–98 %)
- serological detection of trichomonads by means of ELISA (sensitivity 77 %)
- detection of antibodies in the serum.

Toxoplasma gondii:

- serology (antibody detection in the serum)
- direct detection (special laboratory):
  - microscopy of histological sections after staining with Giemsa or with fluorescence-labeled antibodies
  - reproduction in animals (e. g., mouse) (duration: two to four weeks) or cell culture
  - PCR (preferred method).

Malaria (various species of *Plasmodium*):

- Plasmodia are detected microscopically in the infected erythrocytes by means of Giemsa stain. For this purpose, the laboratory requires a thick blood film (a dried drop of blood on a microscopic slide).

Serological Detection and Antibody Detection

Serological Method

General Remarks

Significance, disadvantages, and limitations. The detection of antibodies (Ab) in the serum is the most important method for recognizing viral infections. It also allows one to assess the status of immunity after many infectious diseases.

Many different methods are available, and they produce results within a few hours.

One disadvantage of serology is that antibodies become detectable only two to three weeks after the infection, at the earliest. With an incubation time of two weeks, however, the first antibodies may already be present at the onset of the main symptoms. Another disadvantage of serology is that a second blood sample is required for the detection of an infection that has occurred recently; this has been slightly offset by the increasing use of IgM antibody tests.

The latter approach, however, has created new problems. We have already seen that there are many persistent or reactivated infections; therefore, the exact time of infection can often not be determined—not even with the IgM antibody capture method.

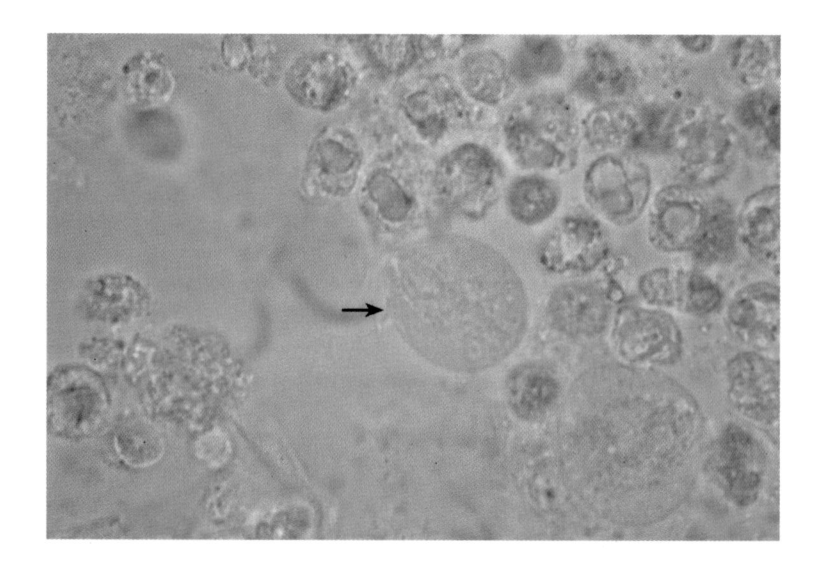

Fig. 3.**5** Trichomonad (arrow) in a microscopic wet mount. Magnification 1000×.

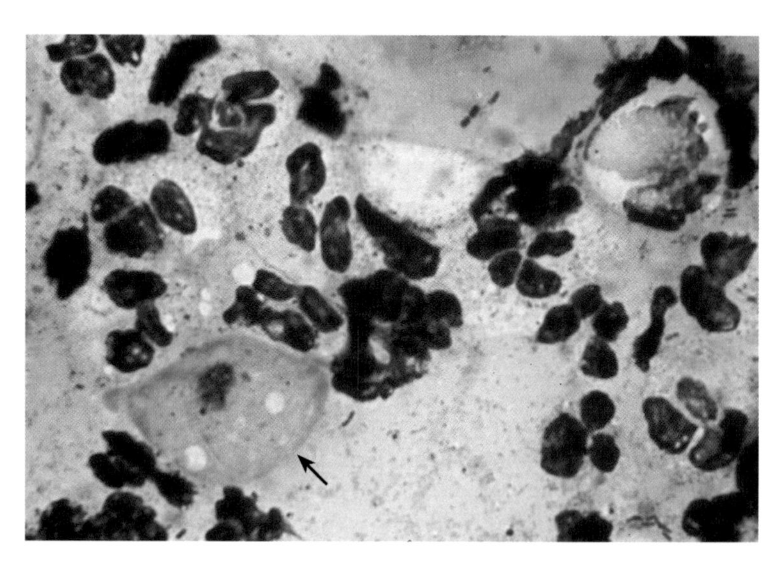

Fig. 3.**6** Trichomonad (arrow) after Giemsa staining. Magnification 1000×.

This is true, in particular, for cytomegalovirus infections and toxoplasmosis.

IgM antibodies are not only produced upon first contact with a new antigen (Ag); they can be detected as long as the antigen is present.

In principle, all systemic and intense local infections result in the production of specific antibodies. Hence, in theory, these infections should be detectable by serological means. However, this looks slightly different in practice, for serological tests have not been developed for all pathogens. Of course, there are reasons for that.

Viruses are difficult to detect by culture methods, but they are good antibody inducers because they possess only a few antigens on their surface and one is dealing with systemic infections in the majority of cases.

It is easier and quicker to detect bacteria by culture methods than by serological means. They are far more complex than viruses and express many more antigenic groups on their surface. These groups are very similar to the antigenic groups of other bacteria or substances (e. g., food) and thus give rise to cross-reactions. In addition, bacteria are superficial pathogens and often do not lead to an intense stimulation of the immune system.

Serology plays a *major role* as a diagnostic means in the following **viral infections**:

- rubella
- measles
- cytomegalovirus (CMV) infection
- diseases caused by Epstein–Barr virus (EBV)
- chickenpox (varicella–zoster virus, VZV)
- mumps

- hepatitis A, B, C, and D
- AIDS (HIV)
- erythema infectiosum (parvovirus B19).

Serological methods are available for the following viruses, but they are only used in *special cases* because of the considerable expense:
- polioviruses
- coxsackie viruses
- echoviruses.

So far, serology does *not* play a role in papillomavirus infections.

Among the infections caused by **bacteria and protozoa** serology plays a *major role* in the following diseases:
- syphilis
- toxoplasmosis
- borreliosis
- *Chlamydia pneumoniae* infections
- as a supplement to pathogen detection in cases of *Chlamydia trachomatis* infections.

Up to now, serology is completely useless for diagnosing *Listeria* infections.

Serological detection methods are available in **mycology** as well. Interpretation of the results is difficult because of the high contamination with *Candida*. Very high titers, however, lets one suspect a widespread or systemic mycosis. Occasionally, serology may be an important supplement to the culture method.

Different Serological Detection Methods

Titer Levels and Objective

In more recent tests, results are measured as optical density (OD) rather than titers. The manufacturer must therefore define for each test a cutoff extinction value that represents the boundary between positive and negative antibody detection.

The various serological detection methods have different sensitivities and specificities. In the case of titers, values may range from 1 : 4 to 1 : 20 000. The enzyme tests always yield very high titers, while direct fluorescence tests yield moderate titers (1 : 200 to 1 : 1000) and complement fixation tests low titers (1 : 10 to 1 : 160). In addition, the same tests carried out in different laboratories will yield different values. Hence, increases in titers can only be evaluated when they are found by the same examiner within the same test run. This applies in a similar way to extinction values.

Every laboratory has to comment on the findings and make an assessment. General printouts of so-called normal values are of no practical use. The laboratory must be provided with a clear objective so that the appropriate tests can be carried out.

It is important to ask and answer the following questions:
- anamnestic titer (IgG antibodies only)
- florid infection (including IgM antibodies).

In case of a florid infection, then ask and answer the following questions:
- primary infection (e. g., in the case of cytomegalovirus infection)
- reactivated infection (e. g., in the case of cytomegalovirus infection)
- fresh infection (e. g., in the case of toxoplasmosis)
- chronic infection (e. g., in the case of toxoplasmosis).

Complement Fixation Test (CFT)

Indication. This is a universal test that has been in use for a long time for detecting most of the viral infections. It detects all group-specific and type-specific antigens. Usually, the serotype is not recognized by this test.

Test principle. The test is based on measuring the consumption of complement; complement is only fixed—and thus becomes enzymatically active—when an antigen–antibody complex has formed. In a second step, the consumption of complement is made visible to the naked eye by adding antibody-coated erythrocytes.

The patient's serum must first be heat inactivated (two hours at 56 °C) in order to destroy its own complement. It is then diluted by a factor of two in a geometrical series.

In step 1, a known amount of antigen (usually two to four units) and two units of complement are added to each serum dilution. This is followed by incubation for one to two hours at room temperature or 37 °C, during which the complement-fixing antigen–antibody complexes form.

To make the reaction in step 1 visible, sheep red blood cells coated with antibodies to sheep erythrocytes are added in step 2. If the patient's serum contains *antibodies* against the antigen used in the test, a complex forms during step 1 and complement is fixed. Hence, there is *no hemolysis* in step 2.

If the patient's serum does not contain antibodies—or if the patient's serum has been diluted to a point where there are not enough antibodies left to form a complex (determination of the titer)—complement has not been consumed and can thus bind the antibody-coated sheep red blood cells added in step 2. This activates the enzymatic activity of complement, and the erythrocytes are hemolyzed. Hence, *hemolysis* means that *no antibodies* are present in the serum.

The test indicates the complement fixation ability of an antigen–antibody complex; if enough antibodies are present in the serum, the serum can be diluted further (titration) and is still able to bind a constant amount of complement.

Also important is the type of antibodies participating in the reaction. IgM antibodies fix more complement molecules than, for example, IgG antibodies. This means that the test yields high titers shortly after an infection (IgM antibodies disappear from the serum within several weeks), and that after several weeks and months this titer steadily declines and may even become negative.

Assessment. The complement fixation test is therefore well suited for determining a current or recent infection, but not for answering the question whether an infection occurred many years ago, i. e., whether immunity had already existed. The sensitivity depends on the antigen used, namely, on the methods of virus preparation, which differ markedly from virus to virus.

A high titer in the CFT (1 : > 80) always lets one suspect an infection that only occurred recently. Here too, however, the best evidence is the detection of newly formed antibodies or an increase in the titer to at least four times the original titer (two steps of titration), with the testing of both serum dilutions in the same assay. If the tests have been carried out by different examiners on different days, a fourfold rise of the titer does not mean anything because the range of results from different laboratories is still high.

Hemagglutination Inhibition Test (HAI Test)

Indication and assessment. This is the standard test for determining rubella antibodies. If not performed properly, it may yield false results. There is often no guarantee for its reliability in the lower titer range, and only higher titers (in the case of rubella, 1 : 32) are recognized as permissible by health authorities. A good laboratory, however, may also include lower titers as being unambiguously specific for rubella.

Test principle. The serum of the patient must be pretreated very carefully prior to the actual test. On the one hand, so-called inhibitors—which include, for example, lipoproteins, which occur at various levels in every serum—must be removed by adsorption to kaolin or heparin–manganese chloride; otherwise they may simulate antibodies where there are none, for these inhibitors are able to bind certain antigens, such as rubella antigen. On the other hand, depending on the type of erythrocytes used, the serum must be pretreated with erythrocytes in order to remove so-called agglutinins that may agglutinate the erythrocytes.

Again, serial dilutions of the serum are prepared for the test. To each dilution, four units of antigen (viral hemagglutinin) are added. After incubation for one to two hours at room temperature, erythrocytes are added. *Failure to agglutinate* indicates the *presence of antibodies.*

Solid-phase Erythrocyte Aggregation Test

Indication. This test is used, for example, for detecting rotaviruses in stool samples of newborns. It involves reverse passive hemagglutination on a solid phase.

Test principle. U-shaped wells of a microplate are coated with virus-specific antibodies. If the sample contains viruses, they will bind to the antibodies. In the next step, erythrocytes are added which are also coated with virus-specific antibodies and will therefore bind to the immobilized viruses, thus preventing sedimentation of the erythrocytes to the bottom tip of the well.

A variation of this test is the hemadsorption–immunosorbent technique developed for the determination of rubella-specific IgM antibodies. In this method, the wells of a microplate are coated with antibodies to human IgM. If the patient's serum contains rubella-specific IgM antibodies, these will firmly bind to the wells, and the subsequent addition of rubella antigen and erythrocytes will not lead to sedimentation of the erythrocytes.

Many other variations of this method are possible.

Hemolysis-in-Gel Test

Indication. This test is used for rubelladiagnosis. It allows one to determine even the specificity of lower titers in the hemagglutination inhibition test.

Test principle. Erythrocytes and antigen are poured onto an agar plate, and the patient's serum is filled into a depression in the agar. The appearance of a ring of hemolysis indicates the presence of rubella-specific antibodies.

Neutralization Test (NT)

This test hardly plays a role in identifying infections in gynecology and obstetrics. It is used for enteroviruses. The test is very expensive because neutralizing antibodies in the patient's serum need to be detected by means of cell cultures (if present, the corresponding virus fails to elicit a cytopathic effect).

Immunofluorescence Tests (IFT)

Indication. Both the number and the quality of commercially available fluorescence tests have markedly increased in recent years. These tests make it possible to detect and identify pathogens (or their components) directly, both in the microscopic smear preparation and after multiplication in cell culture. They can also be used for detecting antibodies in the patient's serum. It is an advantage that they can be performed quickly (one to three hours), though their subjective evaluation is a disadvantage.

Tests are available for the following infections:

- syphilis
- *Chlamydia* infections
- cytomegalovirus infections
- EBV infections
- herpes simplex
- gonorrhea
- HIV infections
- toxoplasmosis
- pertussis.

Test principle. We distinguish between *direct* and *indirect* immunofluorescence tests (see below). For the detection of antibodies in the serum, the indirect test is usually used because it is more sensitive than the direct test, and also because the detection of antibodies against different pathogens requires only one fluorescence-labeled antiserum. Recently, the use of monoclonal antibodies in both tests has increased considerably because of their higher specificity.

Direct immunofluorescence test. It is used for the direct detection of pathogens (e.g., chlamydiae and herpes viruses) in the material collected from the patient. The swab material on the microscopic slide is fixed with acetone or ethanol so that the antibodies can penetrate into the cells. The cells are overlaid with a fluorescence-labeled antiserum and then incubated. The antibodies penetrate into the cells and form complexes with the pathogen; as a result, they can no longer be removed during the subsequent washing procedure. The preparation is then inspected using a fluorescence microscope.

Indirect immunofluorescence test. It is particularly suited for the detection of antibodies in the patient's serum, and especially for detecting IgM antibodies.

Step 1 is carried out exactly like the procedure in the direct immunofluorescence test, except that the antiserum (or *primary antibody*) is not labeled with a fluorescent dye. To make the antigen–antibody complexes visible, a second serum (or *secondary antibody*) is added in step 2. This serum is derived from an animal and contains fluorescence-labeled antibodies against human antibodies. The secondary antibodies react with the primary antibodies bound to the pathogen in the cells; as a result, the pathogen can be detected using a fluorescence microscope.

The advantage of the indirect immunofluorescence test is that it is far more sensitive than the direct one because each antibody molecule derived from the patient can bind several molecules of labeled anti-human antibody. The same labeled anti-human antiserum can be used to detect different antigens. In addition, it is possible to detect selectively IgM antibodies against the pathogen by using a secondary antibody specifically directed against the μ chain of human IgM.

Enzyme Immunoassays (EIA/ELISA)

Indication. Ever since the introduction of monoclonal antibodies, enzyme immunoassays (EIA)—such as enzyme-linked immunosorbent assays (ELISA)—have gained in importance as their specificity and sensitivity have been considerably increased. These tests can be used for detecting antigens as well as antibodies.

They are particularly suited for screening the sera from many patients.

Test principle. For the detection of antigen, pretreated microplates coated with primary monoclonal antibodies are used. The plates are overlaid with the solution containing the patient's swab material. If the antigen is present, it will bind firmly to the immobilized antibodies.

After washing, a secondary monoclonal antibody against the antigen is added; this antibody is coupled to an enzyme. A substrate subsequently added will be converted by the immobilized enzyme, and this reaction is made visible in yet another step by adding a second enzyme system with the appropriate color substrate.

The tandem arrangement of several enzyme systems leads to an amplification of the test, thus increasing its sensitivity. By using a color reaction, this test can be read with the naked eye. If a photometer is used, the results can also be printed out numerically.

Enzyme immunoassays are also used for detecting antibodies.

Indirect ELISA. Antigen is adsorbed to a microplate. If the patient's serum contains antibodies, they will bind to the immobilized antigen. The patient's antibodies are then detected by means of anti-human antibodies labeled with an enzyme (alkaline phosphatase, peroxidase).

For the detection of IgG, IgA, or IgM antibodies to *Chlamydia*, the following material may be used as antigen: elementary bodies of *Chlamydia* adsorbed to a plastic comb (ImmunoComb test), or cell cultures infected with *Chlamydia* (IPAzyme).

Competitive ELISA. Enzyme-labeled specific antibodies compete with the patient's antibodies for the binding sites present on the antigen fixed to the microplate.

Detectable pathogens. Tests are available for the following pathogens:

Antigen detection:
- chlamydiae
- gonococci.

Antibody detection:
- CMV
- hepatitis A virus
- hepatitis B virus
- hepatitis C virus
- HSV
- HIV
- EBV
- rubella virus
- measles virus
- *Toxoplasma.*

Special Detection Methods

Radioimmunoassay (RIA)

The principle of the test is similar to that of enzyme immunoassays, but with the antigens or antibodies adsorbed to test tubes. The detection of antibodies takes place by determining the amount of radioactivity bound.

This test has been widely used for the diagnosis of hepatitis B. Its disadvantage is the use of radioactivity.

Western Blot

Indication. This is a very expensive but extremely specific test. It is used to detect the various antibodies against individual proteins of the pathogen; these antigens are produced systematically during an infection. The type and number of bands thus provides some idea about the duration of an infection. Among other uses, the test has been employed to confirm the detection of HIV antibodies.

Test principle. The pathogen is disintegrated by gentle treatment into its individual components, which are then separated from each other by means of gel electrophoresis based on their molecular weights. Each of the resulting bands contains one protein of the pathogen, and the bands form a very distinct pattern. The bands are then incubated with the patient's serum. When antibodies to a certain protein are present in the serum, an antigen–antibody reaction occurs in the corresponding band.

The respective complexes are then made visible by means of an enzyme test.

If several bands are positive, the specificity of the immune response is confirmed.

Detection of Specific IgM Antibodies

Test principle. IgM antibodies are formed only when antigen is present. After the decline of a florid infection, the IgM antibodies rapidly disappear from the blood. Detection of specific IgM antibodies is therefore evidence of an infection that is coming to an end or one that has recently occurred.

As the serologic tests are usually performed after the appearance of clinical symptoms, an increase in titer—the best evidence for a fresh infection—is often not recorded; but it is only the detection of specific IgM antibodies that can give some idea about its reality.

Basically, **three methods** are available, and these can be combined with each other:

Separation of the heavy IgM antibodies from the lighter IgG antibodies:

- gradient centrifugation (ultracentrifuge)
- column chromatography.

The fraction containing the IgM antibody pool is then used separately in the corresponding test (hemagglutination inhibition test, immunofluorescence test, ELISA).

- Immunological detection of IgM antibodies.

This test is based on the use of specific antibodies against the μ chain of human IgM. An example is the hemagglutination immunosorbent technique for detecting rubella. Other methods work with antigen-coated microplates; the antibody bound to these plates is then detected by using labeled anti-μ serum or antibody. The method is similar to ELISA.

In all these tests, however, interference with rheumatoid factors must be taken into account. To exclude such interference, rheumatoid factors that might be present must first be eliminated by adsorption to aggregated IgG.

The specificity of the test can be increased by combining the separation of IgM antibodies with the use of anti-μ antibodies.

Disadvantages: the immunological detection of IgM antibodies is not entirely without problems. The specificity of the test is not so clear-cut; unfortunately, false results do occur. This applies to both negative and positive test-results.

Absorption Tests

Here, antibody classes or complexes are first separated from interfering molecules in order to increase the specificity of their detection.

Determination of Avidity

The strength of binding between antigen and antibody (avidity) permits some insight into the actuality of IgM antibody production. If IgM antibodies are detected, the avidity allows one to distinguish between a fresh infection and a persistent infection. The longer the infection persists, the stronger the binding between antibody and antigen and the more difficult to break it by urea treatment.

Detection by Molecular Biology Methods

Polymerase Chain Reaction (PCR)

Indication. The PCR method makes it possible to amplify minute amounts of genetic material. The reaction can thus be used for detecting very tiny amounts of pathogens. Prerequisite is the preparation of pathogen-specific DNA primers.

Test principle. Step 1 of the chain reaction is called *denaturation*. Here, the two strands of the pathogen's DNA are separated from each other by heat (94 °C), thus yielding two long single strands.

During step 2, called *annealing*, the separated strands bind to two primers. These are short synthetic oligonucleotides, i. e., segments of single-stranded DNA of approximately 20–30 bases in length. They are selected in such a way that one primer is complementary to the end of one strand of the target sequence while the other primer is complementary to the end of the other strand. The primers hybridize with the fitting sequences in the denatured DNA, thus defining the target sequence.

The annealing temperature depends on the primer's length and base composition (GC contents) and is usually between 40 °C and 60 °C. Once the primers bind to the single strands, the two short segments of double-stranded DNA thus created serve as starting blocks for the enzyme *Taq* polymerase during step 3, called *extension*.

Beginning at the 3' end of each primer, the heat stable *Taq* polymerase now adds, at a temperature of approximately 72 °C, the building blocks complementary to the template and links these with each other. It elongates the primers in the direction of the target DNA segment and thus completes the single strands to double strands. At the end of the first cycle, the original double strand has given rise to two new double strands that are identical to the old one. This cycle consisting of three individual steps can now be repeated several times in a row.

In each subsequent cycle, the newly formed DNA segments provide the templates for the formation of the new strands. A chain reaction has been created.

In theory, about one million copies of the target DNA segment can be obtained after 20 cycles, and about one billion copies after 30 cycles. This is sufficient material to be detected with the traditional methods, such as a color reaction.

Today, PCR is performed fully automatically in thermal cyclers: these are devices that repeatedly run through a certain temperature program (94 °C, 40–60 °C, 72 °C). A cycle usually lasts for less than three minutes. Thus, about one billion of copies of a certain DNA segment can be produced within less than two hours.

The PCR components include the following: the two primers each labeled with a biotin molecule, the enzymes *N*-uracil glycosylase (added to prevent carry-over) and *Taq* polymerase, and the four nucleotides A, C, G, and U.

Each DNA strand newly formed by PCR receives at its end a primer and thus also becomes labeled with biotin. The heat-sensitive *N*-uracil glycosylase loses its activity due to the high temperatures required for the PCR and thus no longer poses a threat to the newly formed strands.

After denaturation of the amplified DNA strands, part of the PCR solution is transferred to the well of a microplate, at the bottom of which a capture probe is anchored by a protein. Capture probes are short single-stranded DNA segments which act as genetic probes, like the primers used in the chain reaction. They are, however, complementary to an area in the middle (rather than the end) of the amplified DNA of the pathogen.

Within a short period, the capture probe catches the complementary PCR products from the solution, and double-stranded areas are formed. Thus, single-stranded DNA with base sequences complementary to the capture probe is fixed to the bottom of the microplate. Unbound strands are rinsed off.

Subsequently, an avidin–enzyme complex is added, which—due to the high affinity of avidin to biotin—quickly forms a very stable binding with the biotin-labeled end of the DNA. After further washing steps and the addition of certain reagents, the solution will turn blue. The color reaction is stopped by the addition of acid, and the color changes to yellow.

The color change to blue or yellow shows that DNA of the pathogen was present in the starting material.

The intensity of the color change to yellow can be evaluated by photometry. It provides a measure for PCR products present in the solution.

Detectable pathogens. The PCR method can be widely used for the detection of pathogens or their DNA. It is highly specific and very sensitive. Prerequisite is, however, that the corresponding DNA primers for pathogen-specific DNA segments can be produced. In principle, every pathogen can be detected by this method. Few tests are so far commercially available. Far more common are homemade tests that are produced by the investigators themselves.

Among the pathogens inducing infections relevant to gynecology, the following ones have already been detected by means of PCR:

- *Chlamydia trachomatis*
- papillomaviruses
- *Neisseria gonorrhoeae*
- hepatitis B viruses
- hepatitis C viruses
- *Treponema pallidum*
- *Candida* albicans
- *Toxoplasma gondii*
- *Borrelia burgdorferi*
- HIV
- cytomegaloviruses
- Herpes simplex virus.

DNA Chips

These are used for verifying resistances and mutations. The first DNA chips (for HIV) became commercially available in 1996. Single-stranded DNA fragments of known genes (gene probes) are anchored with one end to a small piece of glass so that they can be accurately located. The DNA to be tested is amplified by means of PCR and labeled with a fluorescent dye. In a temperature-controlled chamber the test DNA hybridizes with the chip DNA. The fluorescent sites of successful hybridization are detected with a laser beam. The method makes it possible to determine the location of the sequence within the genome.

Diagnostic Gene Chips

DNA diagnostic procedures using gene chips (gene arrays) permit to identify genetic characteristics that are relevant for individual patients. Early detection of diseases, groups with increased risks, and improved follow-up of treatments become possible this way. We distinguish between resequencing chips, polymorphism chips, and gene expression chips.

Diagnosis of Prenatal Infections

Normally, only an infection of the mother during pregnancy is recorded, and the risk for the child is concluded from this. However, not all children are infected if a maternal infection exists. Pregnancies are sometimes terminated without being at risk.

This approach is especially alarming when the risk for the fetus is low. This is true, for example, for rubella in the fourth month, and also for toxoplasmosis. Thus, prenatal diagnostics is not primarily for detecting infections in the child, but rather for excluding an infection and thus maintaining the pregnancy. In the case of treatable infections, it is used for improvement of the treatment.

Detection of Pathogens in the Amniotic Fluid

For a long time, pathogens could rarely be cultured reliably from the amniotic fluid; one of the very few exceptions has been, for example, cytomegaloviruses. With the introduction of polymerase chain reaction, the possibilities for detecting antigens have considerably expanded. This method can now be used in the case of toxoplasmosis (with some limitation), rubella, and cytomegalovirus infection.

Detection of Antibodies in the Umbilical Blood

Advances in ultrasound techniques and puncture techniques have made this method safer.

By puncturing the umbilical cord of the child, blood can be collected for the detection of antibodies. If specific antibodies of class IgM can be detected here, this is evidence for an infection of the child.

The earliest point in time of fetal blood collection is week 20 of pregnancy, because only then can one expect to find sufficient amounts of IgM antibodies. Better is week 22 of pregnancy. The umbilical cord is punctured under ultrasonic guidance directly in the region of the placental insertion, and 1.5 mL to 2 mL of blood can be collected.

Combination of Both Methods

The rate of detection of an infection of the child is limited based on the IgM antibodies present in the fetal blood; among other things, it depends on the amount of antibodies produced. Combining the search for antigen in the amniotic fluid by means of PCR and the search for IgM antibodies in the blood of the child will therefore be the best approach.

4 Anti-infectives (Antibacterials, Virostatics, Antimycotics, Antiparasitics, Antiseptics, Immunoglobulins)

Antibacterials

Definitions

Strictly speaking, **antibiotics** are antimicrobial agents produced by fungi or bacteria. However, the term often includes their semisynthetic derivatives or even completely synthetic **chemotherapeutics** with an antimicrobial effect (Table 4.**1**).

As more and more compounds are now manufactured chemically, the term **anti-infectives** is increasingly preferred. This term must not be confused with disinfectants (antiseptics) (Table 4.**8**).

Ideally, anti-infectives should only be directed at the pathogens of an infection. Their activity is essentially based on the specific inhibition of bacterial enzyme systems. It is possible to develop always new derivatives through chemical modification of the antibiotic molecules, with the derivatives getting better and better with respect to effectiveness and tolerance.

As microorganisms develop counterstrategies (e. g., mutation, selection, exchange of genomes), the search for new compounds and derivatives continues.

Unfortunately, all known anti-infectives interact also with the host organism, although usually only to a minor extent. Sulfonamides or β-lactam antibiotics can cause allergic reactions, aminoglycosides may have nephrotoxic and ototoxic effects, and erythromycin may cause gastrointestinal symptoms, depending on the dose.

In addition to undesired reactions in the host organism itself, the bacterial population changes to various extents, depending on both the antibi-

Table 4.**1** Antibacterials and their sites of action

Group of compounds	Site of action	Compounds (representative trade names)
Penicillins	Cell wall synthesis	Penicillin G, benzathine–penicillin V, amoxicillin, piperacillin
Penicillins + β-lactamase inhibitors	Cell wall synthesis	Amoxillin + clavulanate (Augmentin), ampicillin + sulbactam (Unasyn), piperacillin + tazobactam (Zosyn)
Cephalosporins (i. v. or p. o.)	Cell wall synthesis	Cefuroxime (Zinacef), cefotiam (Spizef), ceftriaxone (Rocephin), ceftazidime (Fortum)
Carbapenems	Cell wall synthesis	Imipenem + cilastatin (Primaxim), meropenem (Merrem)
Tetracyclines	Protein synthesis	Doxycycline (Vibracin)
Aminoglycosides	Protein synthesis	Gentamycin (Garamycin), amicacin (Amikin), tobramycin (Tobrex)
Macrolides	Protein synthesis	Erythromycin (Erythrocin, Staticin), roxithromycin (Xoxin), azithromycin (Zithromax)
Lincosamides	Protein synthesis	Clindamycin (Cleocin)
Glycopeptides	Cell wall synthesis	Vancomycin (Vancocin)
Fluoroquinolones	DNA gyrase activity	Ciprofloxacin (Cipro, Ciloxan), moxifloxacin (Avelox), ofloxacin (Floxin, Ocuflox), levofloxacin (Levaquin)
5-Nitroimidazoles	Nucleic acid synthesis	Metronidazol (Flagyl)
Sulfonamides	Folic acid synthesis	Trimethoprim + sulfamethoxazole (Co-Trimoxazol, Bactrim)

otic agent and its target pathogen. These changes involve primarily the local flora and the selection of resistant pathogens.

Hence, anti-infective therapy should always be well thought out, and it requires a clear diagnosis.

At the start of the treatment, the clinical condition of the patient is crucial; the severity of the disease and the pathogens that might be involved will determine which compound should be chosen. Any material for microbiological diagnosis must be collected prior to administering the first dose. Pathogens found after one to three days should be taken into account when deciding on further treatment.

Determination of Antibiotic Effectiveness In Vitro

The in-vitro effectiveness of an antibiotic is established by determining the minimal inhibitory concentration (MIC) using the serial dilution test. The MIC is defined as the concentration resulting in complete growth inhibition within 24 hours; it depends on the seeding density of the pathogen, the culture medium, and the incubation time.

In the normal routine, however, the disc diffusion test is used; it is less expensive. Agar plates are inoculated with the pathogen isolated from the patient, and individual filter discs soaked with different antibiotics are placed on the culture. The effectiveness of the antibiotic is then deduced from the size of the field of inhibition around the disc. This test is only moderately accurate and depends on many parameters, e. g., bacterial seeding density, culture medium used, thickness of the agar layer, stability of the antibiotic, and the antibiotic's ability to diffuse in agar.

Although the determination of resistance in vitro will provide a rough idea about the activity of anti-infectives, the process is much more complex in vivo and does not always agree with the testing in vitro.

Resistance

We distinguish different types of resistance. In the case of natural or intrinsic resistance, a bacterial species is not at all sensitive to a certain antibiotic agent; for example, penicillin is completely ineffective against *Pseudomonas aeruginosa*. In addition, there is acquired resistance, which includes mutational resistance and secondary resistance. The latter is due to the selection of resistant variants during antibiotic therapy.

Bacteria may acquire resistance by means of chromosomal mutation or by the uptake of plasmids from other bacteria. In the latter case, we talk about transferred resistance.

Mutations causing resistance to antibiotics may occur spontaneously, although they are promoted by the presence of antibiotics. In hospitals, resistance acquired through plasmids plays a larger role than chromosomal resistance. Transferred resistance frequently occurs particularly in gram-negative rod-shaped bacteria. For example, the multiple resistances of *Salmonella* can be transmitted to originally sensitive *Escherichia coli* strains, and this may take place in the intestinal tract, on the mucosae, or on the skin. Conversely, the loss of acquired transferred resistance is also possible.

β-Lactam Antibiotics

These all contain one β-lactam ring. We distinguish four subgroups: penicillins, cephalosporins, carbapenems, and monobactams.

Mechanisms of Resistance to β-Lactam Antibiotics

The two essential mechanisms of resistance are the production of β-lactamases, which hydrolyze the β-lactam ring, and the production of alternative enzymes, which have a reduced affinity to penicillins and take on the function of carboxypeptidases.

Of special importance among the β-lactamases of gram-positive bacteria is the penicillinase of staphylococci. The β-lactamases of gram-negative bacteria include classes A to D, with the chromosomal class A and the plasmid-coded class C being the most important ones clinically.

There is also production of penicillin-binding proteins in gram-positive bacteria.

Penicillins

Properties and Spectrum of Activities

Penicillins represent a well-tolerated group of compounds that may be administered without reservations during pregnancy. They have a bactericidal effect on the multiplication of bacteria by inhibiting cell wall synthesis. The initially narrow spectrum of penicillins has been expanded by altering the side chains. Due to the skeletal structure of 5-aminopenicillanic acid, however, they are not resistant to penicillinase or β-lactamases. By combining them with β-lactamase inhibitors, the spectrum has been expanded for certain pathogens. The half-lives of penicillins are short (apart from a few exceptions) and found to be approximately one hour. For this reason, they must be administered at least three times daily.

The most important **penicillins** are:

- *Penicillin G.* Parenteral administration only (i. v. or i. m.). Depot formulations have a prolonged activity. Very effective against streptococci of group A, gonococci, treponemes, sensitive staphylococci (only 20–60 %), clostridiae, and other anaerobes (but not all of them).
- *Phenoxymethyl penicillin (penicillin V).* This is an acid-resistant penicillin and can therefore be administered orally. It has the same mode of action as penicillin G, but is less potent.
- *Penicillinase-resistant penicillins.* They have only one indication—namely, penicillinase-producing staphylococci—because their activity in sensitive strains is only one-tenth of the activity of penicillin G.

Three compounds are important: dicloxacillin, flucloxacillin, and oxacillin.

Aminopenicillins (ampicillin, bacampicillin, amoxicillin). The spectrum corresponds to that of penicillin G, and there is an increased activity against streptococci, in particular enterococci, and also listeriae. Gonococci and many *Enterobacteriaceae* are affected as well.

Ampicillin was the first broad-spectrum penicillin to be developed. It is preferred during pregnancy because of its broad spectrum, good tissue permeability, and the long-time experience with this compound.

Amoxicillin is better resorbed than ampicillin. It is effective also against species of *Chlamydia* and *Borrelia.*

A major disadvantage of this group of antibiotics is the lack of β-lactamase stability; many staphylococci, enteric bacteria, or other opportunistic pathogens are therefore not affected. Here, an antibiogram provides valuable information.

Another disadvantage is the high rate of exanthemas, ranging from 5–20 %. Only very few exanthemas are caused by allergies, whereas exanthemas are very common when mononucleosis is present simultaneously.

Combinations of aminopenicillins with β-lactamase inhibitors. β-Lactamases are enzymes that open the β-lactam ring of β-lactam antibiotics (penicillins and cephalosporins) and thus destroy their activity.

The preferred location of β-lactamases is the periplasmic space of many gram-negative bacteria. Here, the enzymes serve as part of the bacterial defense system.

The genes coding for β-lactamases may be located on the chromosome or on an episome, i. e., they occur naturally in certain bacteria and can be transferred to other bacteria.

In order to expand the effectiveness of β-lactam antibiotics, β-lactamase inhibitors have been developed. These usually represent rudimentary β-lactam rings that irreversibly bind to β-lactamases and thus inactivate the β-lactamases of the bacterial cell.

The spectrum of penicillins, and also that of cephalosporins, can be considerably expanded in this way.

Common β-lactamase producers include opportunistic pathogens, such as *Staphylococcus aureus*, many enteric bacteria, and certain anaerobes from the *Bacteroides* group.

Three different β-lactamase inhibitors are available today:

- clavulanic acid
- sulbactam
- tazobactam.

They can be administered either as a supplement to the antibiotic or in a fixed combination with the antibiotic, for example:

- amoxicillin + clavulanate
- ampicillin + sulbactam
- piperacillin + tazobactam.

Ureidopenicillins. They are available for parenteral administration only. Their activities are slightly broader than that of ampicillin. Some opportunistic pathogens, such as species of *Pseudomonas*, *Klebsiella*, and *Serratia*, should therefore be more affected; however, studies have not clearly confirmed this. In addition, these antibiotics are not β-lactamase stable.

Examples: azlocillin, mezlocillin, and piperacillin.

Cephalosporins

They are among the most frequently prescribed antibiotics due to their broad spectrum and good tolerance.

Bacteria resistant to cephalosporins include enterococci, listeriae, chlamydiae, and methicillin-resistant *Staphylococcus aureus* strains (MRSA).

Initially, cephalosporins were only available for parenteral administration. Meanwhile, there are also several effective preparations that can be taken orally.

They are subdivided into four groups (first to fourth generation cephalosporins) (Table 4.2), and their spectrum of activity has shifted more and more from gram-positive to gram-negative pathogens and also to opportunistic pathogens.

Properties and Spectrum of Activities

Like the penicillins, cephalosporins belong to the β-lactam antibiotics and inhibit the synthesis of the cell wall (peptidoglycan synthesis).

They differ in their mode of action from the penicillins. They have a different affinity for the bacterial binding proteins, they can penetrate through the bacterial cell membrane, and they are β-lactamase stable.

Through alterations of the side chains, the spectrum of cephalosporins has been increasingly expanded, in particular with respect to gram-negative bacteria. However, this has resulted in some loss of activity with respect to gram-positive bacteria, and the effectiveness against staphylococci has decreased.

Cephalosporins play an important role in gynecology because they are very effective and well tolerated. They may be administered during pregnancy.

One disadvantage of cephalosporins in gynecology is their ineffectiveness against *Chlamydia* and *Listeria*. Enterococci commonly found as colonizing pathogens are also resistant to cephalosporins; they are therefore more often detected in association with this therapy, but this plays only a minor role clinically.

First Generation: Cephalothin Group

These are very effective against gram-positive bacteria, such as streptococci, staphylococci, and also gonococci, whereas their effectiveness against gram-negative bacteria varies.

Second Generation: Cefuroxime Group

These preparations are largely stabile against β-lactamases. They are highly effective against gram-positive bacteria (e. g., staphylococci), but they also show an increased activity against many gram-negative rod-shaped bacteria. They are effective against gonococci, in particular against β-lactamase-producing gonococci. *Klebsiella pneumoniae* is highly sensitive as well. By contrast, pseudomonads, enterococci, mycoplasma, and chlamydiae are resistant.

Today, the most commonly used compounds are cefuroxime and cefotiam.

Table 4.**2** Cephalosporins

Group	Generic name	Representative trade name
First generation	Cefazolin	Ancef
Second generation	Cefamandole Cefoxitin Cefuroxime Cefotiam	Mandol Mefoxin Zinacef Spizef
Third generation	Cefotaxime Ceftriaxone Cefadizime	Claforan Rocephin Opticef
Fourth generation	Ceftazidime Cefepime Cefpirome	Fortaz Maxipime Cefrom

Cefamandole, cefoperazone, cefotetan, and moxalactam are hardly used anymore because of their adverse effects on coagulation and other problems. Cefoxitin is very effective against isolated strains of the *Bacteroides fragilis* group, but less effective against *E. coli* and *Klebsiella*. It has been used in gynecology for a long time.

Third Generation: Cefotaxime Group

This group has an even broader spectrum, especially with respect to gram-negative bacteria. Some preparations are also fairly effective against the opportunistic pathogen *Pseudomonas*. The half-lives of these compounds vary, ranging from one hour for cefotaxime to eight hours for ceftriaxone, depending on their binding to proteins, among other things

Ceftriaxone is the preferred antibiotic for meningitis because of its pharmacokinetic properties.

Fourth Generation

This group has the broadest spectrum of activity. Ceftazidime and cefepime are effective also against pseudomonads. They are less effective against gram-positive bacteria and anaerobes.

Oral Cephalosporins

Their main indications are infections of the skin and soft-tissue infections when it is suspected that streptococci and staphylococci may be involved. These compounds belong to the most commonly prescribed oral antibiotics (Table 4.3).

For example, cefuroxime axetil is very effective against streptococci of groups A and B, gonococci, *Staphylococcus aureus*, and many other

Table 4.**3** Oral cephalosporins

Generic name	Representative trade name
Cefalexine (cephalexin)	Keflex
Cefaclor	Ceclor
Cefadroxil	Duricef
Cefuroxime axetil	Ceftin
Cefixime	Suprax
Cefpodoxime proxetil	Vantin
Ceftibuten	Cedax

gram-negative bacteria. Two doses of this drug are sufficient for gonococci infection; for other infections twice daily for five days or more.

Carbapenems

Of all β-lactam antibiotics, carbapenems have the broadest antibacterial activity, even against opportunistic pathogens and anaerobes. Only mycobacteria, *Enterococcus faecium*, and MRSA strains are resistant. Carbapenems are well suited for monotherapy in the case of severe, unclear infections. Although well tolerated, they do have a noteworthy side effect: if taken for a long period, they promote the selection of multiresistant pathogens and of fungi, in particular.

Carbapenems include:
- imipenem + cilastatin, a fixed combination of antibiotic and inhibitor
- meropenem
- ertapenem.

Monobactams

Particularly effective against *Enterobacteriaceae* (with exception of *Citrobacter* and *Enterobacter*) combination with other drugs or in case of allergy to penicillin.

Other Antibiotics

Tetracyclines

Their bacteriostatic effect is based on the inhibition of protein synthesis, and their activity depends on the medium and its pH. They have long half-lives (approximately 12 hours) and are therefore administered only once a day; moreover, they are effective orally. They diffuse passively through the plasma membrane and cannot diffuse back. The resulting intracellular concentration of the drug is advantageous in cases of intracellular infections (e.g., with *Chlamydia*).

Because these drugs are incorporated into teeth and bones, they must not be administered during pregnancy and breast-feeding. They also interact with oral contraceptives, and security is impaired by bacterial hydrolysis of conjugated estrogens in the intestine. Anticonvulsives affect the activity of tetracyclines.

Tetracyclines have a relatively broad spectrum of activity. Because of their extensive use, resistances have increased especially with respect to gram-negative bacteria. They are therefore unsuitable for monotherapy of severe infections. However, they are effective against many gynecologically important pathogens, such as gonococci (although not all of them), *Treponema pallidum*, listeriae, mycoplasma, and chlamydiae.

Antibiotics of this group include:
- tetracycline
- oxitetracycline
- doxycycline
- minocycline.

Doxycycline is preferred because it can be administered orally, is well resorbed independently of food, and is well tolerated due to its low metabolism.

Aminoglycosides

They, too, inhibit protein synthesis, and they are bactericidal against a wide range of gram-negative bacteria, in particular.

The bactericidal effect is due to the production of nonfunctional proteins that become incorporated into the bacterial cell membrane and thus change permeability. Recently, aminoglycosides have been used less often because of their limited therapeutic range and because new, less toxic compounds with a comparable spectrum have become available.

Aminoglycosides are very effective against staphylococci, *Klebsiella pneumoniae*, *Escherichia coli*, *Proteus vulgaris*, and other enteric bacteria. They are less effective against streptococci and anaerobes. As combination antibiotics, they play a major role in severe infections. They must be administered parenterally. Because of their nephrotoxicity, they have to be individually adjusted for patients with renal insufficiency.

They should be avoided during pregnancy because of their nephrotoxic and ototoxic potential.

The trend today is to use a single dose, whereas it has been recommended in the past that the daily dose be divided into three doses while the patient is under therapeutic drug monitoring. The single dose reduces the risk of nephrotoxicity, and the postantibiotic effect (PAE) of the higher initial concentration raises the drug's effectiveness.

The most important examples, for parenteral administration only, are:

- gentamicin
- tobramycin
- netilmicin
- amicacin.

Other compounds include:

- neomycin, a topical antibiotic for skin infections or, in cases of liver coma, for suppression of the intestinal flora
- spectinomycin, an aminocyclitol antibiotic, has a broad spectrum but relatively low activity. It is used only for single treatment (intramuscular injection) in the case of gonorrhea.

Macrolides

Macrolide antibiotics (Table 4.4) inhibit protein synthesis.

Erythromycin has been known for a very long time. It has a bacteriostatic effect when used in therapeutic doses and a bactericidal effect in very high doses. It is very effective against streptococci, gonococci, listeriae, *Chlamydia trachomatis, Mycoplasma pneumoniae* (but not *Mycoplasma hominis*), and *Ureaplasma urealyticum.*

It is effective, though to variable degrees, against staphylococci. During pregnancy, it is the preferred drug for the treatment of sensitive pathogens (e. g., *Chlamydia*) when other antibiotics are contraindicated. Because of common gastrointestinal problems in 10–20% of patients, more recent macrolides are preferred.

Other macrolide antibiotics include *josamycin* as well as the modern macrolides *roxithromycin* and *clarithromycin.* The latter two can be administered in lower doses because of their increased effectiveness; they are therefore better tolerated. A macrolide antibiotic with very long half-life is *azithromycin*; it needs to be administered only once a week or only as a single dose.

Today, the main indications for macrolides are chlamydiae, mycoplasma, and legionellae, i. e., the pathogens of atypical pneumonia.

Spiramycin, yet another macrolide, is rarely used today. However, it still is the preferred drug for treating toxoplasmosis (see antiparasitics, p. 50) during the first trimester, because there is virtually no passage of this drug through the placenta.

Table 4.**4** Macrolides

Generic name	Representative trade name
Erythromycin	Erythrocin
Josamycin	Wilprafen
Spiramycin	Rovamycin
Roxithromycin	Xoxin
Clarithromycin	Biaxin
Azithromycin	Zithromax

Lincosamides

Examples are *lincomycin* and the gynecologically important *clindamycin, a* derivative of lincomycin. Both inhibit protein synthesis. They are effective against staphylococci and anaerobes. Gonococci as well as all aerobic, gram-negative rod-shaped bacteria (*Enterobacteriaceae*) and mycoplasma are resistant.

Lincosamides can be administered both orally and parenterally. In 5–20% of patients, the intestinal flora may change, which is associated with soft stools and/or pseudomembranous enterocolitis and should be taken into account.

Clindamycin is also available as a gel for topical application in the vaginal region, where it may be used for treating various bacterial disorders, including bacterial vaginosis. The vaginal preparation is the drug of choice for treating purulent vaginitis (plasma cell vaginitis).

Glycopeptides and Lipopeptides

These are soluble, complex, high-molecular-weight compounds with excellent activity against gram-positive bacteria, but they lack activity against gram-negative bacteria. Two preparations have been approved: *vancomycin* and *teicoplanin.* They have systemic activity when administered parenterally. Oral administration of vancomycin is only indicated as a secondary therapy in the case of severe antibiotic-associated colitis. It is excreted through the kidney.

Vancomycin is a high-molecular-weight glycopeptide with a bactericidal effect particularly on the synthesis of the bacterial cell wall. It is especially effective against staphylococci, streptococci, and *Clostridium difficile.* It is an important bactericidal antibiotic reserved for staphylococcal infections and also the preferred drug in cases of pseudomembranous enterocolitis and infections with methicillin-resistant *Staphylococcus aureus* (MRSA) strains.

Oxazolidinones

These represent a completely new class of entirely synthetic antimicrobials.

Linezolid is very effective against staphylococci, including MRSA strains, also against benzylpenicillin-resistant pneumococci (*Streptococcus pneumoniae*) and enterococci (*Enterococcus faecalis* and *E. faecium*), and other gram-positive bacteria. They have a half-life of five to seven hours.

Fluoroquinolones

Properties. Fluoroquinolones are synthetic antibacterial compounds derived from nalidixic acid, and they have a particularly broad spectrum of activity. Chemically, they are fluorinated 4-quinolones that interfere with DNA synthesis by inhibiting DNA topoisomerase (DNA gyrase).

Since their introduction in 1962, continued development has turned these compounds into the most active and versatile class of anti-infective agents. As they are well resorbed when administered orally, oral treatment of infections with multiresistant opportunistic pathogens has become possible. Most fluoroquinolones are well suited for the treatment of urinary tract infections because their main route of excretion is through the kidney. This route of excretion must be considered in cases of renal insufficiency; another route is through the liver. These compounds have much longer half-lives than penicillins, and administering the more recently developed compounds once daily is therefore sufficient.

Fluoroquinolones are extremely effective against *Enterobacteriaceae*, in particular. They are therefore well suited for treating intestinal diseases, including diarrhea picked up while traveling in tropical countries. They are not the first choice for infections with gram-positive bacteria (streptococci and staphylococci). More recently developed compounds (moxifloxacin and gatifloxacin) are more effective against chlamydiae and even against anaerobes. Lactobacilli are not inhibited by quinolones, which is an advantage.

Table 4.**5** Fluoroquinolones

Group	Compound and activity	Representative trade name
First generation	Norfloxacin Pefloxacin	Noroxin Peflacin
Second generation	Ciprofloxacin, i.v. and p.o.: urinary tract infections and soft tissue infections; one of the most commonly used fluoroquinolones worldwide	Ciloxan
	Ofloxacin, i.v. and p.o.: urinary tract infections and soft tissue infections	Floxin
	Enofloxacin Flerofloxacin	
Third generation	Levofloxacin, i.v. and p.o.	Levaquin
	Sparfloxacin	Zagam
Fourth generation	Moxifloxacin: well resorbed orally; long half-life of 11–12 hours; very effective against *Streptococcus pneumoniae* including many resistant strains, *Haemophilus influenzae*, legionellae, chlamydiae, mycobacteria, *Staphylococcus aureus*, *Enterobacteriaceae*, and anaerobes	Avelox
	Clinafloxacin Gemifloxacin	
	Gatifloxacin	Tequin

Indications. Fluoroquinolones are indicated in cases of complicated urinary tract infections with opportunistic pathogens, soft tissue infections with opportunistic pathogens or several pathogens of various sensitivities, and *Chlamydia* infections. They are effective, although with limitation, against opportunistic pathogens having a high natural resistance (e.g., pseudomonads). However, they promote resistances even here, although not as quickly as other antibiotics.

Due to their extensive use, the development of resistances has increased in all relevant bacterial species.

Contraindications. During pregnancy and breastfeeding, fluoroquinolones must not be administered. In growing animals, particularly in the beagle, damage to cartilage tissue has been observed, although at very high doses—many times higher than the therapeutic dose.

Fluoroquinolones are subdivided into four groups (first to fourth generations) (Table 4.**5**).

Nitroimidazoles

These chemotherapeutic agents are the preferred drugs for treating infections with anaerobic bacteria and infections with protozoa:

There are four different nitroimidazoles, although only two of them (metronidazole and tinidazole) are still being used:

- metronidazole
- ornidazole
- tinidazole
- nimorazole.

In protozoa and obligate anaerobic bacteria, they are converted to the active form by reduction of the nitro group. The reduced metabolite then inhibits nucleic acid synthesis by binding to the DNA.

Nitroimidazoles are suited for oral, intravenous, rectal, and vaginal administrations. However, preparations are not available for all these forms of administration. Excellent tissue penetration ensures that these compounds reach high concentrations.

They are the preferred drugs in cases of trichomoniasis, bacterial vaginosis, and—as a supplement—in cases of severe infections involving anaerobes. Due to the long half-lives of eight to 12 hours (exception: three hours for nimorazole), they are administered only once a day or, at the most, twice a day.

Risks. This group of compounds poses a special problem. Based on theoretical considerations, a certain risk of carcinogenesis due to the production of reduced metabolites cannot be excluded; nevertheless, the reduced metabolites are required for the effectiveness of these drugs. Various studies using experimental animals did not provide a clear-cut answer. In none of the cases was the life span of the animals reduced; rather, it was prolonged when very high doses were administered over a long period.

On the other hand, several studies reported an increased incidence of certain tumors. In addition, a dose-dependent mutagenic effect of this group of compounds was demonstrated in experiments with bacteria. For this reason, it is recommended that the duration of treatment be short and administration during pregnancy restricted.

Indications. Trichomoniasis, infections with anaerobes, pseudomembranous enterocolitis associated with *Clostridium difficile* or induced by antibiotics, and Crohn disease.

Sulfonamides

Properties. Sulfonamides (or sulfa drugs) are synthetic chemotherapeutics derived from sulfanilamide. Their bacteriostatic effect on proliferating pathogens is based on the inhibition of folic acid synthesis. They are very effective against streptococci (but not enterococci) and chlamydiae, while their effectiveness against *Enterobacteriaceae*, staphylococci, and gonococci is moderate and variable.

Sulfonamides are rarely used today because of the increase in resistances and allergies and because more effective and less toxic antibiotics are available.

Possible uses. Treatment of toxoplasmosis with sulfadiazine in combination with pyrimethamine, or in general as part of the combination antibiotic *Co-Trimoxazole*.

The latter preparation is a fixed combination of *trimethoprim* with the sulfonamide *sulfamethoxazole*. It has a broad spectrum of activity and is preferentially used for treating urinary tract infections.

If possible, this drug should not be administered during pregnancy—especially not during the last four weeks of pregnancy and during breast-feeding—because of the risk of hyperbilirubinemia in the child. It can be administered orally and parenterally.

Risks associated with *trimethoprim*. During pregnancy, this compound should not be used unless there is an absolute indication. As with sulfasalazine and the diuretic triamterene, there have been reports that this inhibitor of dihydrofolate reductase may increase the risks of cardiovascular defects and facial cleft formation.

Amoxicillin and cephalosporins do not carry such risks.

Trimethoprim should be administered only after careful consideration of the risks, and even then only together with a multivitamin preparation.

Chloramphenicol

Originally derived from *Streptomyces venezuelae* and now produced synthetically, this compound is very effective and has a broad spectrum of activity. However, it is rarely used today because of its bone marrow toxicity. Another side effect is the gray syndrome observed in newborns, which is potentially fatal. Chloramphenicol is therefore contraindicated during the last trimester and during breast-feeding.

Rifamycins

These semisynthetic compounds are derived from substances produced by a strain of *Streptomyces mediterranei*. They act by inhibiting RNA polymerase. They are indicated for the treatment of tuberculosis, in the first place. Recently, they

Table 4.6 Scopes of application of various antibacterials

Class of compounds	Indication/effective against
Penicillins (amoxicillin)	Streptococci, *Listeria*, premature amniorrhexis, prophylaxis, *Chlamydia*
Penicillins + β-lactamase inhibitors	Salpingitis, premature amniorrhexis, prophylaxis
Cephalosporins (i. v. or p. o.)	*Staphylococcus aureus, Escherichia coli, Klebsiella*, abscesses, prophylaxis
Macrolides	*Chlamydia, Mycoplasma* during pregnancy
Aminoglycosides	Rarely used, only as a supplement in cases of very serious infections
Tetracyclines (doxycycline)	*Chlamydia, Mycoplasma*
Fluoroquinolones	Urinary tract infections, (*Chlamydia*)
Metronidazole	Anaerobic bacteria, *Trichomonas*, abdominal infections
Clindamycin	Purulent vaginitis, *Staphylococcus aureus*, puerperal sepsis
Sulfonamides	Toxoplasmosis, urinary tract infections
Glycopeptides (vancomycin)	Rarely used, e. g., methicillin-resistant *Staphylococcus aureus* strains
Carbapenems (imipenem)	Extremely severe infections

have also been used in combination with other drugs for treating infections caused by gram-positive or intracellular bacteria. Rifamycins pose problems because they rapidly lead to resistance and have severe effects on the liver (hepatic enzyme induction, thus causing faster elimination of other substances and liver toxicity).

Fosfomycin

This small molecule is produced by *Streptomyces* species. It acts by inhibiting cell wall synthesis and has a broad spectrum of activity against gram-positive and gram-negative bacteria. It is effective orally as well as parenterally and is excreted through the kidneys. Gastrointestinal side effects are common, and so are allergies. This drug is especially suited for treating infections caused by *Staphylococcus aureus*.

Antibiotics Reserved for Special Cases

Quinupristin/Dalfopristin

Marketed under the name Synercid, this preparation contains quinupristin and dalfopristin (30 : 70). These streptogramins are produced by various *Streptomyces* strains and are related to macrolides and lincosamides. Together, the three types of protein synthesis inhibitors have been termed the macrolide–lincosamide–streptogramin (MLS) group of antibiotics. They bind to bacterial ribosomes at various sites, thus interfering with protein synthesis.

This antibiotic is administered by intravenous injection and is reserved for severe, potentially life-threatening infections with multiresistant opportunistic pathogens. Above all, it is active against gram-positive cocci, e. g., methicillin-resistant *Staphylococcus aureus* (MRSA) strains and vancomycin-resistant *Enterococcus faecium* (VREF) strains. It is not effective against *Enterococcus faecalis*.

Undesired Effects of Antibiotics on the Intestinal Flora

Antibiotic-associated Diarrhea (AAD)

It is well known that virtually all effective antibiotics may cause diarrhea. However, there are differences with respect to how often this happens.

Diarrhea is observed relatively often (10–20 %) with β-lactam antibiotics, e. g., cefixime, amoxillin + clavulanate, ampicillin + sulbactam, and clindamycin. It is less often observed (2–5 %) with fluoroquinolones, macrolides, and tetracyclines.

The symptoms are variable and range from soft stools to colitis. *Clostridium difficile* is the cause of diarrhea only in 10–20 % of patients. However, it is detected in the majority of patients with colitis.

Pseudomembranous colitis, in particular, is typical for infections with *Clostridium difficile*. Other signs of such an infection are leukocytosis, hypoalbuminemia due to the loss of protein caused by enteropathy, and the presence of leukocytes in the stool. The detection of toxins (toxins A and B) by ELISA or tissue cultures is evidence for the presence of this pathogen. However, the tests are not always successful; it is therefore recommended that several stool samples be examined.

Among the risk factors are advanced age (60-year-olds are 20 times more often colonized by this pathogen than 20-year-olds) and admission to hospital (20% to 30% of admitted patients become colonized).

The preferred **therapy** is 3 × 500 mg metronidazole (p. o. or i. v.) for 10 days or vancomycin (p. o. only; i. v. is not effective in this instance).

Prevention is achieved by well-thought-out antibiotic therapy, observance of hygienic rules (washing hands after contact with the patient), and the use of gloves. Symptomatic patients with stool incontinence should be accommodated in single-bed rooms.

Tetracyclines interact with oral contraceptives. The safety of contraceptives is compromised by the reduced bacterial hydrolysis of conjugated estrogens in the intestine. Anticonvulsives interfere with the activity of tetracyclines.

Virostatics

It is difficult to inhibit viruses as they do not have a metabolism of their own but use extensively the enzyme systems of their host cell. Some viruses, however, bring their own starter enzyme with them; for example, HIV has reverse transcriptase, and herpesviruses have thymidine kinase. The first virostatics were analogs of DNA building blocks. As a result of extensive scientific activity in the fight against HIV infections, virostatics have now been developed that interfere, for example, with the assembly of virus particles (virions). Other compounds inhibit viral replication in the host cell.

DNA Analogs That Inhibit DNA Replication

(Effective against HSV, CMV, and HIV)

- Herpes simplex viruses and varicella–zoster virus:
  - Aciclovir (acycloguanosine) has a fairly selective activity in cells infected with herpesviruses, because the viral thymidine kinase converts this drug 200 times more efficiently into its high-energy monophosphate than cellular enzymes do. This makes the compound highly effective at the site of infection. Aciclovir is the preferred drug in cases of severe herpesvirus infections; it is available for oral, intravenous, and topical therapies. At high doses, it is also effective against the varicella–zoster virus. It may be administered during pregnancy or to the newborn in cases of severe infections. Systemic administration (p. o. or i. v.) is more effective as the uptake of the agent after topical application is only moderate. Thymidine kinase-negative strains may develop during long-term use, but they disappear once aciclovir has been discontinued.
  - Valaciclovir is the valine ester of aciclovir. When taken orally, it is rapidly resorbed and almost completely converted into aciclovir plus L-valine by the valaciclovir hydrolase present in intestine and liver. Because valaciclovir is well absorbed in the gastrointestinal tract, its bioavailability is much better (54%) than that of aciclovir (10–30%).
  - Famciclovir is similar to aciclovir but has a slightly longer half-life.
  - Ribavirin, also a guanosine analog, increases the mutation rate and should only be used as a supplement. It is also active against other viruses, e. g., HCV.
  - Foscarnet (phosphonoformate) is fairly toxic when taken orally; it should be used only topically.
- Cytomegaloviruses:
  - Ganciclovir, a guanosine analog, is used only for severe diseases because it is relatively toxic.
  - Cidofovir, a deoxycytosine analog, is only used for CMV retinitis because it is very toxic.
- Human immunodeficiency virus:
  - Zidovudine (azidothymidine, AZT) inhibits the reverse transcriptase of HIV (nucleotide reverse transcriptase inhibitor, NRTI). AZT-resistant mutants may occur during therapy, but they disappear some time after discontinuation of the drug.
  - Didanosine (dideoxyinosine, DDI).
  - Lamivudine in combination with AZT is also effective in hepatitis B.
  - Stavudine is used for combination with didanosine but not with AZT; it increases the risk of lactic acidosis during pregnancy.
  - Zalcitabine (dideoxycytosine, DDC) is contraindicated during pregnancy.
  - Carbovir.
  - Abacavir.

Nonnucleoside Reverse Transcriptase Inhibitors (NNRTI) (Effective Against HIV)

- Nevirapine is used during pregnancy and childbirth.
- Efavirenz is contraindicated during pregnancy.
- Delavirdine is contraindicated during pregnancy.

4

Protease Inhibitors: Inhibition of Virion Maturation and Assembly (Effective Against HIV)

- Saquinavir may be administered during pregnancy in combination with ritonavir.
- Indinavir.
- Ritonavir.
- Amprenavir may be administered during pregnancy.
- Lopinavir + ritonavir may be administered during pregnancy.

Table 4.7 Compounds and numbers of preparations available for treating fungal infections

Topical antimycotics	Number of preparations on the market in many countries
Amorolfin*****	1
Amphotericin B*	7
Bifonazole**	11
Ciclopirox olamine/ciclopirox****	9
Clotrimazole**	71
Croconazole**	2
Econazole**	12
Fenticonazole**	4
Isoconazole**	1
Ketoconazole**	2
Miconazole**	19
Naftifine******	3
Natamycin*	5
Nystatin*	43
Oxiconazole**	7
Terbinafine******	1
Tioconazole**	4
Systemic antimycotics	**Number of preparations**
Amphotericin B	2
Caspofungin	1
Fluconazole	7
Flucytosine	1
Itraconazole	5
Ketoconazole	2
Terbinafine	1
Voriconazole	1

* Polyenes
** Imidazoles
*** Triazoles
**** Pyridones
***** Morpholines
****** Allylamines

Other Compounds for Treating Virus Infections

- Interferon alpha-2a or alpha-2b (inhibition of viral protein synthesis at the level of translation) in cases of hepatitis B and C, and cytomegalovirus infections.
- Neuraminidase inhibitors, e.g., zanamivir in cases of influenza; topical application by means of inhalation.
- Inhibitors of viral penetration, e.g., amantadine in cases of influenza.
- Antisense preparations, e.g., fomivirsen in cases of cytomegalovirus infections.

Special Compounds for Eliminating Genital Warts (HPV)

- The resin podophyllin is obsolete because it is a mixture containing four cytotoxic lignans as well as other mutagenic and carcinogenic substances, such as quercetin and kaempferol.
- Podophyllotoxin or podofilox, on the other hand, is the purified active ingredient of podophyllin. It inhibits mitosis and is available on the market as an alcoholic preparation (0.5%) and as a cream (0.15%). *Pregnancy:* for safety reasons, podophyllotoxin should not be used during pregnancy and breast-feeding because of its antimitotic property. So far, neither teratogenic nor embryo toxic potentials have been detected after topical application in animal experiments.

Antimycotics

Mechanism of Action

All antimycotics (Table 4.7) interfere at various sites with the synthesis of ergosterol, thus causing defects in the fungal cell membrane. Depending on the dose, they are fungistatic and many of them also fungicidal (particularly amphotericin B). An exception is ciclopirox olamine, which binds irreversibly to the cell wall, cytoplasmic membrane, and mitochondria of fungi and therefore is fungicidal.

While most fungal infections are localized processes that can be treated fairly well with topical antimycotics, infections at deeper locations or systemic infections (usually only in patients with a weakened immune system) still pose a therapeutic problem. For most of the intravenous preparations available today, this is primarily due to the narrow range between effectiveness of the drug and manifestation of side effects.

Modern oral antimycotics, such as fluconazole, itraconazole, and voriconazole, make systemic treatment easier. In addition, amphotericin B is better tolerated when administered as deoxycholate.

Polyenes

They are effective against yeasts only. They are always used for topical and intestinal treatment, but some of them may be administered intravenously.

- Amphotericin B for intravenous infusion: amphotericin B deoxycholate, amphotericin B liposomal complex, amphoterin B cholesteryl sulfate complex; formulations are also available for topical application. It is active against *Candida* and other fungi, except dermatophytes.
- Nystatin: it is available as suspension, coated tablets, powder, ointment, and vaginal tablets. It is very effective against *Candida albicans* and other *Candida* species.
- Natamycin: this compound is available as a cream, powder, lozenge, coated tablets, suspension, and vaginal tablets and or as a special galenic preparation.

Imidazole Derivatives

These are effective against yeasts (*Candida*), dermatophytes, and molds as well as gram-positive cocci and *Corynebacterium minutissimum* (erythrasma). Depending on the compound, they act only topically or also systemically.

Imidazoles for topical application only include:

- clotrimazole: well tolerated broad-spectrum antimycotic
- miconazole: broad-spectrum antimycotic for topical and systemic application
- econazole related to miconazole; available for topical treatment
- isoconazole
- terconazole
- tioconazole
- bifonazole: only fungistatic for yeasts, fungicidal for dermatophytes; suited for cutaneous mycoses, erythrasma, pityriasis versicolor
- fenticonazole.

Imidazoles for systemic (oral) and topical application include:

- ketoconazole, the first oral imidazole preparation available.

Triazoles

They are for oral and intravenous application and include:

- fluconazole: effective especially against yeasts; water soluble.
- itraconazole: effective also against dermatophytes; lipid soluble.
- voriconazole: effective also against *Aspergillus.*

Pyridones

- Ciclopirox olamine.

Pyrimidines

Flucytosine or 5-fluorocytosine is a fluoridated pyrimidine; its activity is based on its conversion in the fungal cell to the cytostatic compound 5-fluorouracil. It has a very broad spectrum of activity and is intended for systemic treatment by means of tablets or infusion, both of which are relatively well tolerated. There is a risk that secondary resistance develops. The effectiveness of flucytosine is increased by combination with amphotericin B.

Other Compounds

Dyes

- Pyoktanine (dahlia violet)
- gentian violet (crystal violet), 0.5–2 %
- brilliant green
- potassium permanganate solution.

These are only occasionally used in dermatology because of their moderate activity and their color.

Systemic Treatment of Fungal Infections

Oral or intravenous administration of antimycotics is necessary in cases of severe systemic fungal infections (candidiasis, aspergillosis, cryptococcosis) and generalized mycoses (histoplasmosis, blastomycosis, coccidiomycosis).

- *Candida albicans:* fluconazole or itraconazole
- aspergillosis: amphotericin B, amphotericin B + deoxycholate, voriconazole, possibly itraconazole.

Antiparasitics

Malaria

- Quinine: for initial treatment of cerebral and complicated falciparum malaria.
- Chloroquine: for prophylaxis (permitted during pregnancy) and for therapy of tertian malaria and quartan malaria.
- Mefloquine: for prophylaxis (one tablet per week) and therapy (three to four tables per day); its long half-life of approximately 20 days makes it possible to administer a single dose or a one-day dose for treatment, or one dose per week for prophylaxis.
- Proguanil: for prophylaxis in combination with other drugs.
- Doxycycline: for prophylaxis.
- Atovaquone/proguanil.
- Halofantrine.

Risks During Pregnancy:
Based on the long-term experience with this drug, chloroquine is permitted during pregnancy. Unfortunately, it is hardly effective anymore because resistance has developed in falciparum malaria in Africa. All other antimalarial drugs are contraindicated during pregnancy. The risk is low, however, and the intake of one of these drugs does not justify an abortion. If the risk of malaria is high, both risks must be carefully considered. If in doubt, prophylactic treatment should take place (after the 12 th week of pregnancy).

It has been reported that, after taking mefloquine, there was a four to five times higher rate of stillbirths, but no increased incidence of malformations or neurological disorders.

Toxoplasmosis

Effective compounds against *Toxoplasma gondii* include:

- sulfadiazine
- chloroquine
- spiramycin
- clindamycin.

Anthelminthic Drugs

- Among the benzimidazoles, mebendazole is used for treating infections with nematodes and echinococci, while albendazole is used for treating infections with nematodes, trichinae, echinicocci, and microsporidia.
- Ivermectin: effective against all nematodes.
- Praziquantel: oral administration is well tolerated. For treating infections with trematodes (fluke disease), such as schistosomiasis: one-day treatment with 60 mg/kg body weight; infections with cestodes, such as neurocysticercosis: 15-day treatment with 60 mg/kg body weight/day; teniasis (*Taenia solium*, *Taenia saginata*): a single dose of 10 mg/kg body weight.

Anthelminthic drugs and pregnancy: see also p. 234.

Mebendazole is contraindicated during the first trimester because an increase in congenital defects has been reported.

Pubic Lice, Head Lice, and Mites

- Permethrin is used preferentially in the United States as a single-dose treatment; it should not be administered during pregnancy.
- Lindane emulsion, mesulfen; they should not be used during pregnancy, if possible.
- Pyrethrins: may be used during pregnancy.
- Malathion.

Antiseptics

An overview of various compounds is provided in Table 4.**8**.

Antiseptics only reduce the number of microorganisms; they do not eliminate them.

There is no ideal disinfectant for mucosae. Polyvidone iodine is still the best-proved remedy so far, although it is not free of side effects.

Acidifying substances (e. g., vitamin C-containing vaginal tablets) help the lactobacillus flora to recover.

There are four vaginal antiseptics available: dequalinium chloride, nifuratel, polyvidone iodine vaginal tablets, hexetidine. They are indicated for infections restricted to the vagina or for bacterial imbalances (mixed flora). They can be used to remove pathogenic bacteria (such as *Staphylococcus aureus*), highly resistant bacteria (such as methicillin-resistant *Staphylococcus aureus* [MRSA] strains, which increasingly occur in certain hospitals and senior homes), or *Enterococcus faecium* which one does not yet wish to treat, or cannot reach, by oral antibiotic therapy. There is no doubt that disinfectants are also advantageous in cases of mixed infections with various pathogens (bacteria, fungi, protozoa).

Table 4.8 Antiseptics

Preparations	Scope of application	Comments
1. Phenyl derivatives		
Carbolic acid solution		
Hexylresorcinol solution		
Chlorhexidine	Disinfection of skin	
Hexetidine	Disinfection of vagina	
2. Aldehydes		
Formaldehyde	Treatment of vagina Room disinfectant	Not recommended Very rarely necessary
3. Acids		
Boric acid 2–3 %		Not recommended
Salicylic acid 0.1–0.3 %	Disinfection of vagina	
Acetic acid 0.5–3 %	Diagnostic agent	
Ascorbic acid	Treatment of bacterial vaginosis	High acceptance
4. Oxidants		
Hydrogen peroxide 0.05–0.5 %	Rinsing of wounds infected with anaerobes	Rarely used today
Potassium permanganate 0.01–0.5 %	Disinfection of skin	
5. Halogens		
Polyvidone iodine	Disinfection of mucosae, skin, vagina	
Chloraphore sodium hypochlorite		Not recommended
Chloramine		Not recommended
6. Surfactants		
Benzalkonium	Disinfection of skin	Sometimes ineffective, toxic
Dequalinium chloride	Disinfection of vagina	
7. Salts of heavy metals		
Mercury compounds		
Silver nitrate, silver proteinate	Ophthalmic prophylaxis in newborns	Ineffective against chlamydiae
8. Acridine and quinoline derivatives		
Ethacridine 0.1–0.5 %	Disinfection of wounds	Not recommended, sometimes ineffective
9. Alcohols		
Ethanol (70 %)/propanol (10 %)	Disinfection of skin	
10. Bipyridines		
Octenidines (Octenidine hydrochloride)	Disinfection of skin, puncture sites, catheters	

Immunoglobulins

Prophylaxis

The organism can temporarily be put in a condition of immunity by supplying specific antibodies.

This plays a major role in cases of infection by pathogens for which there is no chemotherapy, such as viral infections.

Even in cases of certain bacterial infections associated with toxin-producing pathogens (e. g., tetanus, gas gangrene, botulism, diphtheria), the timely supply of antiserum can save lives.

Immunoglobulin preparations are available for the following infections:

- rubella
- varicella
- hepatitis B
- hepatitis A
- measles
- mumps
- rabies
- cytomegalovirus infection
- tetanus
- gas gangrene
- botulism
- diphtheria.

The amount of antibodies supplied and the time they are administered will decide on the success of immunoprophylaxis. In general, the protective effect is the better, the earlier antibodies can be supplied after the infection.

In cases of droplet infection through the nasopharyngeal space, protection can still be achieved after three to five days. In cases of direct inoculation of the pathogen through needles (hepatitis B) there are only a few hours left for prophylaxis.

It is also important whether the immunoglobulin can be administered intravenously, in which case it becomes immediately effective, or intramuscularly, in which case maximal titers in the blood are reached only after 24 hours. With intramuscular injections, only about half of the supplied antibodies become available for protection.

After pathogen exposure, administration of immunoglobulin may lower the risk of infection, but it cannot prevent it completely. Particularly during pregnancy, one should always examine whether an infection took place after all, and the remaining risk should then be discussed with the patient (this applies particularly to rubella).

Special immunoglobulin preparations *(hyperimmunoglobulin preparations)* have very high titers against the pathogens in question. With the exception of hepatitis A and measles, such preparations are available for all of the above-mentioned infections—though no longer for rubella since 2002.

Therapy

Indications and effectiveness:

- congenital immunoglobulin deficiency syndrome
- secondary immunoglobulin deficiency syndrome (radiation, cytostatics, burns, trauma, neoplasms, malnutrition)
- idiopathic thrombocytopenic purpura (ITP)
- HIV stages III and IV in children.

More difficult is the assessment of the effectiveness of immunoglobulin therapy in patients with an intact immune system and severe bacterial infection (sepsis).

Here, timely administration of an effective antibiotic is the most important measure. Single-case observations on the positive accessory effect of immunoglobulins have been repeatedly reported. Studies that unambiguously prove their effectiveness are not yet available because these infections are fortunately rare, and their symptoms and courses are diverse.

Sufficient dosage is essential for the effectiveness of the therapy. Intravenous injections of, at least, 20–50 g of immunoglobulin per day are required. If sufficient amounts of antibodies against the sepsis-causing pathogen are available, the results are more favorable—as demonstrated in experimental studies. However, even without specific antibodies, the immunomodulatory effects of immunoglobulin lead to a more favorable course of the infection.

Mechanism of Action:

- direct damage to the pathogen
- neutralization of bacterial toxins and viruses
- promotion of phagocytosis and activation of the complement system
- inhibition of various mediators.

Preparations

Standard (polyvalent) immunoglobulin preparations. These are prepared from blood pooled from at least 1000 donors. They contain the average amount of antibodies present in the population from which the plasma has been collected. The advantage lies in the broad spectrum of different antibodies; the disadvantage is the relatively low titer of antibodies against specific pathogens.

Hyperimmune sera. These are preparations obtained from individuals with especially high titers against the pathogen in question. They are recommended for specific prophylaxis. Prophylactic treatment may be performed also with standard immunoglobulin preparations containing defined titers, provided correspondingly higher doses are applied. Normally, administration of such large amounts is only possible by intravenous injection.

Intravenous immunoglobulin preparations. Immunoglobulins for intramuscular injection do not require special pretreatment. However, pretreatment is necessary when the preparation is to be applied intravenously. During manufacture of immunoglobulins from plasma, various steps of purification lead to spontaneous aggregation caused by the Fc fragment. Immunoglobulins for intravenous injection must therefore be pretreated accordingly, for example, by alkylation with β-propionolactone, incubation with acid, or reversible sulfitolysis.

All modern intravenous immunoglobulin preparations have an almost normal half-life of approximately three weeks.

Caution is advised for intravenous administration of immunoglobulins to patients who have complete IgA deficiency and, therefore, carry anti-IgA antibodies (the incidence is 1 : 800), because this may lead to shock.

All immunoglobulin preparations are safe from viral transmission (HBV, HCV, HIV, CMV).

5 Signs of Infection

Immune Responses

Many common symptoms of an infection do not directly result from metabolites of the multiplying microorganism; rather, they represent the body's immune responses to the pathogens or their metabolites.

If these responses are absent, the following may occur:

- in the best-case scenario, there are no symptoms, and the patient is not in danger.
- in the worse case scenario (e.g., when the infection is developing very rapidly and the immune system has been weakened), the body is overwhelmed by the infection and the outcome is usually fatal (e.g., sepsis caused by group A streptococci).

Local Symptoms

Many gynecological infections begin as a local infection. In response to certain mediators, granulocytes and, later, macrophages invade the tissue, and this is associated with the typical signs of inflammation: swelling, reddening, hyperthermia, and pain.

In the region of the vulva, these signs of an infection are easily recognized. Diagnosis is more difficult in the region of the uterus and adnexa. Here, pain is one of the most reliable signs. If a secretion can be collected from the infected region, the increase in leukocytes is easily recognized under the microscope. In many cases, pathogens (fungi, bacteria, trichomonads) can readily be identified microscopically.

When the body is unable to confine the infection to a local area either the pathogen itself, or its toxic substances, will spread, thus causing general symptoms.

Local signs of an infection:

- pain (spontaneous pain, tenderness to pressure)
- reddening (vascular dilation associated with hyperthermia)
- swelling (edema, followed by pus)
- nodules (early manifestation of herpes simplex virus, *Candida albicans*, *Staphylococcus aureus*)
- vesicular lesions (herpes simplex virus, varicella-zoster virus, *Candida albicans*)
- ulcers (herpes simplex virus, though less typically; varicella-zoster virus, syphilis)
- pus (*Staphylococcus aureus*, gonococci, chlamydiae)
- discharge (trichomoniasis, herpes genitalis, bacterial vaginosis, chlamydial cervicitis)
- crepitation (air in the tissue, such as in gas gangrene; much more often, however, this is of no importance after surgical intervention).

Systemic Symptoms

- Pain
- fever
- weakness
- malaise
- tachycardia
- tachypnea
- hypotension
- chills
- pain in the limbs.

Pain

Pain is usually associated with an inflammation. As a warning sign, it is more reliable than fever. Especially in cases of rapidly developing, severe infections (e.g., puerperal sepsis), the best indicators for a life-threatening condition are diffuse pain in the abdominal region and the malaise of the patient. In such a situation, it will be fatal to wait for fever to develop before administering an antibiotic.

Pain is caused by injuries and pathogens, and it is triggered by cytokines. Pain caused by injuries (surgery) or immune diseases (rheumatism, Behçet syndrome, etc.) can be distinguished from pain due to infections based on the patient's history, course of the disease, and parameters of the inflammation.

When caused by local processes, such as wounds and abscesses, the pain is restricted to an area, while it is diffuse when caused by systemic diseases (sepsis).

Local or diffuse pain that cannot be controlled by painkillers should only be treated with more analgesics if infectious processes have been excluded by determining the inflammatory parameters, or if effective antibiotics are administered simultaneously.

Fever

Etiology, Pathogenicity, and Symptoms

Fever is one of the most typical symptoms of an infection. It may be absent, however, when the inflammatory process is minor and locally restricted, or—a bad sign for the prognosis—when the infection is developing so quickly that the immune system is not able to initiate this mechanism of defense.

Fever develops either from exogenous pyrogenic substances, which are directly produced by viruses, bacteria, or other pathogens, or endogenously by means of interleukin-1, which plays a central role in the stimulation of various defense systems.

Fever is brought on when phagocytes contact microorganisms, thus triggering the release of interleukin-1 by means of various mediators. This activates T lymphocytes, B lymphocytes, and granulocytes, induces the production of acute phase proteins in the liver, and stimulates fibroblast proliferation and prostaglandin synthesis.

Fever itself is a useful reaction to infection. Many metabolic processes are accelerated by elevated temperatures. In addition, fever is a measurable parameter that often provides information about the intensity of the infection.

The control centers for body temperature are located in the hypothalamus. Chills lead to a rapid increase in temperature and are characteristic for many bacterial infections. If chills are present, one should always run blood cultures because this is the best way of detecting the pathogen.

Fever is not always an indicator for an infection. Numerous noninfectious diseases and disturbances are also accompanied by elevated temperatures, for example, dehydration, trauma, cerebral thrombosis, malignant diseases, hemolysis, rheumatic fever, periarteritis nodosa, and erythema nodosum.

Elevation of the body temperature by 1 °C (1.8 °F) increases the metabolism by 12% and the heart rate by 15 beats per minute; it also leads to hyperventilation.

There are different patterns of fever. Intermittent septic fever predominates with gynecological infections, as these are mostly soft tissue infections spreading pathogens and toxins. All other types of fever—such as continued fever, remittent fever, and recurrent fever—are rather characteristic of other, nongynecological infections.

Therapy

Since fever frightens the physician and burdens the patient, it is usually reduced by drug therapy. Only extremely high temperatures of above 41 °C (105.8 °F) are dangerous. On the other hand, it has been shown that reducing the fever does not weaken the defense mechanisms of the body. Nevertheless, one should not disregard the fact that elevation of body temperature is a useful defense reaction of the body.

Reasons for reducing the fever:

- protection of the patient from secondary damages by tachycardia, febrile convulsions (in children), hyperventilation, or encephalopathy (only above 41 °C or 105.8 °F)
- the well-being of the patient; many patients feel more comfortable when high temperatures have been reduced.

Options for lowering the temperature:

Antipyretics:

- acetylsalicylic acid (Aspirin), acetaminophen/paracetamol (Tylanol), metamizol sodium (Novalgin)
- cool, wet towels (wet packs around the lower legs).

Drug fever

It is often difficult to decide whether a persistent or recurrent fever is just a flareup of the infection or caused by the drug therapy. Such febrile reactions have been described in connection with many different pharmaceuticals.

Typical is the clinical discrepancy between the general condition of the patient and the intensity of the fever. The exact time when the fever first appeared may be important, since in most patients fever has been observed seven to 10 days after the therapy started.

Discontinuation of all drugs can help clarifying the connection.

Overlooking true infections can be avoided, to a great extent, by observing the patient carefully and carrying out the appropriate laboratory tests (e.g., C-reactive protein in the serum).

Laboratory Values

Leukocytes in the Blood

An increased number of leukocytes in the blood is characteristic for many infectious diseases. There is a dramatic increase in the number of neutrophil granulocytes during most bacterial infections. If the granulocytes are produced fast enough and not in sufficient amounts, there is an increased release of band cells (rod neutrophils) and finally also of metamyelocytes (juvenile neutrophils).

Leukopenia

Less than 4000 leukocytes/μL ($<4 \times 10^9$/L). Leukocyte values of below 500/μL ($<0.5 \times 10^9$/L) are associated with increased susceptibility to infections, but only values of below 100/μL ($<0.1 \times 10^9$/L) are dangerous.

Normal Range

Values of 4000–10 000 leukocytes/μL ($4–10 \times 10^9$/L).

Leukocytosis

More than 10 000 leukocytes/μL ($>10 \times 10^9$/L). During an inflammatory reaction, neutrophil granulocytes are attracted to the tissue by the chemotactic effect of complement factors, such as leukotrienes, and bacterial toxins. This leads to increased granulocyte formation, with their numbers in the blood rising to above 10 000/μL ($>10 \times 10^9$/L). After injury or surgery, leukocyte numbers may rise for several hours, even in the absence of an infection. During pregnancy, some women have leukocyte values of up to 15 000/μL ($<15 \times 10^9$/L). A short-term increase may be observed also during labor, though other signs of an infection are not detected. Values higher than 20 000/μL ($>20 \times 10^9$/L) are highly suspicious of an infectious process.

Differential Blood Count

Gram-positive pathogens usually induce only an increase in neutrophilic granulocytes.

Infections with gram-negative pathogens lead to the agglutination of granulocytes and their rapid elimination from the blood due to the formation of endotoxins. The result is a shift to the left (e.g., band cells) with leukocyte values only slightly increased, or not at all increased, or even decreased.

Differential blood counts are only of limited importance in gynecological infections. Only rarely does one observe immature cells or even leukocytes with toxic granulation. Infections with viruses (e.g., EBV) may lead to an increased proliferation of lymphocytes, and allergic reactions or parasitoses may be associated with a slight increase in eosinophils. In chronic inflammation, lymphocyte values are normal, and monocyte values may be increased.

Thrombocytopenia

A decrease in the number of platelets may have different causes and also occurs in connection with sepsis. It is usually only observed when sepsis is already advanced and is therefore not a premonitory symptom.

In the case of HELLP syndrome ("hemolysis, elevated liver enzymes, and low platelet count," a special form of gestosis) during pregnancy, thrombocytopenia—together with an increase in liver transaminases—is one of the key findings leading to the diagnosis.

Erythrocyte Sedimentation Rate (ESR)

The ESR reflects the tendency of erythrocytes to aggregate, depending on changes in the quantitative and qualitative composition of plasma proteins as well as on the number, size, and shape of the erythrocytes. Dysproteinemias with an increased concentration of high-molecular proteins—such as fibrinogen, immunoglobulins, α_2-macroglobulin, and immunocomplexes—accelerate sedimentation. Erythrocytic factors increasing the ESR include macrocytosis and anemia. Increased plasticity of the erythrocytes, the presence of abnormal erythrocytes (poikilocytes, echinocytes, sickle cells, etc.), and an increase in erythrocyte numbers inhibit sedimentation.

The ESR is useful for the recognition of acute, chronic, and chronically active inflammations and for assessing the course of the inflammation. Diagnostic sensitivity is high, though diagnostic specificity is low.

During the course of an inflammatory process, the ESR responds slowly. Only 24–48 hours after the onset of the acute phase reaction, the sedimentation rate increases; after the acute phase reaction is complete, the half-life of the decrease in sedimentation rate is 96–144 hours.

Table 5.1 Acute phase proteins

Proteins	Reaction times
PMN-elastase C-reactive protein (CRP) Serum amyloid A protein (SAA protein)	Response after six to10 hours, increase by a factor of 100 to 1000
α_1-antitrypsin, Acid α_1-glycoprotein (AGP) Phospholipase A_2 (PLA_2) Inflammatory cytokines: interleukin-1 and -6 (IL-1, IL-6), tumor necrosis factor α (TNF-α) Fibrinogen Haptoglobin	Response after 24 hours, increase by a factor of two to five
Ceruloplasmin Complement C3, C4	Response after 48–72 hours, maximum increase by a factor of two

An increased ESR may be due to:

- small erythrocytes
- chronic infection with persistence of the pathogen, e.g., chlamydial salpingitis
- abscess-forming infection
- inflammation associated with rheumatic diseases
- autoimmune diseases
- malignant diseases
- anemia
- excessive citrate in the assay
- technical error.

Nevertheless, the ESR can be successfully used for the evaluation of infections, since there is hardly any infection without an increased ESR. Normal values for the first hour lie in the range of 15–20 mm, for women over the age of 50 they are between 20–30 mm. After tissue trauma, such as surgery, the ESR usually increases, and this is also often the case during pregnancy.

The ESR plays a major role if the presumed diagnosis is adnexitis. In many patients it is the only pathological laboratory parameter, especially with subacute adnexitis caused by *Chlamydia*. The ESR can also be useful when assessing the course of the infection; it increases more slowly than the number of leukocytes in the blood, and it also declines more slowly. The ESR increases considerably in abscess-forming processes, with values reaching up to 80 mm during the first hour.

The ESR can help with recognizing undetected subacute infections of the uterine tubes, for example, prior to hysterosalpingography.

Acute Phase Proteins

These are proteins produced in the liver upon interleukin-1 stimulation; and they are detected in the serum (Table 5.1).

The most important ones are PMN elastase and C-reactive protein.

PMN Elastase

The polymorphonuclear (PMN) granulocytes invading the tissue during the inflammatory reaction incorporate microbial pathogens and tissue debris in their lysosomes where these are degraded. Depending on the intensity of the inflammation, lysosomal enzymes (e.g., the serine protease elastase) are set free because of degranulation and cytolysis.

In case of excessive stimulation of the granulocyte reaction, there is not enough α_1-proteinase inhibitor to inactivate the elastase thus released; this may cause tissue damage in the lungs, liver, and kidneys, particularly during shock.

The concentration of PMN elastase present in the serum (as a complex with α_1-proteinase inhibitor) is a measure for granulocyte activity during the inflammatory reaction. High concentrations of PMN elastase are observed in cases of postoperative and posttraumatic complications, such as organ dysfunction (e.g., adult respiratory distress syndrome, disseminated intravascular coagulation, and liver and kidney failure), infections (e.g., sepsis), and states of shock.

The most important indications for the determination of PMN elastase include:

- Prediction of postoperative and posttraumatic complications in intensive care patients:

When assessing the course of an inflammation, a value of more than 85 mg/L on day 5 after the onset of the noxious event makes it very likely that the patient will suffer life-threatening complications on days 6–12 (predominantly due to organ failure with or without infection). The determination should be carried out twice a day, and the mean value should be used for assessment.

- Early diagnosis of neonatal sepsis: postpartal values of more than 75 mg/L in the serum of the newborn during days 2–10 after birth indicate a neonatal infection.
- Early recognition (within up to six hours) of lung complications (pulmonary edema) in cases of severe gestosis characterized by edema, proteinuria, and hypertension (EPH gestosis).

C-reactive Protein (CRP)

Of the various acute phase proteins that can be determined in the serum, we have the most experience with *C-reactive protein.* It indicates an infectious process several hours before the appearance of other parameters of infection (leukocytosis, fever). After a short time, however, it returns to normal values. During pregnancy, it may serve as an additional indicator, as the ESR may already have increased physiologically. In addition, CRP can be a valuable tool for diagnosing the beginning of amniotic infection syndrome, associated with premature amniorrhexis. It is also useful for differentiating between pelvic pain syndrome and subacute pelvic inflammatory disease.

Determination of CRP measures only inflammation. Based on its quick responsiveness, dramatic increase in concentration, and positive correlation with the extent of the inflammation, serum CRP is the most important indicator of the acute phase reaction and is a parameter of its clinical course. Values of up to 10 mg/L exclude an infectious disease or tissue necrosis; values above this level indicate an organic disease, even though clinical symptoms may still be absent.

Due to the rapid onset of CRP synthesis in the liver (half-life of increase: five to seven hours, maximum value after approximately 50 hours) and the quick plasma clearance (half-life of decline: two to four hours), plasma concentrations of CRP have a distinct dynamic. By repeating the determination every day, changes in the inflammatory process—caused by either disease or therapy—can be recognized in time. C-reactive protein is therefore especially suited for monitoring infectious and noninfectious states of inflammation. By contrast, the individual CRP value is not very convincing with respect to the differential diagnosis of acute clinical situations. Its discriminatory potential for distinguishing between infectious and noninfectious diseases, and for making the distinction between bacterial and viral infections, is minor, although values of more than 100 mg/L do indicate a bacterial infection.

Acute phase proteins are not specific for an infection, since they occur with every tissue damage and, hence, also after surgical intervention. They are usually increased only at the beginning and normalize during the course of the infection, despite the fact that the infection still exists. In infections associated with severe leukocytic reaction, such as abscess-forming infections, the normal value of CRP in the serum (5 mg/L) is increased markedly ($>$ 200 mg/L), whereas it is only slightly increased in viral infections (20–40 mg/L).

Coagulopathy

Coagulopathy can be caused by bacterial toxins and thus is a typical symptom of severe general infections, such as sepsis. The use of heparin in severe infections is disputed; it should be administered with great caution. Unfortunately, there have been examples where heparin caused more damage than benefits. Substitution with clotting factors and freshly frozen plasma is possible today and should be employed as soon as possible, while being monitored through appropriate laboratory tests.

Liver Values

Elevated liver values may indicate hepatitis, but they may also be associated with poisoning and sepsis. In cases of severe infections, the liver values may rise more than 100-fold. Normalization takes many weeks. Liver disorders should be taken into consideration before administering antibiotics because some chemotherapeutics (e.g., tetracycline, ketoconazole, clindamycin, sulfonamides) may cause temporary disturbances (cholestasis) in case of a previously damaged liver or overdosing.

Kidney Values

Severe systemic infections lead to increased kidney values as a sign of nephropathy. Since most antibiotics are eliminated through the kidneys, the dosage must be reduced in cases of limited renal function; certain substances should not be administered at all, because they are nephrotoxic (e.g., aminoglycosides).

6 Diagnosis of Infections During Gynecologic Examination

Colposcopy

Colposcopy allows for better observation of the epithelium, thus making it possible to evaluate any efflorescence and to detect small parasites. The acetic acid test (3–5 %) should be used not only for assessing the vaginal portion of the cervix, but also when findings on the vulva are not clear (though not in the case of rhagades). Dysplasia, such as Bowen disease and subclinical HPV infections, become visible only this way and can therefore be easily distinguished from lichen simplex or lichen sclerosus.

Measuring the pH of the Discharge

(Special indicator paper for pH 4.0–4.7, Merck.)

This is part of every gynecological examination because it tells something about the bacterial colonization of the vagina. A pH value of < 4.5 means that lactobacilli are present, since only they produce lactic acid and can still multiply at this pH. It also means that the normal protective flora is present, which—depending on estrogen levels—largely keeps the vagina free of germs derived from the perianal region during times of severe strain (Table 6.**1**, Figs. 6.**1**–6.**3**).

Table 6.**1** Significance of the pH value of discharge

Range of pH value	Significance
pH 3.8–4.2	Many lactobacilli, possibly yeast infections
pH 4.3–4.7	Few lactobacilli, slightly mixed flora (may include yeasts), possibly leukocytosis
pH 4.8–5.5	Disturbed vaginal flora (mixed flora) suspected, bacterial vaginosis, trichomoniasis, status post antibiotics (when lactobacilli are no longer present), severe leukocytosis
pH > 6.0	Atrophic vaginitis, amniorrhexis during pregnancy, condition of a girl prior to estrogen production; this is also the pH of cervical secretion

Test for Amines

A drop of 10 % potassium hydroxide solution is added to the discharge collected on a cotton swab or microscopic slide. This intensifies the characteristic fishy odor (amines) in the case of bacterial vaginosis. However, this effect may be limited to specific instances.

Microscopy

For microscopic examination, the discharge is spread onto a microscopic slide and stained and then viewed in oil, or in solution under a cover slip. Alternatively, the discharge is first diluted and then viewed as so-called wet mount. Specific sampling of the discharge is easily performed with the wooden handle of a cotton probe, which is then stirred into a drop of methylene blue solution (0.1 %) on a slide. The mildly microbicidal methylene blue provides a better contrast if the flora is disturbed (with the higher pH resulting in better staining) and prevents contamination of the diluting solution. However, if trichomonads are suspected (yellow discharge), sodium chloride solution should be used instead of methylene blue solution; otherwise the trichomonads lose their vitality too quickly.

A normal light microscope with a 40× objective will suffice (Table 6.**2**, Figs. 6.**4**–6.**7**). Some pathogens (trichomonads and yeasts) are easier to find when using phase contrast; however, phase contrast is of no advantage for bacteria, especially when stained.

Biopsy

A biopsy should always be performed whenever a diagnosis can be established neither clinically nor microbiologically. It is especially important in such cases to exclude any malignancies.

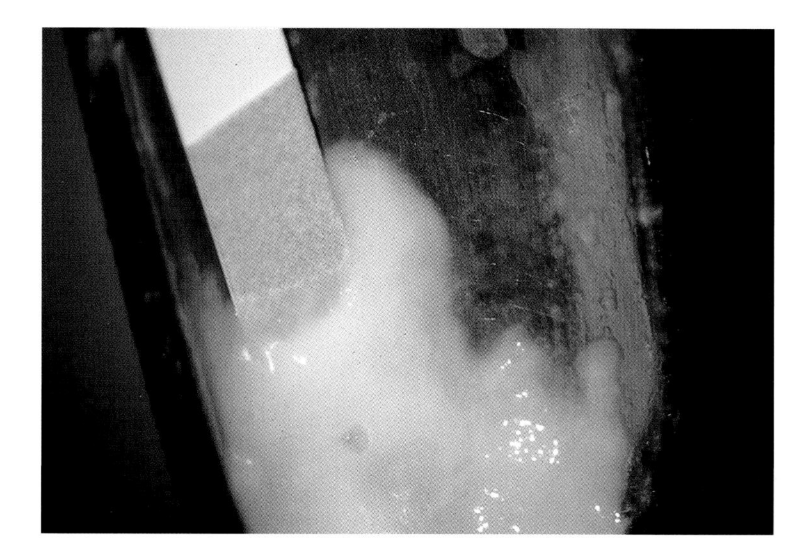

Fig. 6.**1** Normal discharge, with a pH value of 4.0.

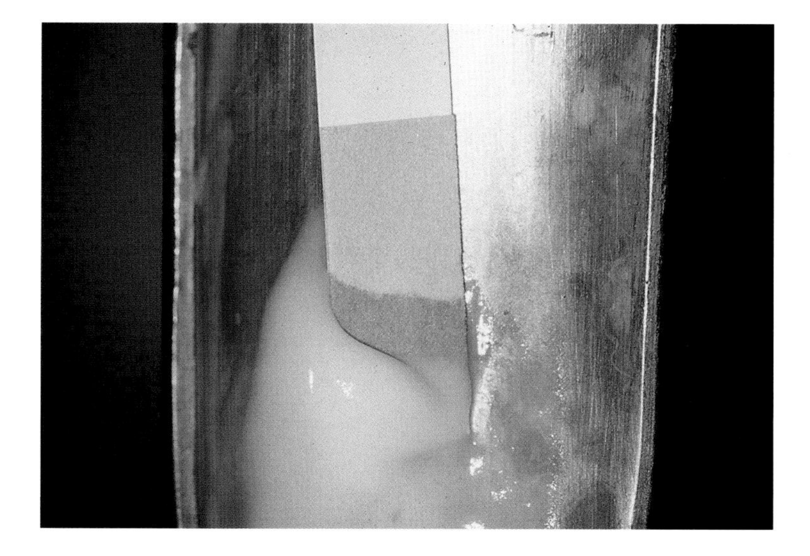

Fig. 6.**2** Discharge from a patient with bacterial vaginosis, with a pH value of 5.0.

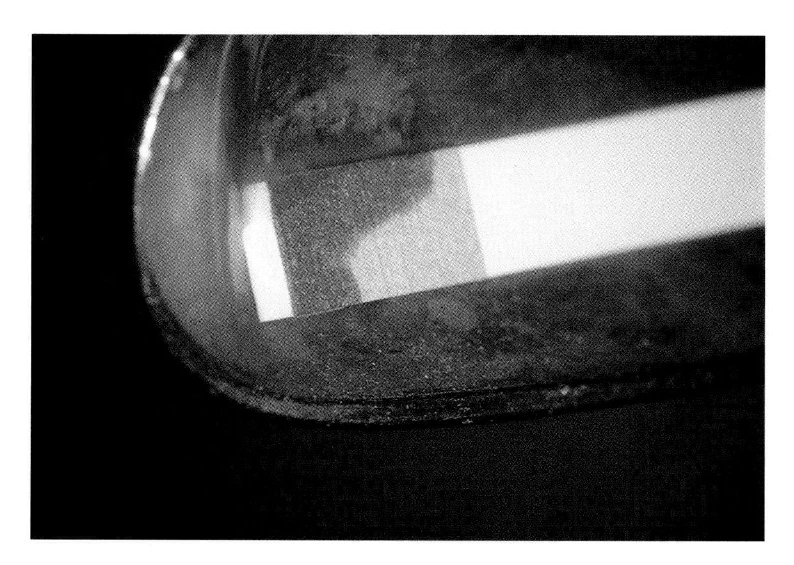

Fig. 6.**3** Amniotic fluid after premature amniorrhexis, with a pH value of 7.0.

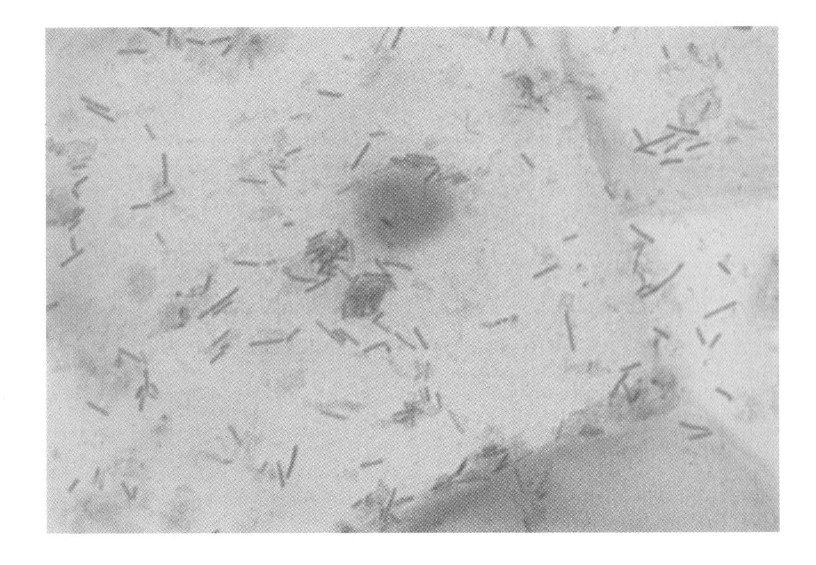

Fig. 6.**4** Normal vaginal flora, with lactobacilli in the microscopic wet mount containing methylene blue.

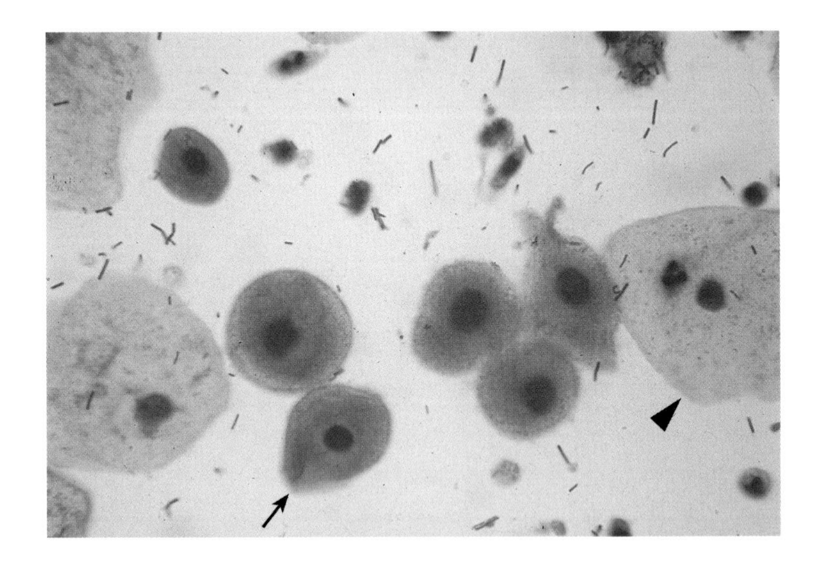

Fig. 6.**5** Discharge in case of mild atrophy, with parabasal cells (arrow) in the wet mount. Superficial cell (arrowhead).

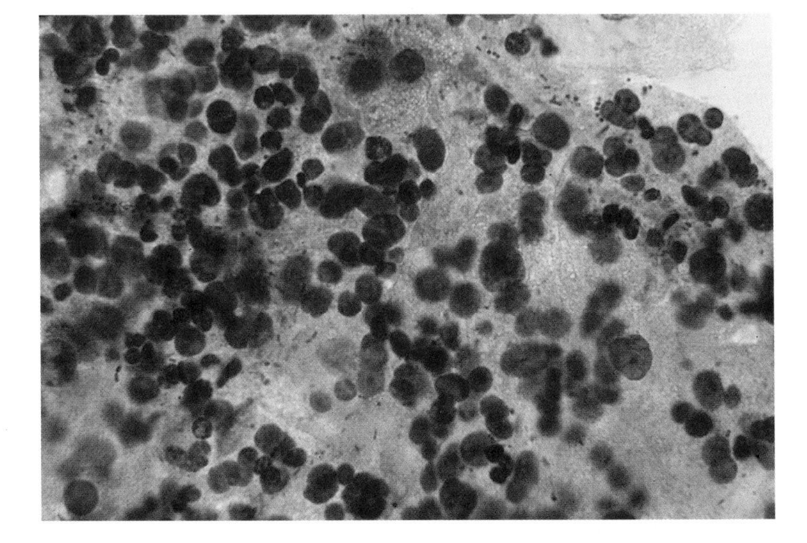

Fig. 6.**6** Discharge with masses of leukocytes.

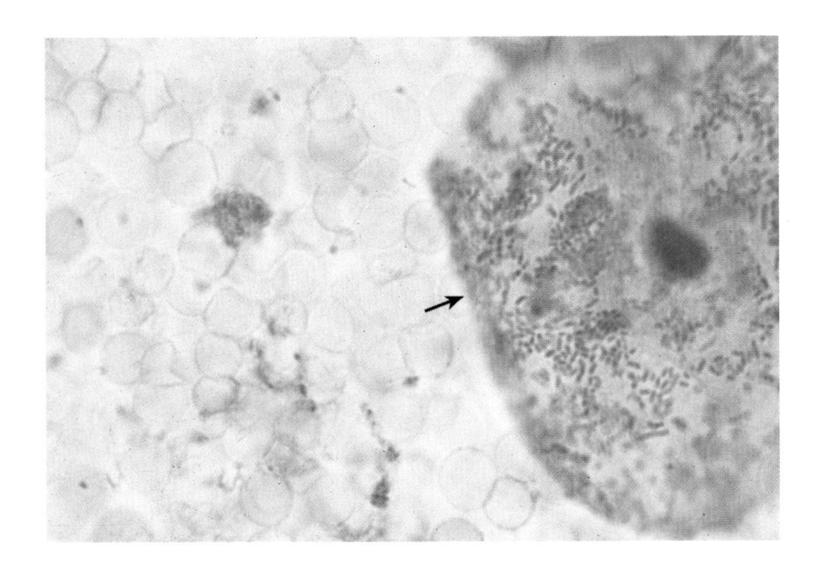

Fig. 6.**7** Discharge in case of bleeding and bacterial vaginosis, with clue cell (arrow). Erythrocytes are visible as empty rings.

Table 6.**2** What can be detected under the microscope?

Diagnosis	Microscopic findings
Normal conditions	Large rod bacteria (lactobacilli), many lactobacilli (very low pH), few leukocytes (20 per field of view), mature epithelial cells
Mixed flora	Lactobacilli plus many small bacteria, various amounts of leukocytes (noteworthy especially during pregnancy because a seemingly mild disturbance of a mixed flora is often involved in premature births)
Absence of bacterial flora	For example, after administration of antibiotics
Leukocytes	This is always a sign of inflammation. If no typical pathogens (yeasts, trichomonads) are visible under the microscope, a smear should be taken for bacterial culture in order to exclude group A streptococci and *Staphylococcus aureus*.
Trichomonads	Jerking flagellar movements of trichomonads (about the size of a lymphocyte) together with plenty of granulocytes (100 per field of view, 40× objective) (Fig. 3.**5**, p. 30, Fig. 7.**106**, p. 118)
Yeast cells	Budding cells are suspicious, while pseudomycelia are almost proof of candidiasis; moderate to high numbers of leukocytes
Bacterial vaginosis	Clue cells (epithelial cells covered with bacteria), masses of small bacteria, lactobacilli absent, few leukocytes (Fig. 7.**119**, p. 125)
Purulent vaginitis (plasma cell vaginitis)	Masses of leukocytes (100–200 per field of view, 40× objective), mixed flora, mature (superficial) and immature epithelial cells (intermediate cells, individual parabasal cells) (Fig. 7.**110**, p. 121)
Atrophic vaginitis	Only immature epithelial cells (intermediate and largely parabasal cells) or leukocytes and little perianal flora (Fig. 7.**123**, p. 129)

Methods of Taking a Vulvar Biopsy

This is a minor intervention performed either with biopsy forceps or with a biopsy punch (Stiefel Laboratories). The sharp cutting cylinder of the punch, which is advanced with slight pressure while being turned, cuts through the collagen fibers of the reticular layer of the dermis and lifts the biopsy tissue above the level of the surrounding skin. It can then be easily grasped with tweezers and cut off at the base (Fig. 6.**8 a–d**). A sample of 4 mm in diameter is sufficient. The biopsy site does not need to be stitched up. Swabbing the wound with Monsel solution is suitable to stop bleeding.

Application of EMLA cream (lidocaine and prilocaine) is adequate for anesthesia. It takes at

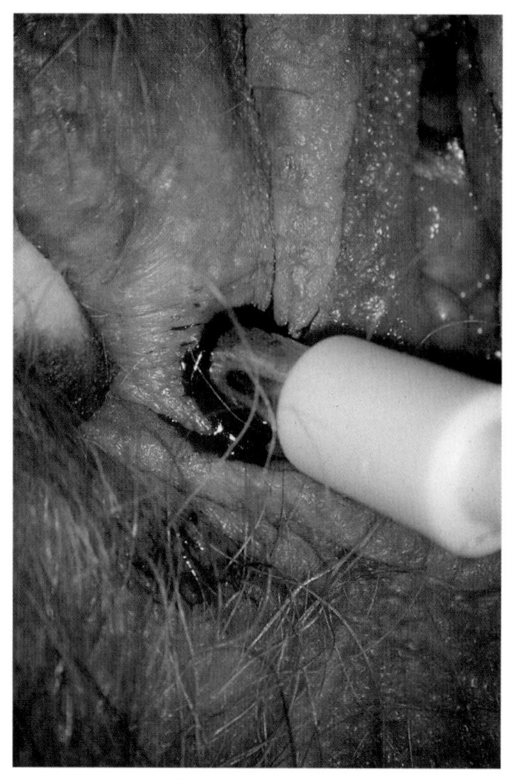

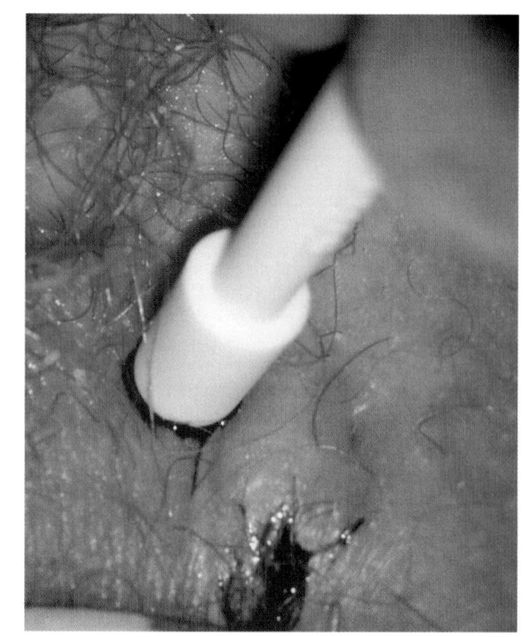

Fig. 6.**8** Taking a biopsy from the vulva:
a Positioning the punch after anesthesia with EMLA cream.
b The punch is advanced by turning it under mild pressure.

least 30 minutes for the cream to become effective. The deeper the biopsy, the longer the waiting period needs to be. For very deep biopsies (up to 6 mm), waiting for 60 minutes suffices in most patients. Anesthesia by infiltration of lidocaine or mepivacaine should only be carried out when less time is available or the biopsy reaches even deeper.

Biopsies from the vaginal fornix or the vaginal part of the uterus do not require anesthesia.

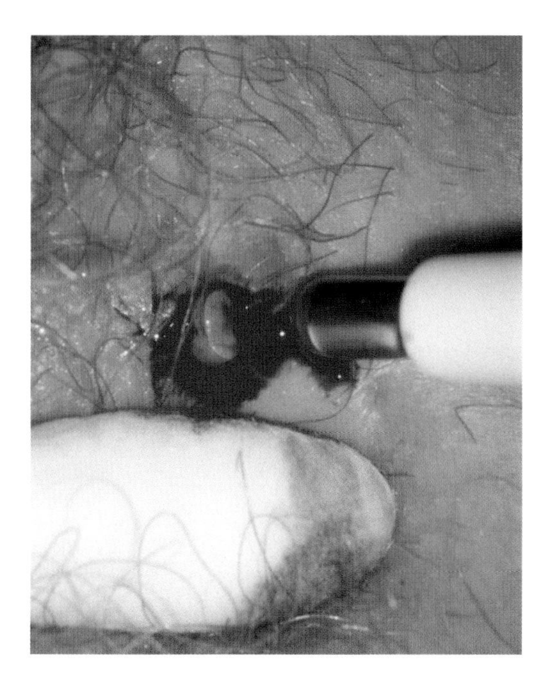

c The cylindrical biopsy tissue remains in place when withdrawing the punch.

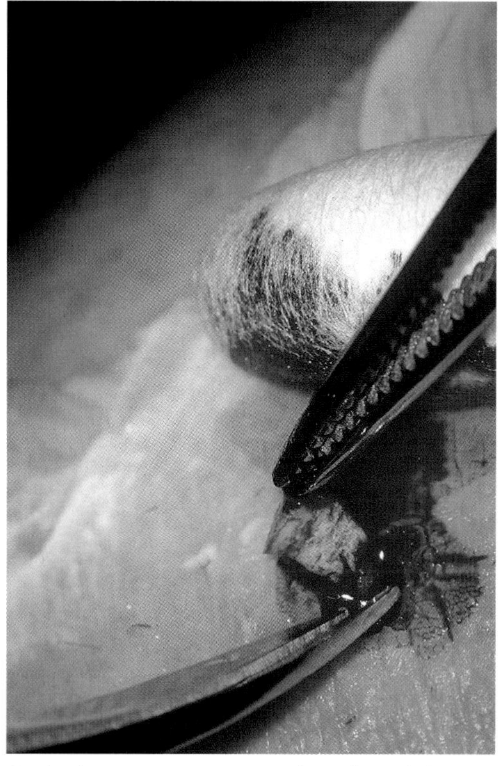

d The biopsy tissue is grasped gently and then cut off.

II Infections and Prevention

7 Gynecologic Infections

Infections of the Vulva (Vulvitis)

Introduction and Pathogenesis

The vulva and, in particular, the vaginal orifice (introitus) are among the most sensitive regions of the body because of their rich supply with sensory nerves. Any disorder and inflammation in this region is therefore experienced as extremely uncomfortable and is often noticed before anything becomes visible.

On the one hand, the external region is quite resistant to most pathogens because of the keratinizing stratified squamous epithelium. On the other, the vaginal orifice with its very delicate epithelium may respond with pain to the mere touch even in the absence of any inflammation. In addition, infections and their treatments may lead to an increase in the sensitivity and tenderness of this region.

Another problem is the close proximity to the anus and, therefore, to large amounts of facultative pathogens (the intestinal flora). These bacteria and their metabolites often generate an unpleasant odor, which may lead to excessive washing behavior. Even without using soap, repeated washing may result in a rough and dry skin—thus causing considerable other problems in the long term, for example, skin lesions, more frequent infections, and allergies. This can be remedied by proper skin care, such as using ointments containing lavender oil.

When discussing the vulva and its susceptibility to infections, the anal region and the properties of the skin in this region should not be ignored. Hence, the prevention of infections in the genital region begins externally, namely, with the vulva and the anal region.

In addition to skin lesions and infections, a number of dermatoses occur in the vulvar region. These, in turn, may promote infections, or they may be confused with infections—or they are actually the cause of complaints (Table 7.**1**).

In some patients, a presumed infection is treated far too long—only because bacteria (e. g., intestinal bacteria) or a harmless yeast species have been detected. For this reason, we discuss here dermatoses and other disturbances together with vulvar infections with which they may be confused.

Infections occur preferentially, when:

- skin lesions—due to intercourse, rhagades (Fig. 7.**1**), excessive skin care, and scratching—promote the invasion of pathogens, e. g., herpesviruses, papillomaviruses, *Treponema*, group A streptococci
- pathogens infect skin appendages (glands, hair follicles), e. g., *Staphylococcus aureus* (folliculitis)
- congestion or the formation of pouches (obstruction of sebaceous glands or Bartholin gland, or synechia of the preputium) create favorable conditions for bacteria to multiply, e. g., *Staphylococcus aureus*, intestinal pathogens, gonococci
- pathogens are able to penetrate the epithelium by means of enzymes, e. g., *Candida albicans*, group A streptococci
- pathogens, or their vectors, actively bore through the skin by means of bites or stings, e. g., ticks, mosquitoes, pubic lice, mites, *Schistosoma*, creeping eruption (larva migrans).

Frequent and long bathing sessions let the skin swell and make it easier for pathogens from the perianal region to attach and penetrate.

Onset and persistence of many infections are also promoted through conditions that weaken or damage the skin, such as allergic noxa, eczema, diabetes mellitus, or mechanical means (scrubbing, rubbing, or scratching), and also by moisture in large skin folds (e. g., erythrasma).

The common misconception that proper hygiene would involve frequent and excessive washings—using all kinds of washing lotions that are marketed as being especially effective—is often the cause of itching chronic vulvitis. Typical pathogens are rarely found in this situation.

Once infections reach the deeper skin layers, they are painful because the vulva is richly supplied with sensory nerves. Redness and swelling are characteristic signs of such infections (Fig. 7.**2**).

If no pathogens can be detected, diagnosis may be difficult. Allergy, eczema, or other dermatological problems should then be considered.

The symptom of pain may be absent in the case of superficial intradermal infections (condylomas, erythrasma, pityriasis [tinea] versicolor). Simultaneous infections with several pathogens are possible.

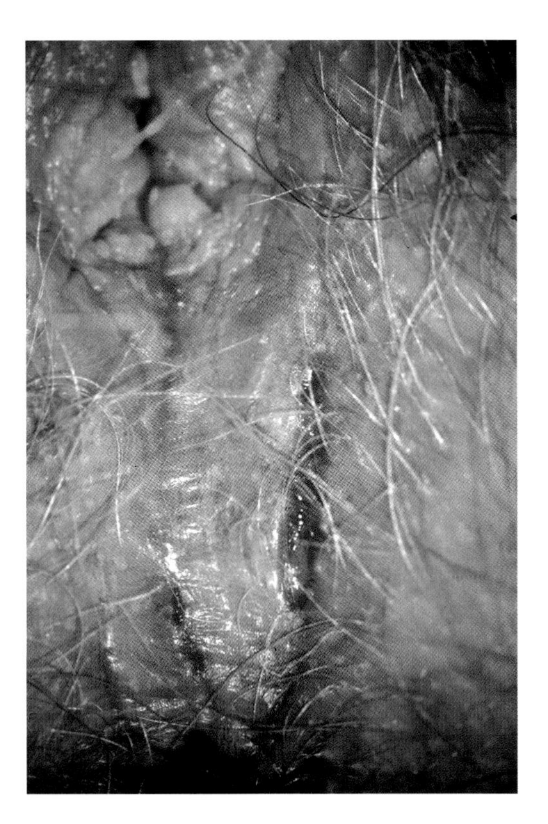

Fig. 7.**1** Vulva of a 25-year-old patient complaining about itching. The perineal region shows dry skin with rhagades.

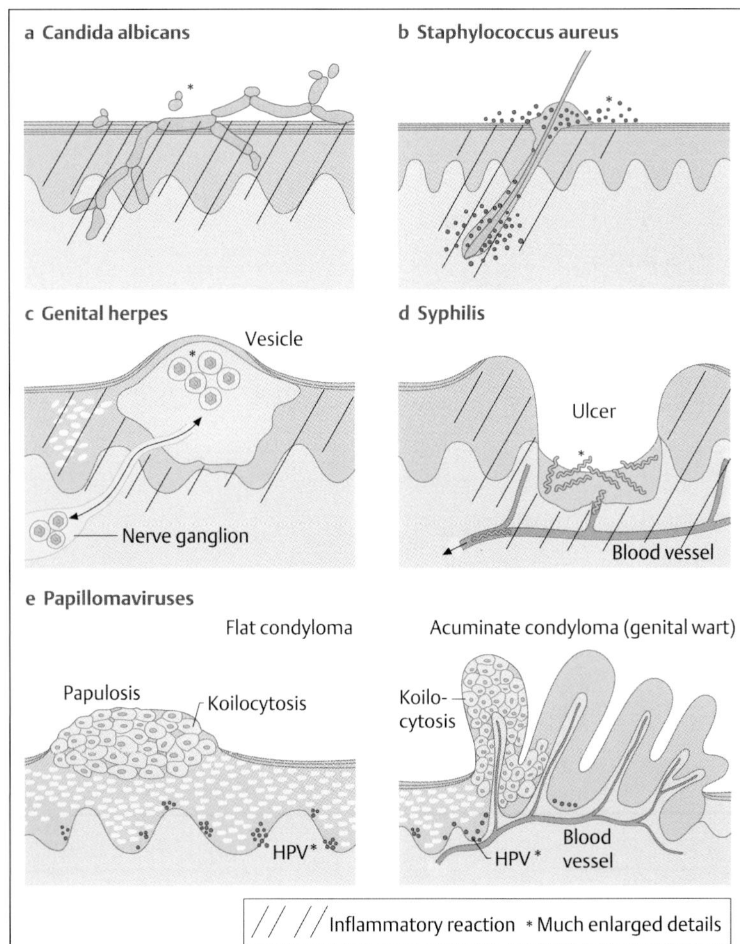

Fig. 7.**2** Schematic illustration of pathogen localization and pathogen spread in various diseases of the vulva. The individual pathogens are shown much enlarged. Areas of inflammatory reaction are indicated by hatching.

Table 7.**1** Diseases of the vulva grouped according to etiology, complaints, and clinical picture

I. Etiology **Infections**	**Dermatoses**	**Benign tumors**	**Malignant tumors**	**Artifacts and others causes**
Candidiasis	Lichen sclerosus	Condyloma	Carcinoma of the vulva	Scratch marks
Papilloma (HPV)	Lichen simplex	Atheroma	Paget disease	Excessive washing
Genital herpes	Erosive lichen planus	Hidradenoma	Melanoma	Injuries
Group A streptococci	Behçet syndrome	Fibroma		Factitial lesions
Staphylococcus aureus	Irritable dermatitis			Skin damage
Trichomoniasis	Eczema			Depression
Plasma cell vulvitis	Allergies			Sexual disorders
Herpes zoster (VZV)	Toxic reaction			Partner conflict
Molluscum contagiosum	Pemphigus vulgaris			
Syphilis*	Pemphigoid			
Lymphogranuloma venereum (LGV)*				
Chancroid*				
Pyoderma fistulans				
Acne conglobata				
Hidradenitis				
Erythrasma				
Pthiriasis				
Schistosomiasis				

II. Complaints **Itching**	**Burning**	**Pain**	**No complaints**
Fungal infection	Genital herpes	Behçet syndrome	Condyloma (HPV)
Lichen sclerosus	Erosive lichen planus	Folliculitis (*Staphylococcus aureus*)	Erythrasma Fibroma
Lichen simplex	Plasma cell vulvitis	Abscess	Malignancy
Pthiriasis	Herpes zoster	Injury	Possibly: factitial lesions
Eczema	Toxic reaction	Pyoderma fistulans	
Dry skin	Group A streptococci Trichomoniasis Irritable dermatitis Skin damage	Pemphigus Acne conglobata Hidradenitis Skin damage	

III. Clinical picture **Flat redness**	**Nodules**	**Pustules**	**Vesicles**	**Ulcers**
Candidiasis Trichomoniasis	Candidiasis Genital herpes	Candidiasis Genital herpes	Genital herpes Herpes gestationis	Genital herpes Behçet syndrome
Erosive lichen planus	Folliculitis	Folliculitis	Toxic reaction	Scratch marks with lichen sclerosus
Irritable dermatitis	Sebaceous cysts	Pyoderma		Injuries (intercourse)
Toxic reaction Plasma cell vulvitis	Acne conglobata Hidradenoma	Varicella Herpes zoster	Varicella Herpes zoster	Carcinoma Syphilis
Erysipelas (group A streptococci)	Molluscum contagiosum		Pemphigus	Chancroid

IV. Whitening of skin
Lichen sclerosus
Lichen planus
Vitiligo
Hyperkeratosis

* Reportable infection

Table 7.2 Options for local treatment of diseases of the vulva

	Type of drug	Preparation
Anti-infective agents	Antibiotics Antimycotics Antiseptics Virostatics	Metronidazole, clindamycin Nystatin, clotrimazole, etc. Polyvidone iodine, hexetidine, dequal-inium chloride, nifuratel Acyclovir, foscarnet
Hormone	Estrogens Cortisol	Estrogen ointment/ovules Topical: e. g., clobetasol, triamcinolone
Removal	Ablation Denaturation	Surgery, laser, electric loop Trichloroacetic acid (> 50 %), podophyl-lotoxin, albothyl
Immunological	Immunomodulators	Imiquimod, tacrolimus
Skin care	Lubricant	Ointments containing lavender oil

Skin Care in the Anogenital Region

The principle source of bacteria in the genital region is the anus, since up to 50 % of the discharged excrement (feces) consists of bacteria. Anyone concerned with the genital region tries to keep this area as clean as possible because of the offensive odor of bacterial metabolites. If the skin is sensitive, this easily causes skin lesions and these, in turn, promote the growth of bacteria.

The best skin care of the anal region consists of lubricating the anus with ointments containing lavender oil prior to having a bowel movement. This not only facilitates defecation and prevents anal lesions, but it also reduces the amount of bacteria colonizing the skin.

Lubricating the vulva and the vaginal orifice with ointments containing lavender oil prior to intercourse prevents injury to the skin if there is a disposition for it, and it diminishes the development of infections. (**Caution:** condoms made of latex are damaged by oil.)

Vulvitis Caused by Fungi

Fungi are the most common cause of inflammation in the external genital region. Hence, they should always be considered in case of any complaints, and they should be excluded as a contributing factor.

Candidiasis

Frequency, pathogen, transmission, and risk factors. Vulvitis caused by fungi is the most common infection associated with an inflammatory reaction of the vulva. In most patients, it is caused by *Candida albicans* (> 90 %) and only very rarely by *C. tropicalis*, *C. crusei*, or other species. Up to 5–10 % of gynecological patients may be affected. Some women rarely have a manifest infection, while others have frequent infections.

The pathogen *Candida albicans* is widely distributed. It is taken up together with food and through human contact. It is thus found in up to 50 % of adults as a colonizing pathogen in the mouth and intestine.

Some of the factors promoting the onset of *Candida* infections are known, e. g., diabetes mellitus, antibiotic therapy, high doses of estrogen, and immunosuppression. However, the majority of women suffering from recurrent *Candida* infections do not have any of the known risk factors.

Skin lesions (Fig. 7.**1**) promote the onset of a fungal infection. On the other hand, fungi are also found as colonizing organisms in various forms of dermatitis and are then not the sole cause of the complaints.

Symptoms. The main symptom is itching; if there is only burning, this rules out fungal infection as a cause. Only very pronounced candidiasis is associated with pain. Some patients just complain of discharge, which means that only the vagina is affected.

Clinical picture. Redness and swelling of the vulva associated with flaky, crumbly discharge (Fig. 7.**3**) are such characteristic symptoms that this picture can hardly be confused with any other forms of vulvitis. More difficult is the diagnosis when there is redness with tiny nodules (Fig. 7.**4**), or pustules with redness (Fig. 7.**5**), or

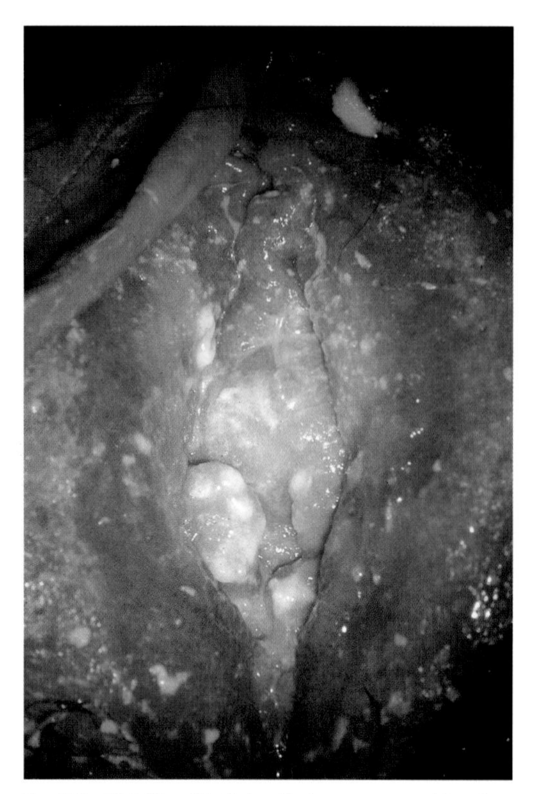

Fig. 7.**3** Vulvitis with flaky discharge, caused by *Candida albicans* in a 43-year-old patient.

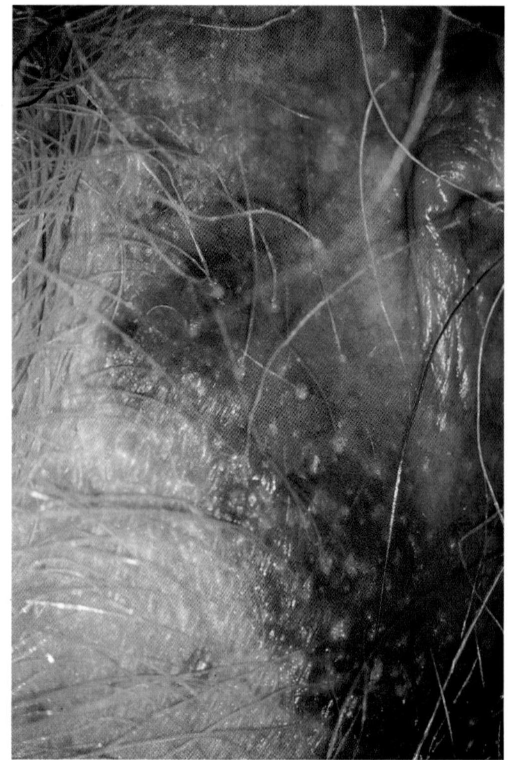

Fig. 7.**4** Vulvitis with nodules, caused by *Candida albicans* in a 40-year-old patient.

even pustules without redness (Fig. 7.**6**). Candidiasis is easier to identify if the vulva shows dry redness (Fig. 7.**7**), or when there are discrete white stipples (Fig. 7.**8**) or discrete tiny rings (remains of pustules) in the region of the vaginal orifice. Fungus-induced pustules persist for many days, in contrast to those induced by herpesviruses. If the vulvar redness is spread over larger areas with irregular boundaries (Fig. 7.**9**), this indicates very severe candidiasis—often in association with a basic disease, such as diabetes mellitus.

Diagnosis:

- *Microscopy.* Diagnosis is most successful when based on microscopic examination of the discharge. Using the wooden handle of a cotton swab, some discharge (including flakes or crumbs, if possible) or the scrapings from pustules or nodules are mixed into a drop of 0.1 % methylene blue solution and then screened for fungal elements.

Because the distribution of yeast cells is usually inhomogeneous, it is better to look for flakes that are then homogenized in the methylene blue solution. These flakes consist of exfoliated epithelial cells that are clumped together by elongated, adhesive yeast elements (pseudomycelia).

Some examiners recommend that 10 % potassium hydroxide solution is used for dissolving the epithelial cells, but this is hardly necessary in the genital region. Staining is not required because viewing the sample under a phase-contrast microscope makes it easy to find yeast cells.

If typical pseudomycelia (treelike aggregations of elongated yeast cells, often attached to each other only by pointed connections; Fig. 7.**10** and Fig. 3.**1**, p. 27) are detected, the diagnosis is confirmed, and further diagnostic steps are superfluous. Microscopic evidence of pseudomycelia is virtually synonymous with the diagnosis of candidiasis. Occasionally, it may be easier to detect these characteristic fungal elements in swabs from the vagina.

The most sensitive method of detection is fluorescence microscopy. After adding a fluorescent dye that specifically stains the walls of yeast cells, the individual budding cells can be recognized between the epithelial cells.

In the absence of leukocytes, the presence of numerous small budding cells lets one suspect colonization with *Candida glabrata*, while fairly large, elongated budding cells indicate colonization with *Saccharomyces*.

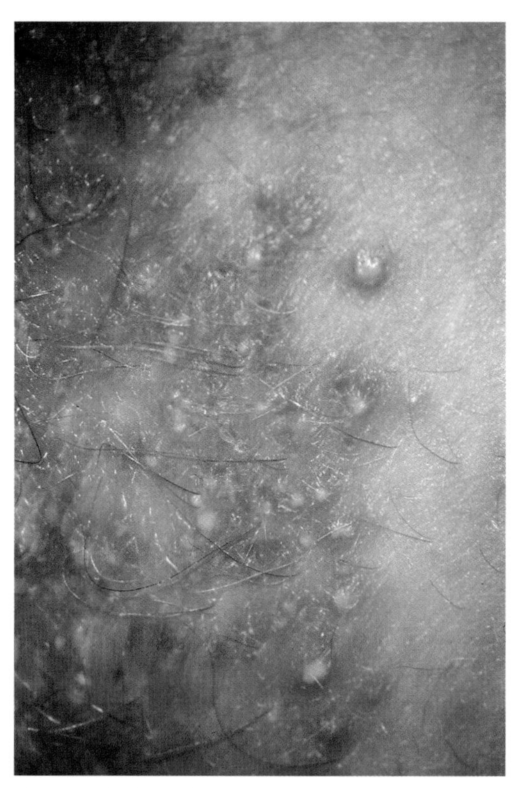

Fig. 7.**5** Vulvitis with pustules and pronounced redness, caused by *Candida albicans* in a 46-year-old patient.

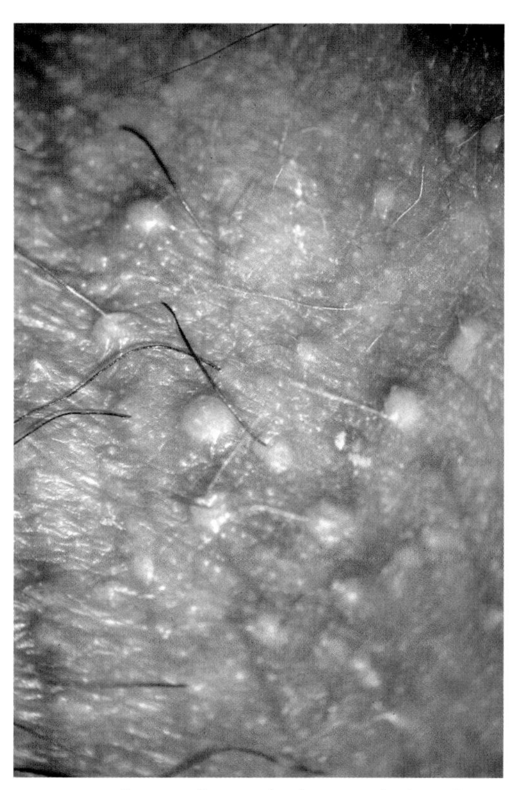

Fig. 7.**6** Vulvitis with pustules but very little redness, caused by *Candida albicans* in a 34-year-old patient.

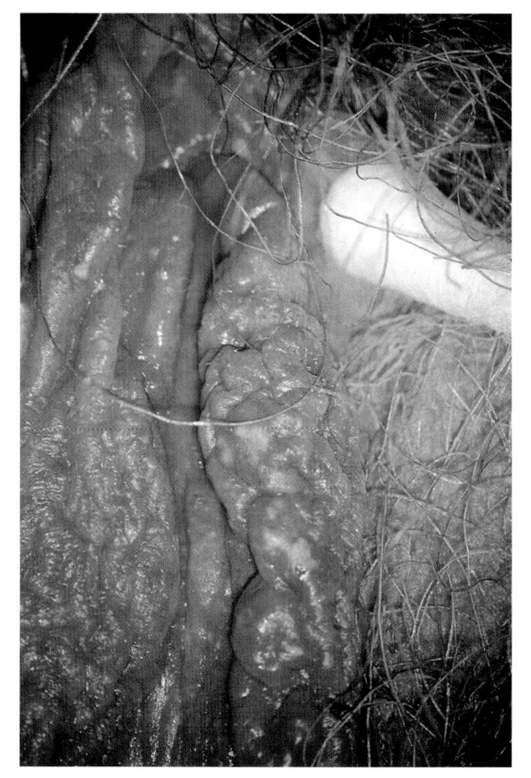

Fig. 7.**7** Dry vulvitis caused by *Candida albicans* in a 43-year-old patient.

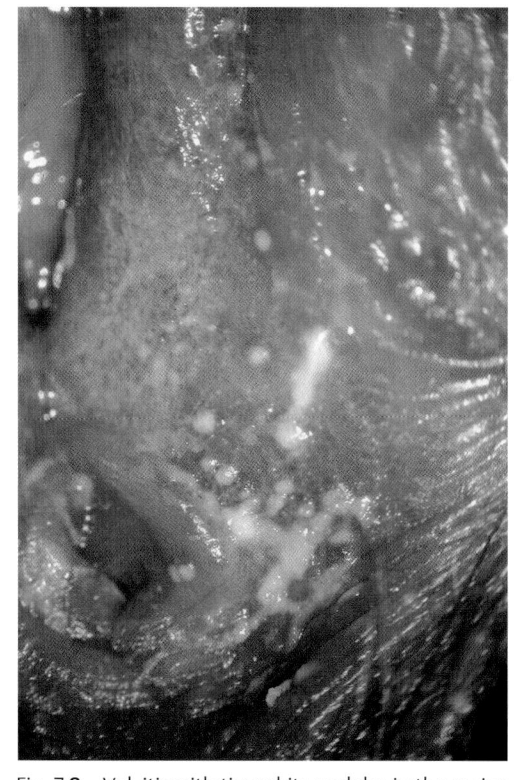

Fig. 7.**8** Vulvitis with tiny white nodules in the region near the vaginal orifice, caused by *Candida albicans*.

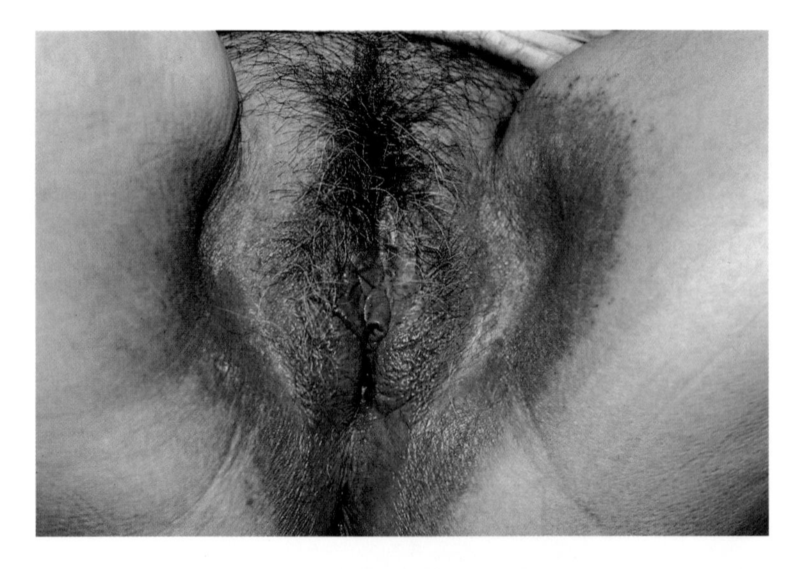

Fig. 7.**9** Severe chronic vulvitis caused by *Candida albicans* in a 54-year-old patient with diabetes mellitus.

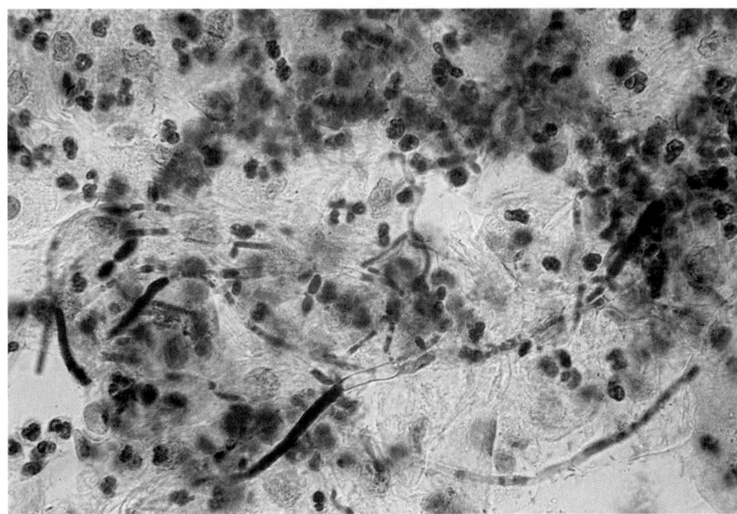

Fig. 7.**10** Micrograph illustrating pronounced candidiasis with pseudomycelia and numerous leukocytes. Discharge stained with 0.1 % methylene blue.

1
2
3
4
5
6
7
8
9
10
11
12
13
14
15

- *Culture.* The material on the cotton swab used for preparing the wet mount may be smeared onto Sabouraud agar or washed out in a tube containing Sabouraud solution (see Table 3.**1**, p. 25).

When taking swabs from a dry vulva, the cotton swab should be *premoistened* in order to make it absorbent. This may be done by briefly inserting it into the vagina, or by dipping it into culture medium or even tap water.

Fungal cultures are required whenever the patient's complaints and the clinical picture suggest a fungal infection but fungal elements cannot be detected microscopically. In addition, cultures for the purpose of a differential diagnosis are indicated whenever only budding cells (but no pseudomycelia) are seen under the microscope and apathogenic yeasts have to be excluded (e. g., *Saccharomyces cerevisiae*, baker or brewer yeast).

Determination of resistance is not required for routine diagnosis.

- *Biopsy.* In inconclusive cases (e. g., hyperkeratosis, adhesive coating, questionable nodules), a biopsy may be helpful (for the method, see p. 61). Fig. 7.**11** shows the clinical picture of candidiasis, while Fig. 7.**12** shows the corresponding histology. The histological preparation (staining with periodic acid–Schiff reagent, PAS) shows in an impressive way that fungi are able to penetrate the epithelium and do not always stay on the surface, where they are easier to eliminate.
- *Serology.* It hardly plays a role in genital candidiasis (only in cases of systemic infections, particularly in immunosuppressed individuals).

Differential diagnosis (Fig. 7.**13**). Apart from other infections, many dermatoses should be considered. A fungal infection often exists in

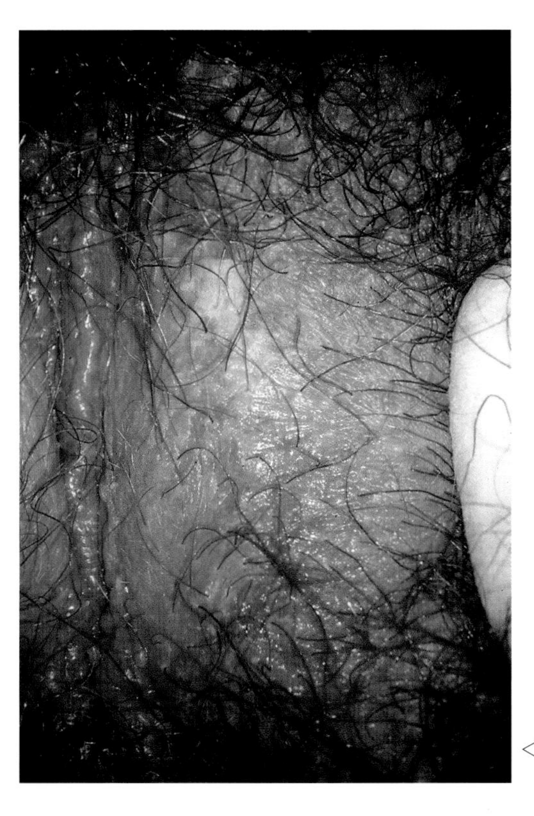

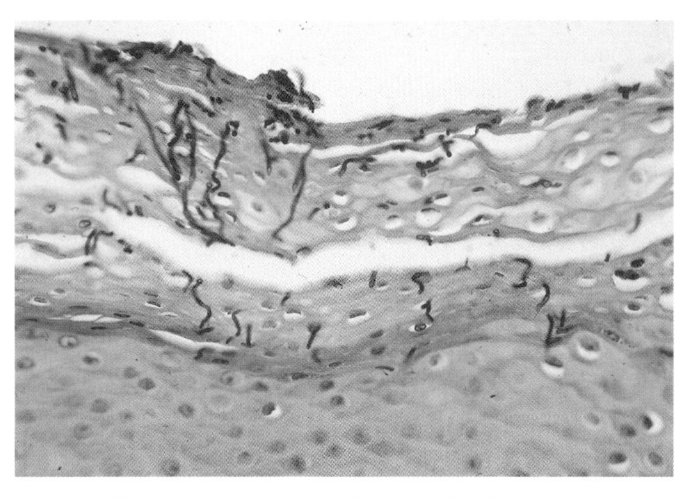

Fig. 7.**12** Histological preparation taken from the skin area shown in Fig. 7.**11**. Fungal hyphens invading the epithelium are easily detected in the PAS-stained cross-section.

◁ Fig. 7.**11** Apparent hyperkeratosis in a 32-year-old patient, identified in the histological preparation as candidiasis.

addition to a dermatosis. The fungal infection then represents an extra burden for the damaged skin to endure:

- folliculitis (*Staphylococcus aureus*)
- genital herpes, where burning is the predominating symptom and the various herpes stages (vesicles, pustules, erosions) are of very short duration, lasting only a few hours or days)
- tinea inguinalis (caused by dermatophytes)
- infection with group A streptococci
- infection with papillomavirus (does not cause any symptoms)
- eczema (contact dermatitis/allergy)
- psoriasis vulgaris
- erosive lichen planus
- lichen simplex chronicus (circumscribed neurodermatitis)
- pinworms in the perianal region (causing itching)
- bowenoid papulosis (easy to identify by using the acetic acid test).

Therapy. Treatment depends on the severity of the disease and on the patient's history and condition. Normally, yeasts are not life threatening for immunocompetent individuals; they are rather a nuisance. Therapy is therefore only necessary when there are complaints of inflammatory reactions, during pregnancy, and when the immune system is suppressed. In about 15% of women without complaints, *Candida albicans* can be detected at low counts in cultures from vaginal swabs.

As illustrated in Fig. 7.**12**, yeasts are able to penetrate into the epithelium even in immunocompetent persons; they are therefore not easily removed by washing. When the immune system is intact, an antimycotic drug will bring quick relieve.

Therapy for Rarely/Occasionally Occurring Fungal Infections

Therapy is normally not a problem here. Short-term topical treatment is the rule, and it should always be a combination of cream for external use and vaginal ovules/tablets for internal use. In the past, treatment for several days (five days) has been the norm, but short-term therapy (one to three days) is gaining acceptance. By simply increasing the concentration of the active component, the same therapeutic results can be achieved—and the patients appreciate the shorter term of treatment.

A single oral dose is also an option. It has the advantage that the drug can reach also those areas left out by topical application. This form of treatment can also be applied during the period.

Antimycotic drugs. See p. 48.

7

Fig. 7.**13** Differential diagnosis of vulvovaginal candidiasis.

	Reddened epithelium	Papules, pustules, nodules	Normal epithelium	White epithelium
Infection	Candidiasis Trichomoniasis Group A streptococci Purulent vulvovaginitis Tinea inguinalis Erythrasma	Genital herpes Herpes zoster Staphyloderma Folliculitis Pyoderma Condyloma Molluscum contagiosum Scabies Syphilis	Worms	
Dermatosis	Erosive lichen planus Psoriasis Eczema Irritable dermatitis Local drug eruption Toxic reaction	Behçet disease Pemphigus		Lichen sclerosus Vitiligo Hyperkeratosis
Other causes	Vestibulitis Atrophy	Injury Scratch marks Sebaceous cysts	Excessive washing Skin damage	Lichen simplex
Dysplasia		Bowen disease Carcinoma Paget disease		

Therapy for Chronic Recurrent Candidiasis

Frequently occurring fungal infections—more than four per year, up to every three to four weeks—due to treatment failure or reinfection (relapses) call for a different approach. The causes and cofactors must be identified because it is quite possible that the fungal infection is only a superinfection. One should also consider that not every itch is caused by fungi and that the fungus detected in the culture may be a harmless colonizing organism.

Approach to Recurrent Candidal Vulvitis

- Typing of *Candida* species: the most severe symptoms are induced by *C. albicans.*
- Exclusion of cofactors: diabetes mellitus, immunosuppression through medication or HIV infection (these are rather rare cofactors).
- Condition of the vulvar epithelium, especially in the perianal region: skin lesions, dryness, rhagades, coarse epithelium, anal fissures, and hemorrhoids (these are common cofactors).
- Examination of anal and oral swabs for gathering information on the extent of the patient's colonization with fungi and also to recognize potential sources of infection.
- Examination and parallel treatment of the patient's partner: swabs from the penis, mouth, or extremities (a common cofactor).
- Consultation about washing habits and sexual habits, including inquiring about symptoms observed in the partner (a common cofactor).
- Inquiring about eating habits: sweets and a diet rich in carbohydrates promote fungal growth in the intestinal tract, which may indirectly increase the transmission of fungi from the anus to the vulva (a less important cofactor).
- Termination of the use of ovulation inhibitors is not recommended, as there is no evidence that candidiasis is promoted by relatively low doses of estrogen. High doses of estrogen create a vaginal milieu that is rich in nutrients and sugars, thus promoting the growth of fungi (there is hardly any candidiasis in the genital region in the absence of estrogen).

Therapeutic Options for Frequently Recurring *Candida albicans* Infections

- Treatment with a systemic antimycotic, e. g., fluconazole. The following therapeutic approach has proved useful: prescription of fluconazole (100 mg tablets, four treatments of two tablets each); the first dose immediately, the second dose after one week, followed by culture after two weeks to rule out the presence of *Candida* in the vagina, the third dose after four weeks, and the fourth dose after eight weeks. The partner should be treated as well (oral dose once or twice).

- Avoiding soaps or other skin care products that may irritate the skin, even though they may be marketed as being particularly gentle (the fungus detected in the culture may represent a secondary colonization).
- Reducing the use of water while intensifying perianal skin care with ointments containing lavender oil (lubrication and protection of the anus *prior to defecation).*
- Regular care of the vulva with ointments containing lavender oil after every washing.
- Inclusion of the partner in the topical or oral treatment (e.g., fluconazole or itraconazole). Regular skin care should include the partner as well (e.g., lubrication of the penis and anal region with ointments containing lavender oil).
- Skin care of the genitals prior to intercourse (lubrication as prevention of microlesions).
- Attempt to eradicate the fungus by simultaneous nystatin therapy: oral treatment (lozenges), intestinal treatment (coated tablets, four times two tablets per day), and topical treatment (vulva and vagina) for 20 days. Intestinal sanitation requires at least 3 g nystatin per day (taken as powder, if possible); however, the success is limited due to frequent reuptake of exogenous fungus.

Approach in Case of Treatment Failure

- If the findings get worse during therapy, one should also consider a possible intolerance or allergy to the base of the antimycotic ointment (see also irritable vulvitis, p. 109).
- Many creams and skin care products contain emulsifiers and preservatives that may cause allergies when used for a long time.
- Changing the drug or switching to oral therapy. Short-term treatment with cortisone cream, followed by regular lubrication with ointments containing lavender oil that are free of emulsifiers and preservatives.
- If one is not dealing with chronic candidiasis: *C. albicans* may represent only a secondary colonization of skin lesions caused by too much washing or rubbing (lichen simplex).
- If one is dealing with a dermatosis: psoriasis (Fig. 7.**93**, p. 111), for example, may look different in the genital region than at the usual predilection sites.
- Biopsy in case of inconclusive findings in order to exclude dermatosis.

Infections Caused by Other Fungi

Other yeast species (see Table 1.**2**, p. 8) play a minor role.

Candida glabrata (Formerly: *Torulopsis glabrata*)

This species can only form budding cells. It is almost always a harmless colonizing organism. *C. glabrata*, which affects more the vagina than the vulva, is often found together with *C. albicans*—and it is the species that remains after therapy (selected species), thus still yielding positive cultures.

Typical for a colonization by *C. glabrata* is the microscopic finding of many small budding cells in the native preparation, without any signs of an inflammatory reaction (very few leukocytes), or the fact that the patient is free of symptoms although the fungal culture is still positive. If symptoms are present but only *C. glabrata* can be detected in the culture, one should search for other causes of the symptoms.

Common antimycotic drugs are rather ineffective against *C. glabrata*, and increasing the dose in an attempt to eliminate this yeast species is not a good idea.

In the presence of chronic systemic diseases and immunosuppression, *C. glabrata* may also be detected in blood cultures.

Dermatophytes (Tinea Inguinalis)

This fungal skin infection is also called tinea cruris, ringworm of the groin, and jock itch. Unlike yeasts, which prefer moist and warm body parts, dermatophytes tend to infect dry skin areas. They rarely occur in the genital region—and if they do, then rather in the perivulvar region.

Pathogen. Usually *Trichophyton rubrum.*

Clinical picture. Round, flat, and red foci of inflammation with distinct margins. Very itchy and spreading (Fig. 7.**14**).

Diagnosis:

- *Clinical picture.* Red patches with distinct margins.
- *Microscopy.* Mycelia form treelike ramifications, exhibiting true bifurcations and septae.
- *Culture.*

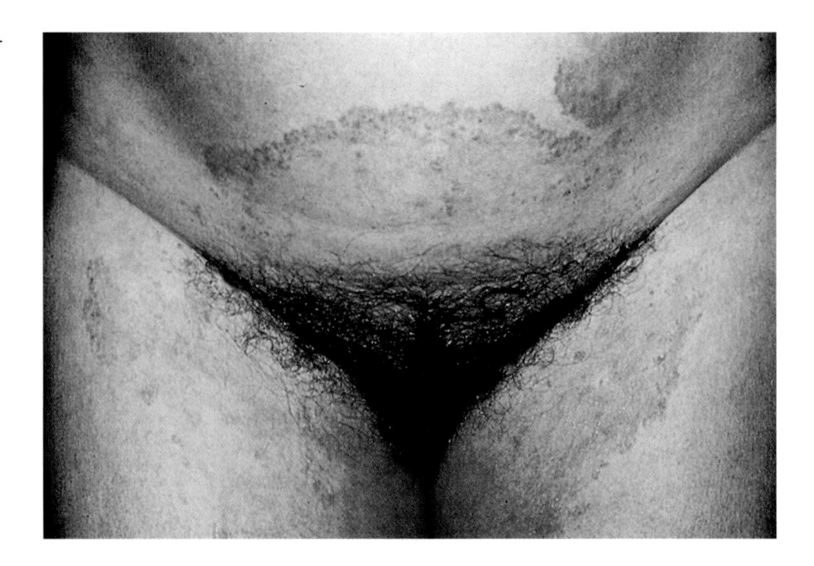

Fig. 7.**14** Tinea inguinalis caused by the dermatophyte *Trichophyton rubrum* mostly in the perivulvar region; the infected area is characterized by distinct margins. (Photograph courtesy of Dr. S. A. Qadripur, Department of Dermatology, University Hospital, Göttingen, Germany.)

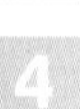

Differential diagnosis:

- candidiasis
- erythrasma
- eczema
- psoriasis.

Therapy. Imidazole preparations (see p. 49).

Vulvitis Caused by Bacteria

Because of the close proximity to the anus, an abundance of bacteria can be cultured from swabs of the vulva. However, most of them are intestinal bacteria and are therefore only contaminating or colonizing microbes.

The most important bacterial species able to cause infection and inflammation of the vulvar skin are *Staphylococcus aureus* and group A streptococci. The clinical pictures may be quite different.

Pyoderma of the Vulva and Surrounding Areas

Pyoderma, a purulent infection of the skin, is caused by pus-forming bacteria. The various forms of pyoderma include:

- folliculitis (*S. aureus*)
- furuncle and carbuncle (*S. aureus*)
- impetigo contagiosa (group A streptococci, occasionally also *S. aureus*)
- vulvitis in young girls (group A streptococci)
- erysipelas (group A streptococci).

Infections Caused by Staphylococcus aureus

Folliculitis

An infection of hair follicles by *S. aureus*. The clinical picture is easily diagnosed by colposcopy when the inflammatory process (nodules, pustules) is associated with hair follicles (Figs. 7.**15**–7.**17**).

Pathogen. *S. aureus.*

Diagnosis. Clinical picture and detection of *S. aureus* in the culture.

Therapy. Antibiotics are administered for five days. Without an antibiogram, a cephalosporin of the second generation is appropriate; with antibiogram and in case of sensitivities, amoxicillin or other antibiotics may be administered. At an early stage, one may also attempt to cure the infection by means of topical application of polyvidone iodine cream.

Differential diagnosis:

- Vulvitis pustulosa caused by *Candida albicans* (pustules are not associated with hair follicles; see Figs. 7.**4**–7.**6**, p. 71).
- Genital herpes (rapid course of stages with vesicles and erosions during the primary infection, see Figs. 7.**31**–7.**38** (pp. 84–86); or temporary groups of vesicles and pustules at a single site only in case of a relapse, see Fig. 7.**42**, p. 88).

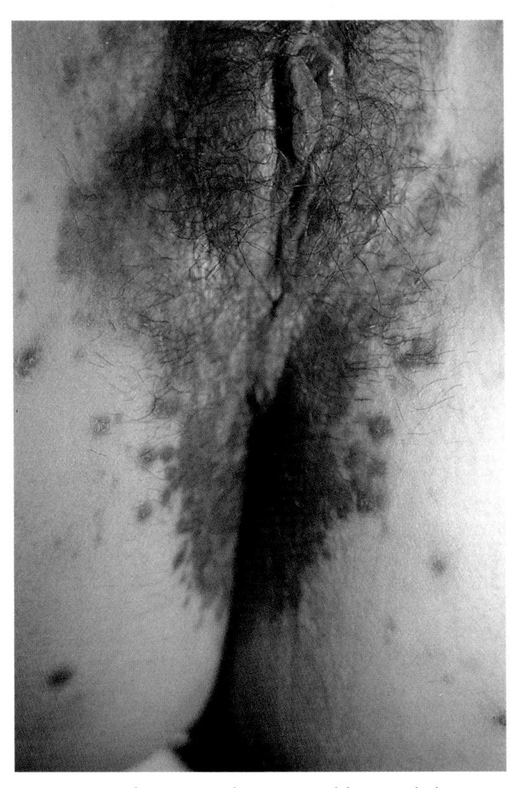

Fig. 7.**15** Vulvitis pustulosa caused by *Staphylococcus aureus* in a 24-year-old patient.

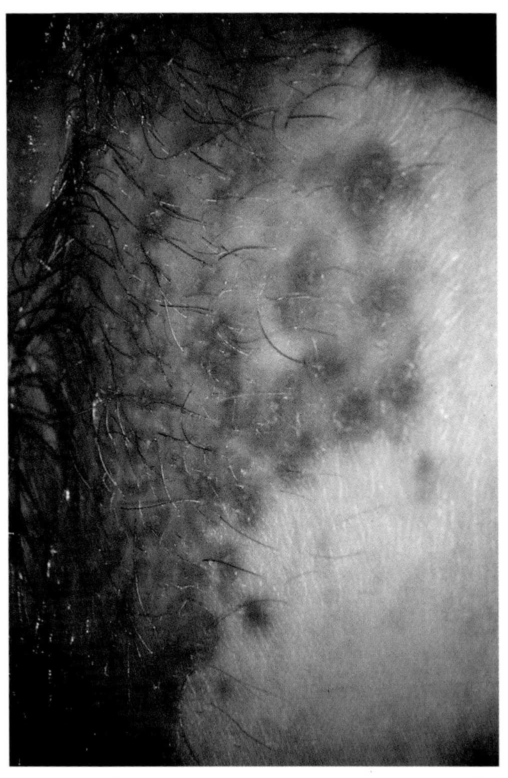

Fig. 7.**16** The same patient as in Fig. 7.**15**; pustules shown at higher magnification.

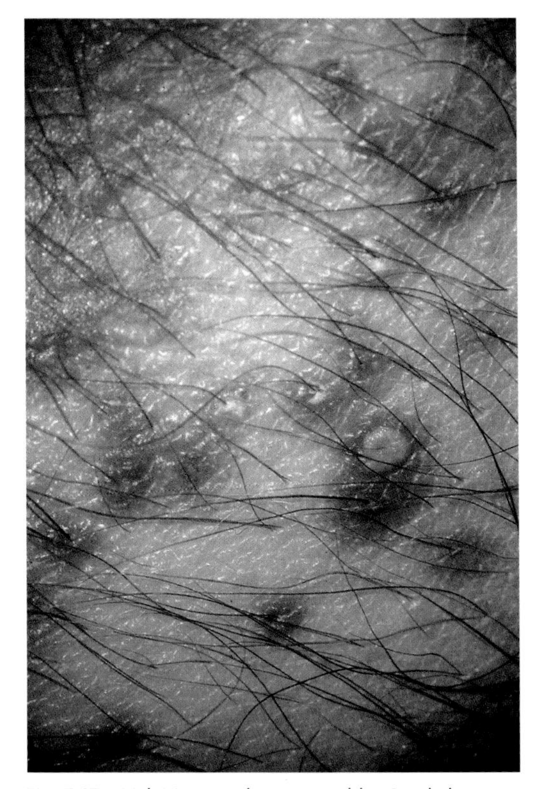

Fig. 7.**17** Vulvitis pustulosa caused by *Staphylococcus aureus;* the pustules are clearly associated with hair follicles.

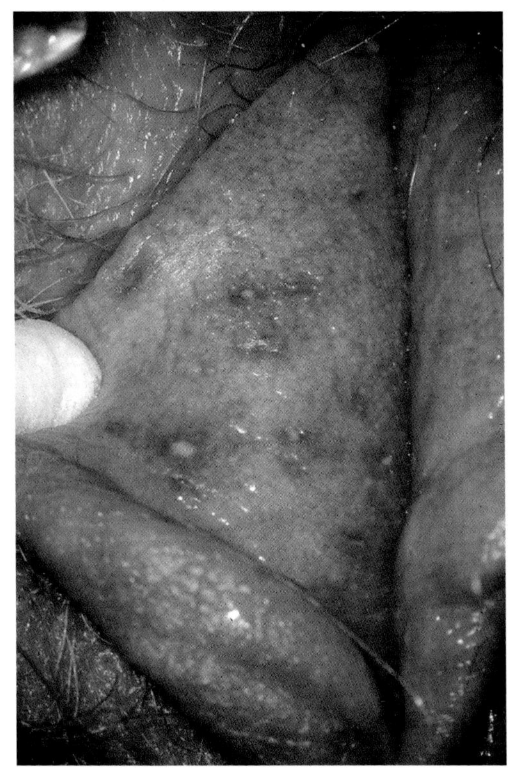

Fig. 7.**18** Vulvitis with pustules of the sebaceous glands caused by *Staphylococcus aureus.*

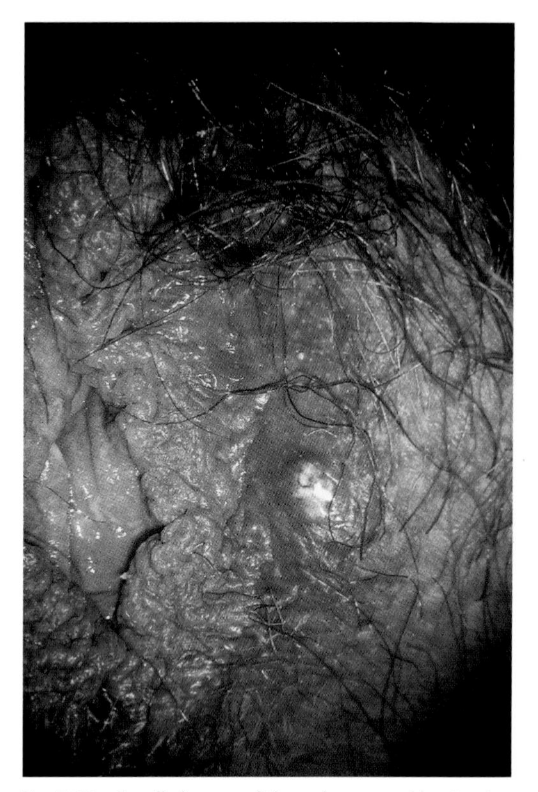

Fig. 7.**19** Small abscess of the vulva caused by *Staphylococcus aureus* in a 45-year-old patient.

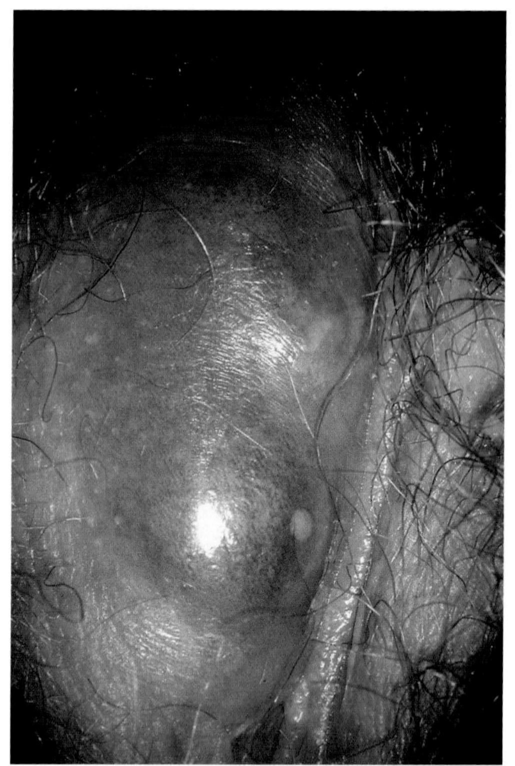

Fig. 7.**20** Abscess in the right labium majus caused by *Staphylococcus aureus.*

▶ Molluscum contagiosum (see Fig. 7. **51**, p. 91; easy to identify by colposcopy).

Furuncle/Carbuncle

This is an infection originating from a hair follicle or sebaceous gland (Figs. 7.**18**, 7.**19**) with central necrolysis of deeper tissues caused by *S. aureus* (Figs. 7.**20**, 7.**21**). It is usually a smear infection promoted by insufficient hygiene, but other causes are also possible, such as basic diseases and immunosuppression. Carbuncle is the most severe form and is always very painful because of its rapid increase in size and the severe inflammatory reaction. It may also occur in young girls (Fig. 7.**23**).

Pathogen. *S. aureus.*

Therapy. The abscess is opened by stab incision (Fig. 7.**21**) after anesthesia with ELMA cream (wait at least 30 minutes until the cream becomes effective). This is followed by skin care with polyvidone iodine cream. Treatment with oral antibiotics is rarely necessary.

Infections Caused by Group A Streptococci

Vulvitis

Pathogen. β-hemolytic streptococci of serogroup A (*Streptococcus pyogenes*).

Transmission and pathogenesis. This infection is promoted by insufficient hygiene and mechanical irritation of the skin, particularly in the absence of estrogens and a lactobacillus flora. It is caused by smear infection with the fingers from the mouth to the genitals (oral–vulva infection) and occurs typically in prepubertal girls (Fig. 7.**22**). It is increasingly seen also in women, perhaps as a result of oral–genital sexual contact.

Clinical picture. The diffuse redness, which spreads over a large area (Figs. 7.**24**, 7.**25**, 7.**27**), is associated with leukocytic discharge (Fig. 7.**28**) and often affects also the perianal region. It frequently occurs in families with children.

Otherwise, this is the typical and almost only type of severe vulvitis in prepubertal girls. Occasionally, there may be a whitish irregular coating (exfoliated epithelial cells) and red nodules

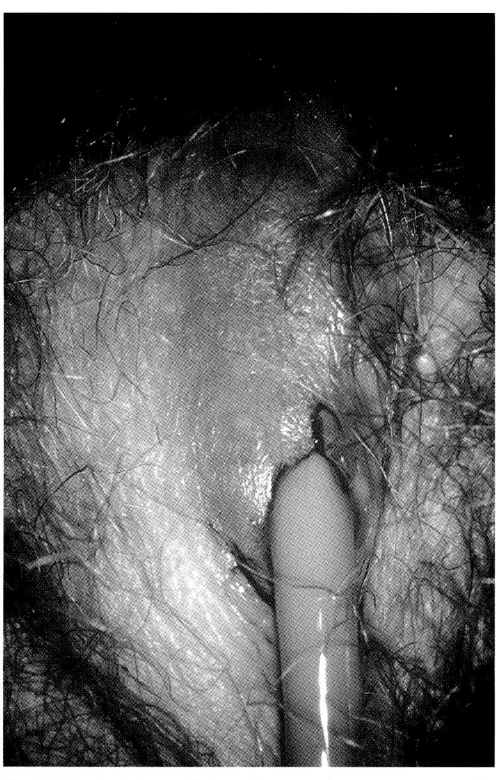

Fig. 7.**21** Incision of the abscess shown in Fig. 7.**20**, with drainage following the incision.

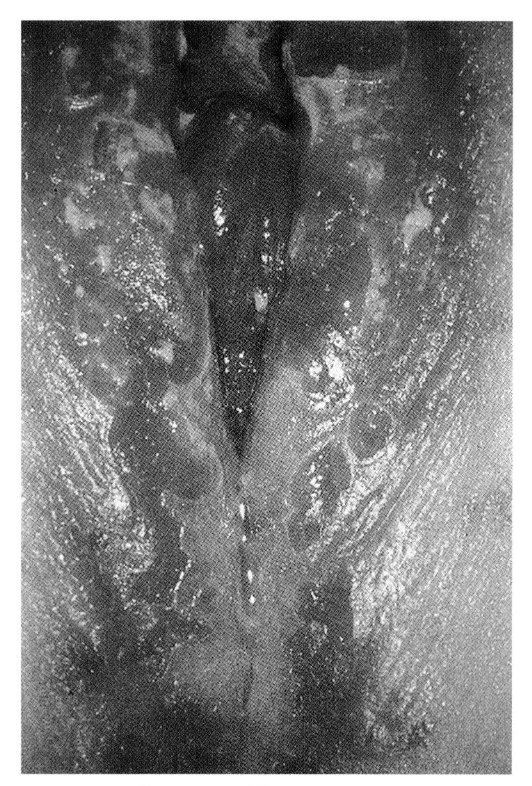

Fig. 7.**22** Vulvitis caused by group A streptococci in a six-year-old girl. This form of vulvitis is typical for children. Transmission most likely occurs by means of the fingers from the frequently colonized nasopharyngeal space to the genitals.

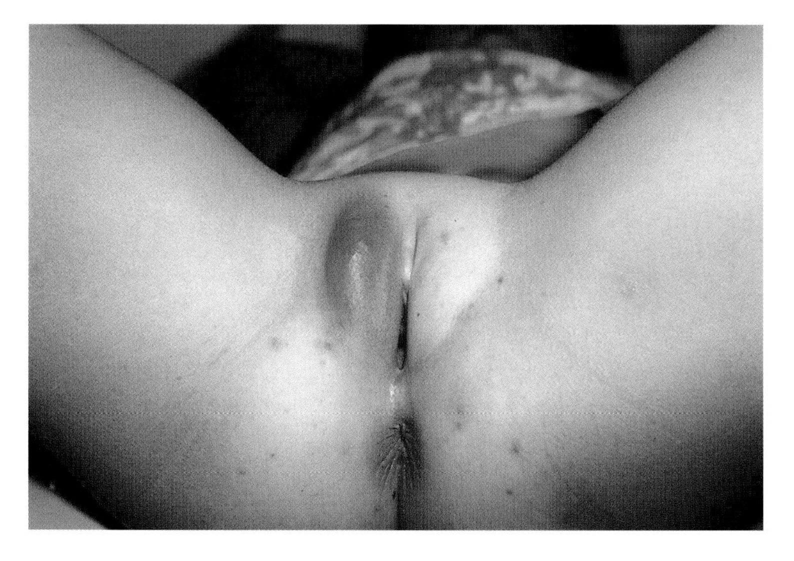

Fig. 7.**23** Large abscess of the right labium majus in a six-year-old girl.

(Figs. 7.**22**, 7.**26**). A fungal infection is therefore often considered initially, thus delaying proper treatment. Ischuria may occur if there is pronounced inflammation and pain. The infection may occur repeatedly in families at risk.

Widespread inflammation with redness reaching to the anus and without a pathogen visible under the microscope is typical for, or prompt the suspicion of, an infection with group A streptococci (Fig. 7.**27**).

Diagnosis:

- *Microscopy.* Wet mounts in 0.1 % methylene blue solution show plenty of granulocytes and cocci (Fig. 7.**28**).
- *Culture*

Fig. 7.**24** Recurrent vulvovaginitis and perianal dermatitis caused by group A streptococci in a 30-year-old patient with two children.

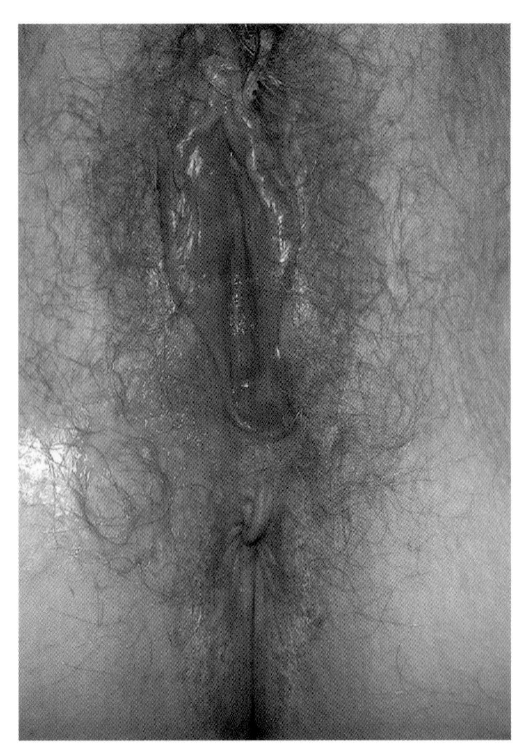

Fig. 7.**25** The same patient as in Fig. 7.**24** after 10 days of treatment with amoxicillin.

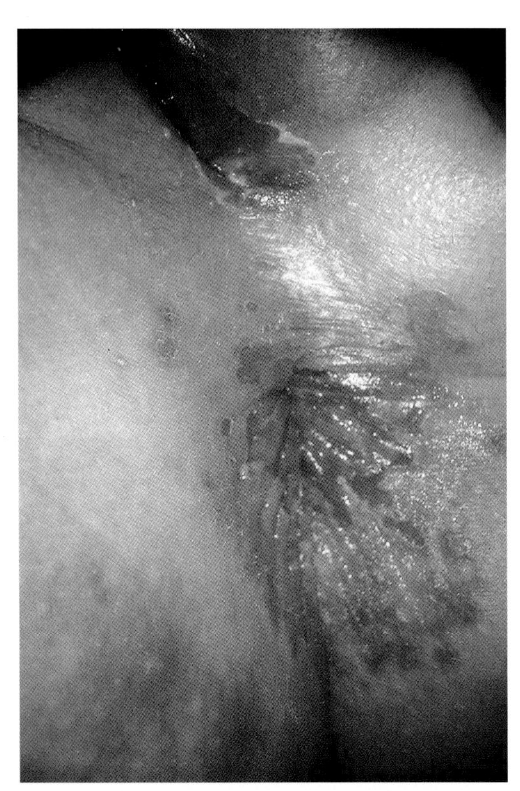

Fig. 7.**26** Perianal dermatitis and vulvitis caused by group A streptococci in a three-year-old girl.

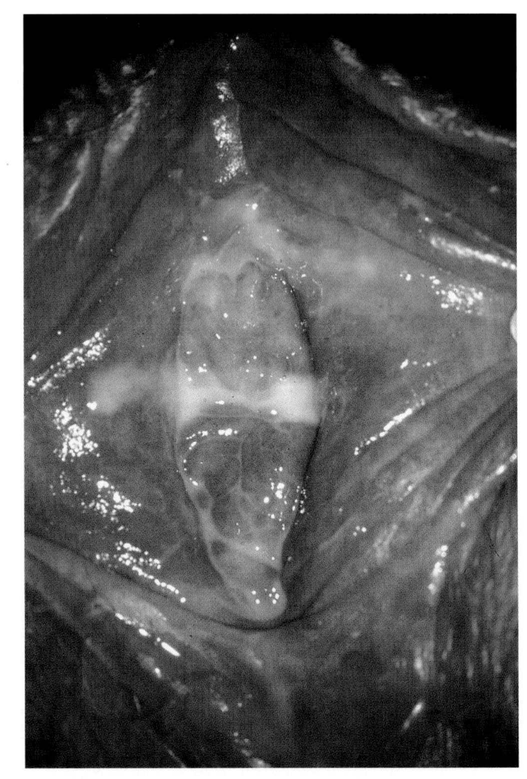

Fig. 7.**27** Pronounced vulvitis caused by group A streptococci in a 38-year-old patient.

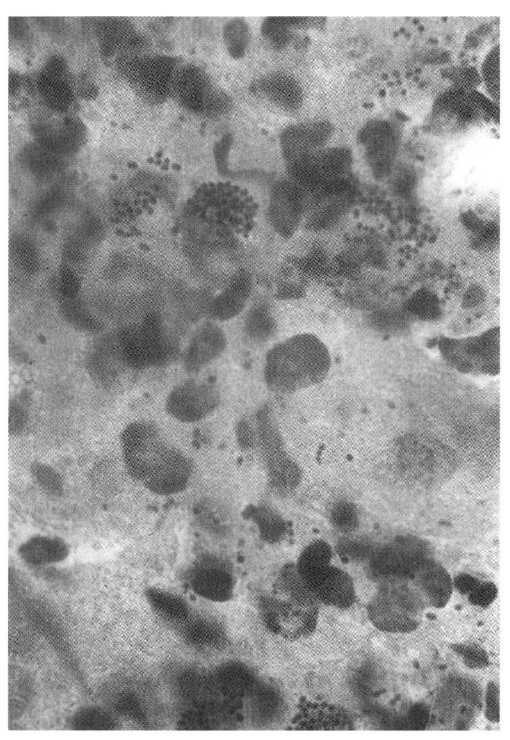

Fig. 7.**28** Micrograph illustrating vulvitis caused by group A streptococcus in a six-year-old girl. The swab material taken from the vulva and stained with methylene blue contains numerous cocci in addition to masses of granulocytes.

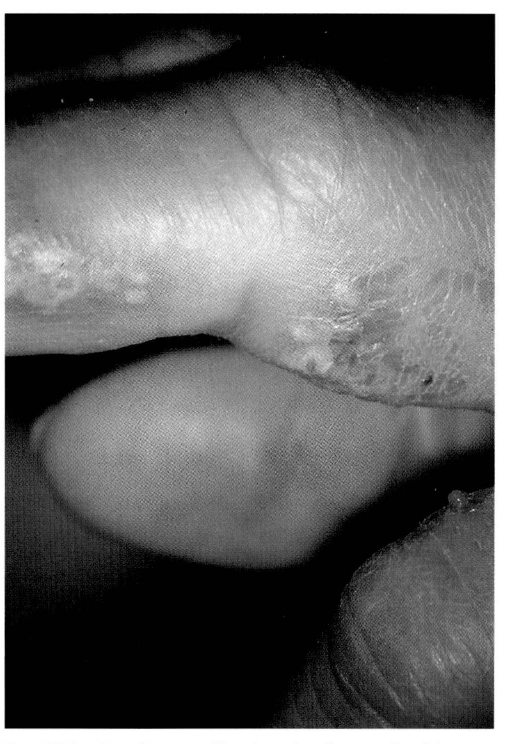

Fig. 7.**29** Pyoderma affecting the finger of a 58-year-old patient suffering simultaneously from malaise, dermatitis, and vulvitis caused by group A streptococci.

- *Antibiogram*, (normally not necessary as resistances are rare).

Therapy. Penicillin, amoxicillin, or cephalosporin for 10 days.

Differential diagnosis. Candidiasis, plasma cell vulvitis, trichomoniasis, atrophic vaginitis.

Special risks. Systemic spreading and the transmission to other persons endanger pregnant women, in particular, because of the perils of puerperal sepsis (see p. 218).

Group A streptococci are the most dangerous bacteria in the genital region.

Impetigo Contagiosa

Caused by group A streptococci, this infection of the skin is almost exclusively seen in children.

Occasionally, it may occur also in women. Group A streptococci are among the most dangerous pathogens in the genital region. There is always the risk of introducing them into the genital region from other sites of the body, especially when fingers are infected (Fig. 7.**29**).

Erysipelas

Clinical picture. This acute superficial skin infection is caused by group A streptococci and, less often, by group G streptococci. The pathogens usually enter the body through small skin lesions. Apart from superficial, circumscribed, and painful redness of the skin (Fig. 7.**30**), the infection causes swelling of the regional lymph nodes as it is spreading through the lymph vessels. There may be fever, malaise, and also shaking chills.

Diagnosis. Diagnosis is based on the clinical picture, since the pathogen cannot be detected in the skin. Detection of group A streptococci from the nasopharyngeal cavity or the genitals may be helpful.

Therapy. Penicillin is administered orally for 10 days, and cephalosporins or macrolides are also an option.

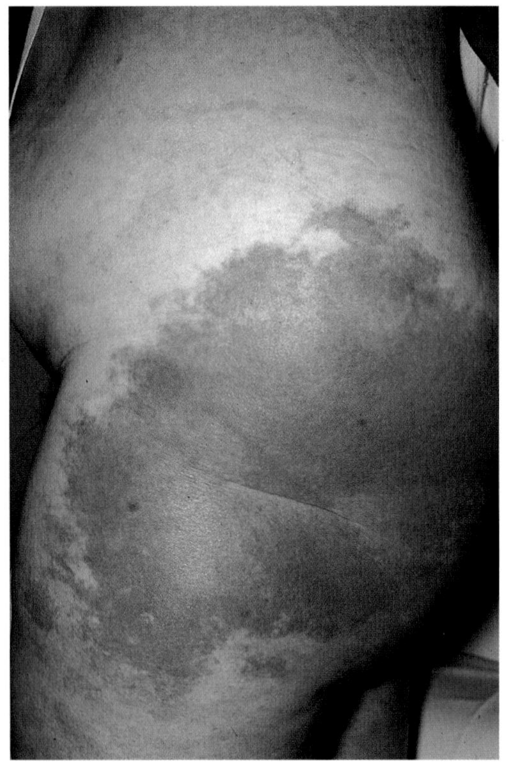

Fig. 7.**30** Erysipelas of the left hip (caused by group A streptococci) after vulvectomy and chronic lymphostasis.

Vulvitis Caused by Viruses

Genital Herpes

Genital herpes is among the most common infections of the genital region. The primary infection with herpes simplex virus is sexually transmitted. Its course is severe, unless there is immunity to herpes simplex virus due to a preceding oral infection. Relapses are much milder, but they may become a nuisance due to the frequency of their occurrence. Transmission of the virus to the newborn can lead to fatal infection.

The clinical picture varies and ranges from asymptomatic secretion of the virus to burning pain and, finally, to very painful and febrile vulvitis, vaginitis, and cervicitis. Lower abdominal pain similar to that of pelvic inflammatory disease may occur as well. The degree of discomfort depends on the frequency and extent of the local inflammatory reaction. Early therapy may prevent both. Because the relapses vary greatly with respect to frequency and symptoms, many recurring herpes attacks are not recognized as such. On the other hand, supposedly herpes virus-induced ulcers may be treated without success, thus leading to doubts regarding the therapy.

Pathogen. Genital herpes is caused by two pathogenic human herpesviruses. These are herpes simplex virus type 2 (HSV-2) and herpes simplex virus type 1 (HSV-1). The viral genome consists of a single molecule of linear double-stranded DNA. It is surrounded by a nucleocapsid that, in turn, is enclosed in a loose lipid-bilayer envelope. Between the nucleocapsid and the envelope is a tegument of amorphous material. The HSV-1 and HSV-2 genomes exhibit about 50 % homology of their nucleotide sequences. Serologically, the two viruses can be distinguished by means of specific monoclonal antibodies against different nucleocapsid antigens and, in particular, antigens of the envelope. Humans seem to be the only natural reservoir of these viruses. HSV-1 is considered the oral type, which is found almost exclusively in nongenital regions, whereas HSV-2 is defined as the genital type.

Transmission and infectivity. The virus is transmitted from person to person through smear infection (direct contact infection). It is rarely transmitted through objects (indirect contact infection) because the virus is not stable. Nevertheless, it is possible in some patients.

Points of entry are the mucosae and small lesions in the keratinized skin. The amount of transmitted virus particles, the point of entry, and the immune status of the afflicted person determine the length of the incubation period and the severity of the disease.

Vesicles (small blisters) filled with virus particles are particularly infectious. Ulcers and erosions also set free many virus particles, and detection of the pathogen is possible from here. Even at the crust stage, the virus can still be detected in cultures or PCR.

Herpes viruses can be set free even when no lesions are visible—for example, in the regions of the cervix, urethra, and mouth—and thus may infect the sexual partner or the newborn. This seems to be the most common form of transmitting the infection to the sexual partner. Petting offers no safe protection from transmission, and a condom provides only partial protection because it does not cover the entire genital region.

Epidemiology. Antibodies to herpes simplex viruses are formed by 80–90 % of adults. About 20 % of adults carry antibodies to type 2. The primary infection by HSV-1 usually takes place in early childhood in the orofacial region at the border between skin and mucosa. The infection is transmitted through direct body contact, normally already in early childhood. About 50 % of all children become infected with the virus and are then seropositive. Only rarely does the infection become clinically manifest (recurrent aphthous stomatitis [canker sore], herpes of the cornea). A second episode of infection begins postpubertal with intimate relationships. It is only now that also HSV-2 becomes evident epidemiologically. Up to 70–80% of adults possess antibodies against HSV-1 and up to 20–30% possess antibodies against HSV-2. Between HSV-1 and HSV-2 there is partial cross-immunity, which prevents the spreading of HSV-2. Up to 70–80% of genital herpes attacks are caused by HSV-2, and 20–30% are caused by HSV-1.

Today, HSV-1 is isolated in about 50% of clinically manifest primary infections. Our own studies during the last 10 years have shown that the portion of HSV-1-induced severe genital infections has increased. Of 55 patients with primary genital herpes who turned up for examination and from whom herpes simplex virus was cultured, type 1 was detected in 37 (67%) (unpublished data). However, this high portion of type 1 is not only connected with the increase of this type in the genital region, but also with the state of immunity of the patient. In women lacking immunity against type 1—namely, those who did not suffer from this infection during childhood—the primary infection with type 2 takes a much more severe course than in women with existing immunity against type 1.

The manifestation index of primary genital infection is not known precisely. It is estimated to be 20–30%.

Pathogenesis. During an active infection, the HSV of genital herpes penetrates along the sensory nerve tracts into the sacrospinal dorsal root ganglion, where is persists in a latent form after larger lesions (or just the primary inflammation) have healed. In this phase, no structural proteins of the virus can be detected in the neurons by molecular biology tests; only the genome and latency-associated regulatory proteins are present. Various stress factors can reactivate the latent infection into a virus-producing infection. Important stress factors include hormonal changes (menstruation-associated herpes), emotional stress (anger, exhaustion, lack of sleep), trauma, UV irradiation of the innervation segment of the mucocutaneous region, infections, and fever (herpes febrilis, also called cold sore or fever blisters).

Clinical picture. Only about 30% of cases of genital herpes are clinically clear and are recognized as such. About 20% do cause complaints but are misinterpreted by the patient—and sometimes also by the physician. Half of all genital herpes patients are more or less asymptomatic. Thus, the actual number of HSV-2-infected patients is, in fact, three times as high as one might assume based on the clinical experience.

The clinical picture is very characteristic, with the infection running its course relatively quickly and in defined stages. Development and duration may vary depending on whether it is a primary infection or relapse, on the one hand, and the state of the patient's immunity, on the other.

We distinguish between two forms of genital herpes:

- the primary infection caused by exogenous infection after sexual contact
- the relapse caused by endogenous reactivation of the persisting virus in the respective nerve ganglion.

Primary Genital Herpes

Pathogens:

- herpes simplex virus type 2 (HSV-2), 50–70% of patients
- herpes simplex virus type 1 (HSV-1), 30–50% of patients.

Transmission. Genital herpes is transmitted through sexual contact with mostly asymptomatic virus carriers, often also through oral–genital contact. Rarely, if at all, it is transmitted by means of objects or by using the same toilette.

Incubation period. Three to eight days, rarely longer (up to 14 days).

Clinical picture. Characteristic features include:

- swelling of the vulva (Fig. 7.**31**)
- spreading of the vesicles over large areas of the genitals and adjacent skin (Figs. 7.**32**, 7.**33**)
- bilateral appearance of symptoms
- long persistence of lesions (up to three weeks)
- painful swelling of inguinal lymph nodes (Fig. 7.**34**), which occasionally persists longer than the efflorescence of the vulva, sometimes over many weeks and even months.

In addition, the rapid course of the first stages (within hours and a few days) is very typical:

- painful swelling and redness of the vulva associated with initially small nodules
- quick transition to intraepithelial clear vesicles
- vesicles becoming opaque and confluent (Fig. 7.**35**)
- transition to lesions, less often to ulcers that develop a red halo (Figs. 7.**36**, 7.**37**)
- crust stage and healing without the formation of scars.

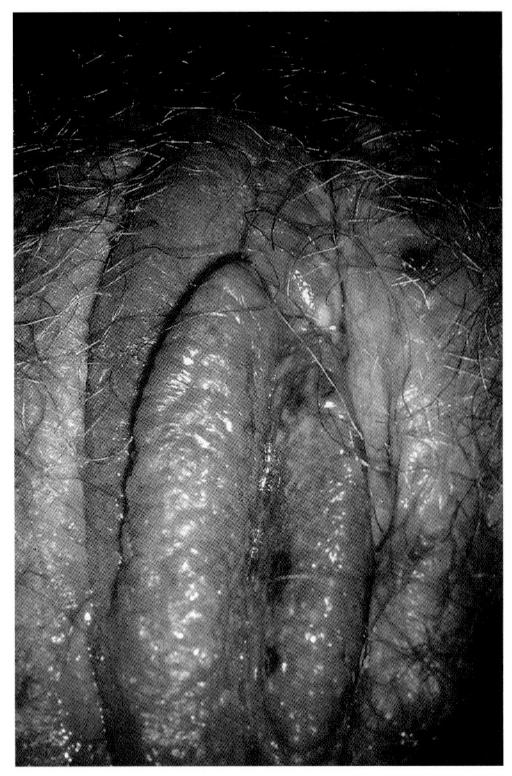

Fig. 7.**31** Primary genital herpes (HSV-1) in a 21-year-old patient with severe swelling of the labia minora.

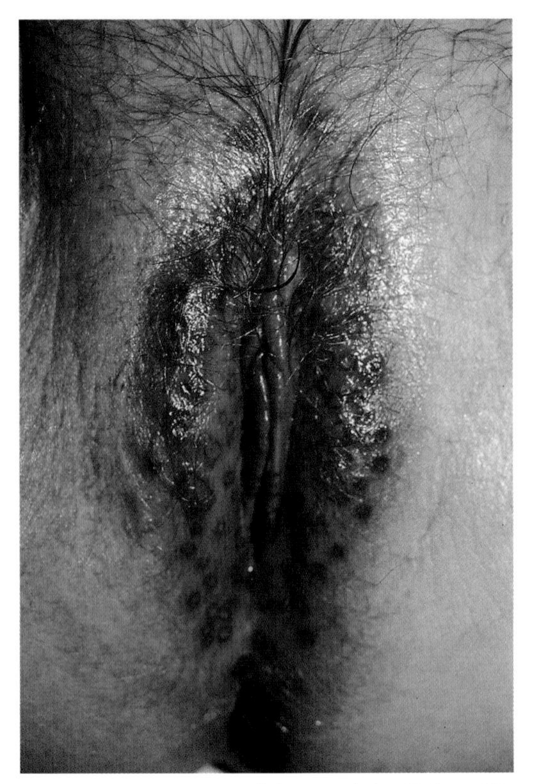

Fig. 7.**32** Primary genital herpes (HSV-2) in a 25-year-old patient.

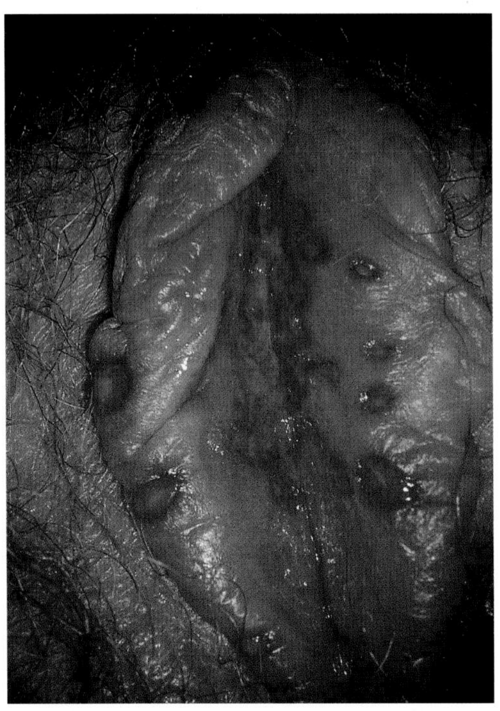

Fig. 7.**33** Primary genital herpes in a 20-year-old patient after eight days of infection. Severe pain, dysuria, and swollen inguinal lymph nodes; no antibodies to herpesviruses, but isolation of HSV-2.

Some of the patients have systemic symptoms like fever, headaches, malaise, or pain in the muscles and lower back.

In patients who already have HSV-1 antibodies, usually due to an oral herpes infection suffered during childhood, local symptoms are less pronounced (Fig. 7.**38**) and systemic symptoms appear less frequently.

About 50% of primary genital herpes infections are not diagnosed during the first visit to the doctor because, initially, there is only burning and pain, while vesicles or eruptions are not yet visible at this early stage. Occasionally, the early stage is confused with candidiasis (fungal infection; see Figs. 7.**5**, 7.**6**, p. 71).

The vagina (see Fig. 7.**101**, p. 115) and the vaginal part of the cervix (portio vaginalis) (see Figs. 7.**143**–7.**146**, p. 141) may be affected in addition to the vulva. Because of the tenderness of the sensitive vulvar region, using the speculum may initially not be an option if the lesions are severe. Extensive primary genital herpes in the vulvar region of a child is rare (Fig. 7.**39**) and only possible through smear infection from mother to child, or through sexual abuse.

Voiding problems in the context of primary genital herpes may be explained by the presence of herpes vesicles in the urethra.

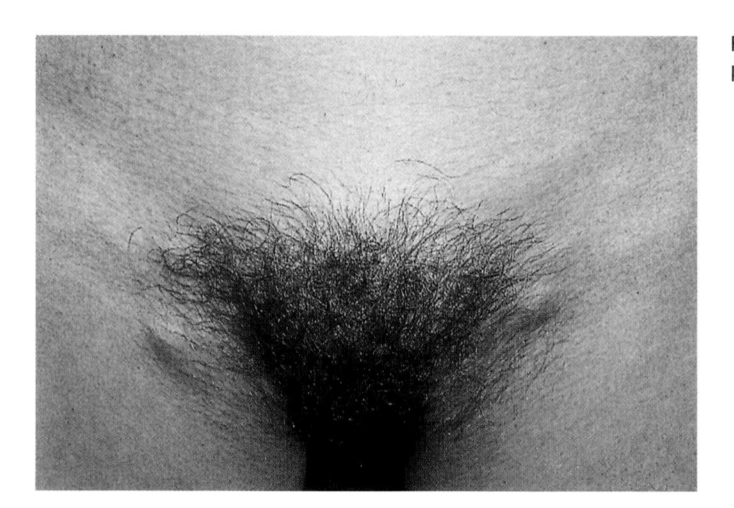

Fig. 7.**34** Swelling of the inguinal lymph nodes in a patient with primary genital herpes.

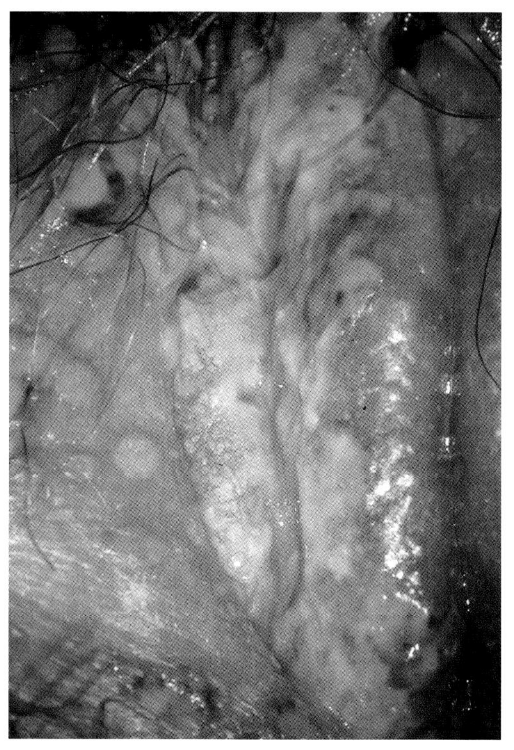

Fig. 7.**35** Primary genital herpes (HSV-1) in a 20-year-old patient with opaque vesicles (pustules).

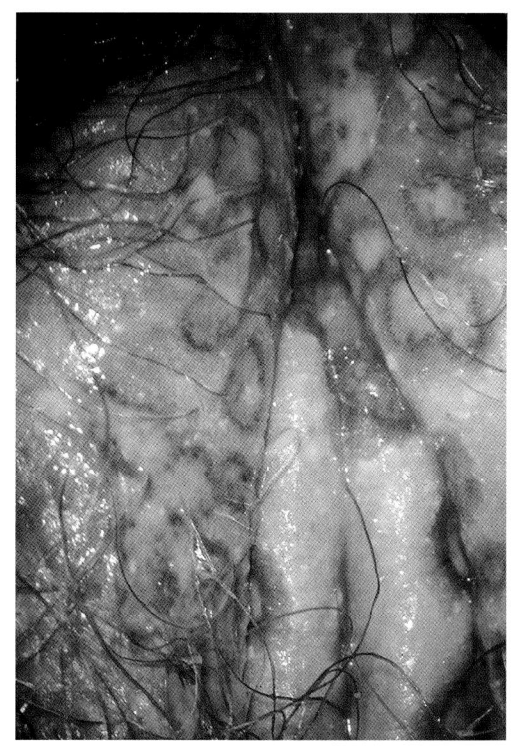

Fig. 7.**36** The same patient as in Fig. 7.**35**, showing confluence of lesions four days later.

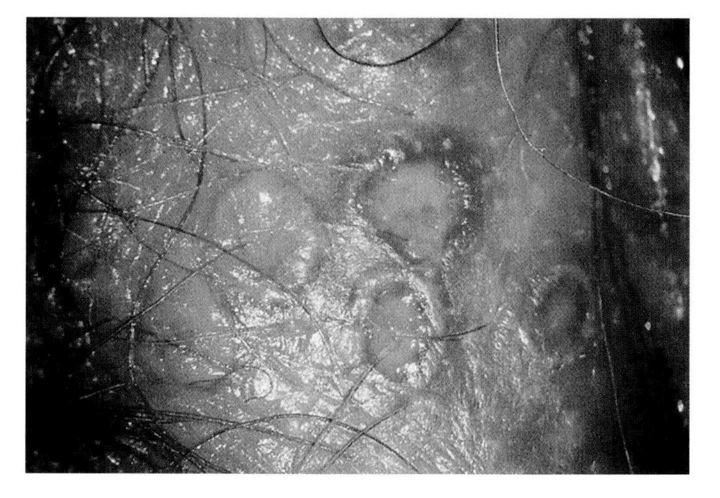

Fig. 7.**37** Primary genital herpes of the vulva in a 42-year-old patient. The course of infection was quick and of medium severity; flat ulcers (greatly enlarged) already present after six days.

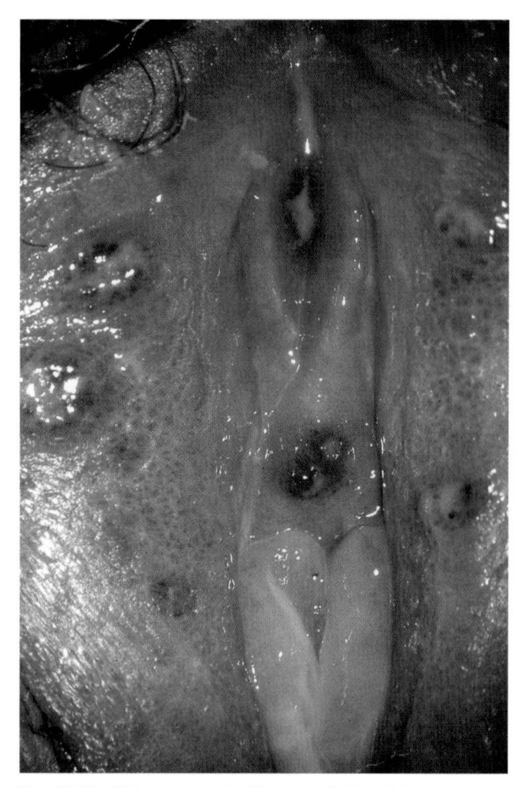

Fig. 7.**38** Primary genital herpes (HSV-2) in a patient with partial immunity due to HSV-1.

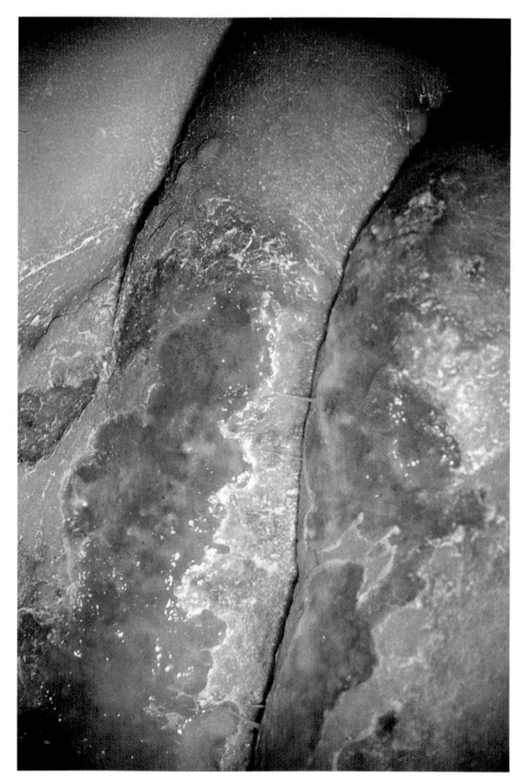

Fig. 7.**39** Primary genital herpes in a six-month-old girl, infected by the mother through oral contact.

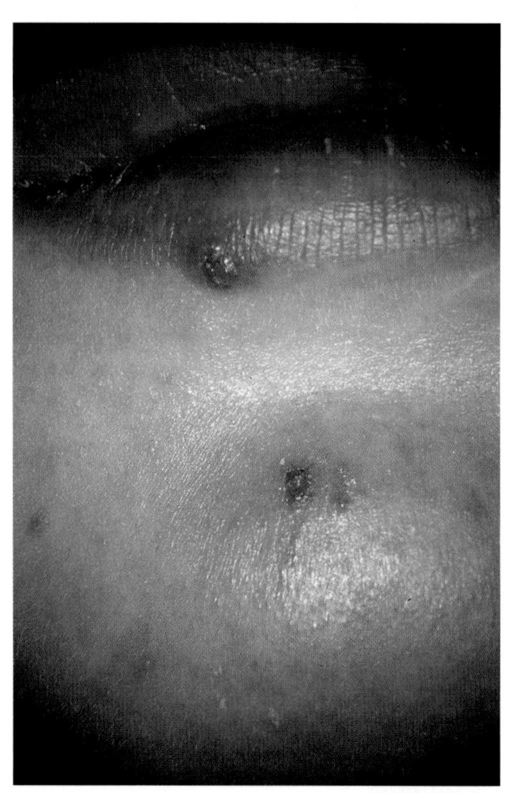

Fig. 7.**40** Discrete lesions of herpes labialis in the presence of pronounced primary genital herpes (HSV-1).

Note. Lesions in the mouth or on the face (Fig. 7.**40**) may occur during primary infection with HSV-1 in the genital region. Because these lesions cause little pain, they usually do not attract much attention and are not recognized as such. Meanwhile, we have repeatedly observed that it was possible to culture the identified virus from both regions.

Diagnosis. Extensive laboratory tests are not required in case of a typical clinical picture and sufficient experience. However, tests are essential in questionable cases and with insufficient clinical experience.

Detection of the pathogen from vesicles or erosions/ulcers is the most reliable means of establishing the diagnosis:

- *Culture and typing.* Up to now, this is the detection method of choice because herpesviruses can be easily and quickly grown in cell cultures. If plenty of virus particles are present, the cell culture will be positive after 24 hours. If there are only a few virus particles, the cytopathic effect in the cell culture will take several days to occur. Confirmation of the diagnosis and determination of the virus type is done by subsequent fluorescence microscopy using type-specific immune sera.

- *Direct antigen test.* An immunofluorescence test for the detection of HSV is available. For this purpose, a swab taken from the base of the vesicle or ulcus is rolled onto a microscopic slide and then fixed with acetone or ethanol. This method has the advantage that cell cultures are not required and transport problems thus do not play a role since the sample is permanently preserved. However, the sensitivity of this test is only 80–95 % as compared with cell cultures. There are also enzyme tests available, which are slightly less sensitive.
- *Molecular biology methods using DNA.* The detection of viral DNA by means of hybridization is about as sensitive as the antigen test. DNA amplification tests (PCR) will be the method of the future. So far, these tests are used if herpes simplex encephalitis is suspected. For routine diagnosis, this method has not yet been established in practice.
- *Serology.* The detection of antibodies in the blood is neither suitable for diagnosis of primary genital herpes nor for recurrent genital herpes. It is, however, useful for determining the immune status or for distinguishing between primary infection and a relapse. In case of genital herpes relapse, IgM antibodies can be detected in the minority of patients; hence, serology is not very helpful. Up to now, many of the commercially available serological tests for distinguishing antibodies against HSV-1 and HSV-2 have not been meeting expectations.

Therapy. Early systemic administration of antiviral substances is crucial. Treatment for at least five days is recommended. In individual patients, the dose will need to be increased and the duration of treatment prolonged as well.

In case of severe pain, additional administration of 100 mg diclofenac for the first one to three days once or twice per day is indicated. Topical application of anaesthetic ointments in the periurethral region one to two hours prior to voiding may facilitate passing urine.

- *Aciclovir* (5 × 200 mg orally for at least five days) inhibits the multiplication of viruses (p. 46); when given early, pain will be alleviated relatively quickly (two to three days), which shows that the treatment is successful.
- *Valaciclovir* (orally 2 × 500 mg), the valine ester of aciclovir. After oral uptake, it is transformed quickly and almost completely to aciclovir and L-valine by valaciclovir hydrolase in the intestine and liver. This significantly improves the bioavailability of valaciclovir (54 %) as compared with aciclovir.
- *Famciclovir* (3 × 250 mg orally for at least five days).

Differential diagnosis:

- candidiasis (confusion is only possible at an early stage, Fig. 7.**6**, p. 71)
- folliculitis (*S. aureus*, see Fig. 7.**15**, p. 77)
- plasma cell vulvitis (see Fig. 7.**56**, p. 93)
- skin lesion (see Fig. 7.**94**, p. 111)
- toxic reaction (see Fig. 7.**91**, p. 110)
- irritable dermatitis (see Fig. 7.**90**, p. 110)
- Behçet syndrome (see Figs. 7.**85**, 7.**86**, p. 108).

Recurrent Genital Herpes

Pathogens:

- herpes simplex virus type 2 (HSV-2), 80–90 % of patients
- herpes simplex virus type 1 (HSV-1), 10–20 % of patients.

Transmission. Recurrent genital herpes is not an exogenous infection but the endogenous reactivation of the virus and thus occurs independently of sexual contact.

Clinical picture. About 85 % of patients with primary genital herpes will experience a symptomatic relapse. Characteristic are circumscribed groups of vesicles (Fig. 7.**41**), pustules and lesions (Figs. 7.**42**–7.**44**), or crusts (Fig. 7.**45**). Generalized symptoms occur less often than with the primary infection. This also applies to the swelling of regional lymph nodes and neuralgic symptoms. Relapse frequencies vary; depending on the HSV type, there may be 12 and more relapses per year, with HSV-2-induced relapses being more frequent than those induced by HSV-1.

The location of recurrent genital herpes symptoms may change from superior to inferior locations and from the front to the back (e. g., to the buttocks, Fig. 7.**46**), whereas the affected side of the body remains the same in most patients.

Deep lesions expanding over larger areas due to recurrent genital herpes occur only in the presence of immune suppression (Figs. 7.**47**, 7.**48**). In such patients, diagnosis is considerably hampered and can be established only by means of laboratory tests (detection of the virus and simultaneous detection of species-specific antibodies).

In contrast to the primary manifestation, herpes relapses in the genital region are preceded by prodromal symptoms, such as hyperesthesia, neuralgiform pain, and malaise. It is especially the recurrent herpes that causes serious emotional, sexual, and psychosocial conflicts within an existing partnership.

Fig. 7.**41** Recurrent genital herpes in a 19-year-old patient with fresh cluster of vesicles.

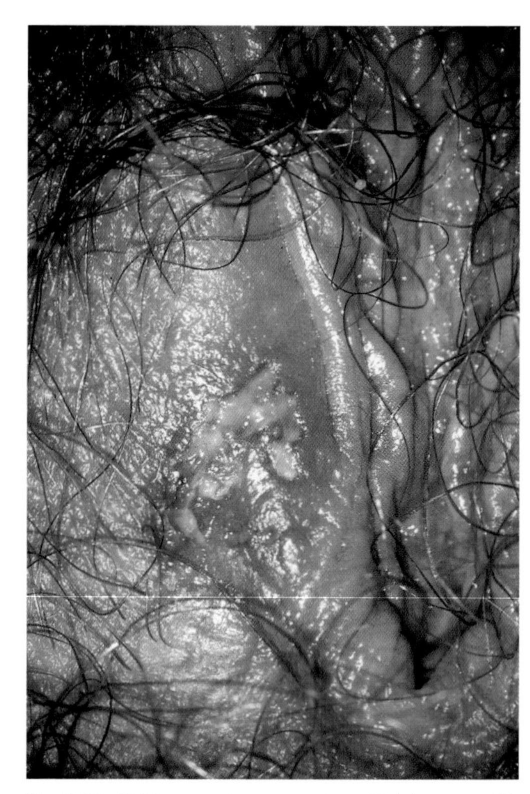

Fig. 7.**42** Widespread recurrent genital herpes with lesions turning opaque (pustules) and small vesicles.

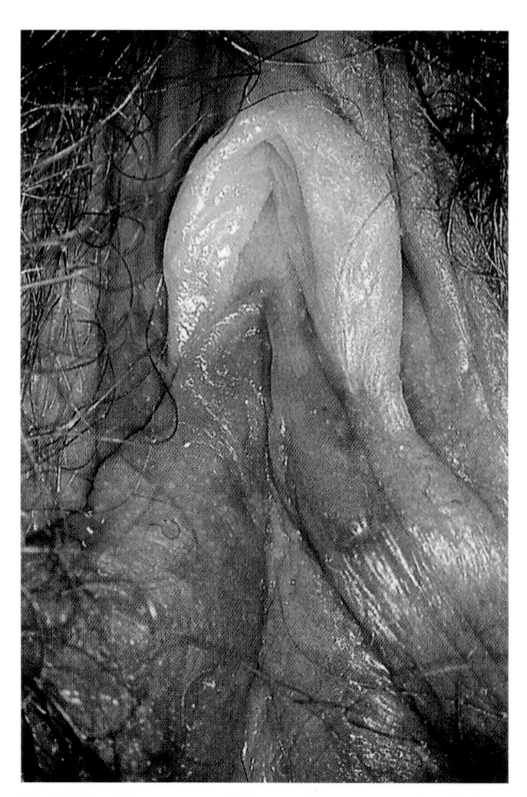

Fig. 7.**43** Discrete vesicles and tiny pustules below the clitoris on the left.

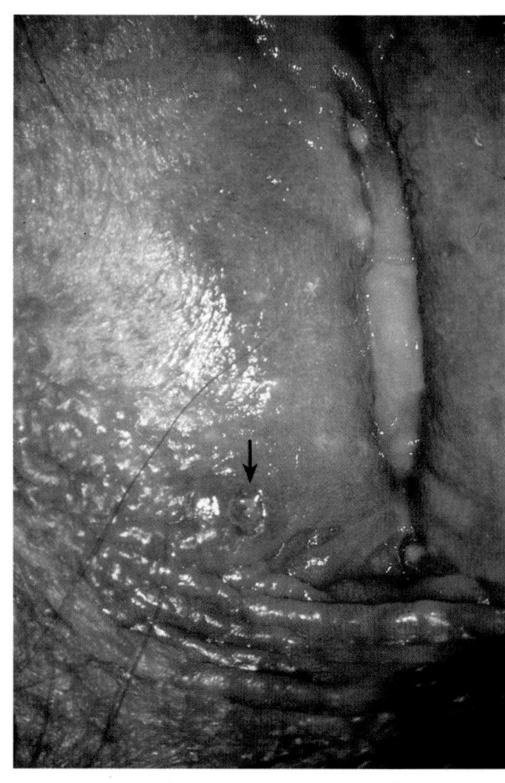

Fig. 7.**44** Very discrete recurrent genital herpes in a 32-year-old patient.

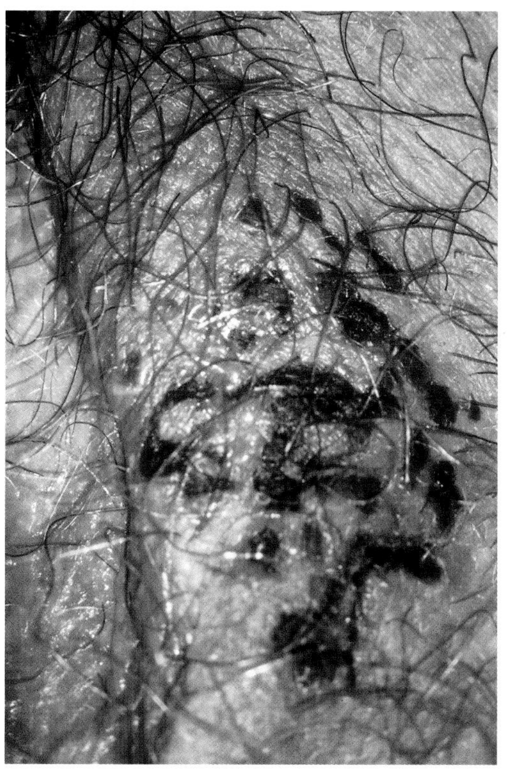

Fig. 7.**45** Widespread recurrent genital herpes at the crust stage in a 37-year-old patient.

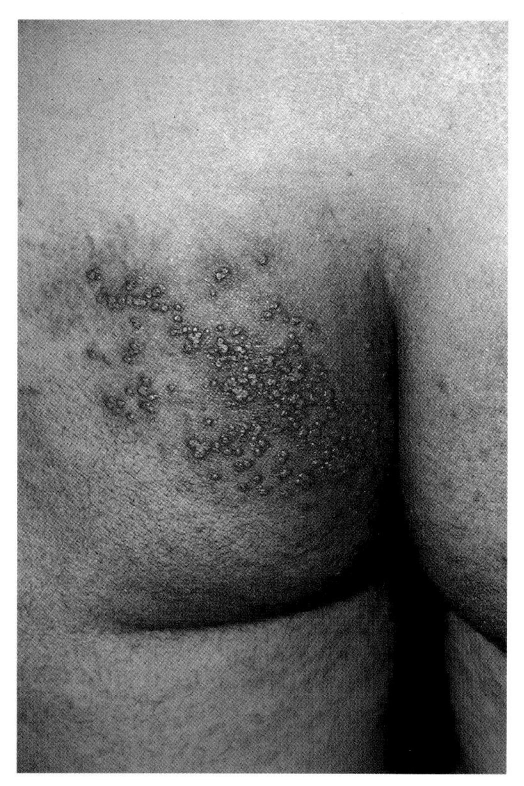

Fig. 7.**46** Unusually widespread recurrent herpes glutealis in a 33-year-old patient.

Herpes is often confused with recurrent cystitis, particularly when the urethral orifice is affected (Fig. 7.**49**).

Figure 7.**49** shows urethral herpes in a patient who has been repeatedly treated with antibiotics against cystitis for 10 years. Occasionally, when the bacteriological culture from the urine was negative, her complaints were brushed aside as being psychosomatic. The virus culture revealed HSV-2. Immediate intake of aciclovir tablets has to a great extent freed this patient from her burden.

Foci of herpes may also be present in the vagina (Fig. 7.**101**, p. 115) and on the portio vaginalis (Figs. 7.**143**–7.**148**, pp. 141–142). Due to the low sensitivity of these areas, herpes infections that occur only here are detected only by chance. There may be occasional heavy discharge, at the most, and herpes will only be identified as its cause if the vagina is thoroughly examined and the corresponding detection procedures are employed.

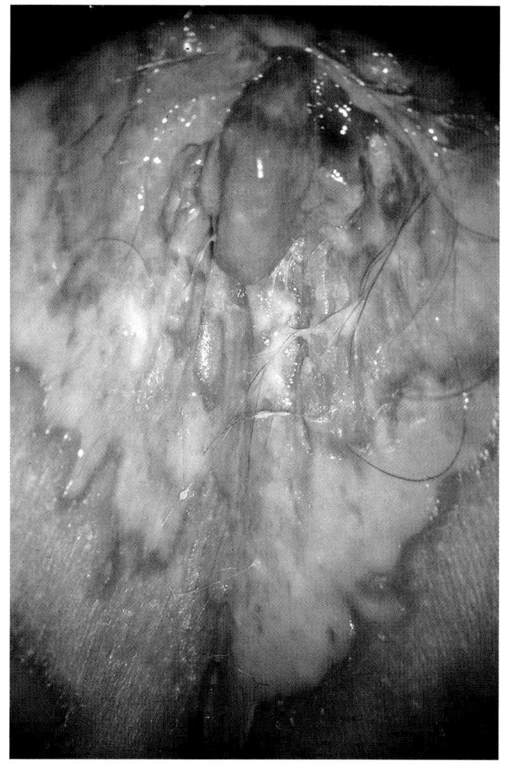

Fig. 7.**47** Florid recurrent genital herpes in a 48-year-old patient with hemolytic uremic syndrome after kidney transplantation.

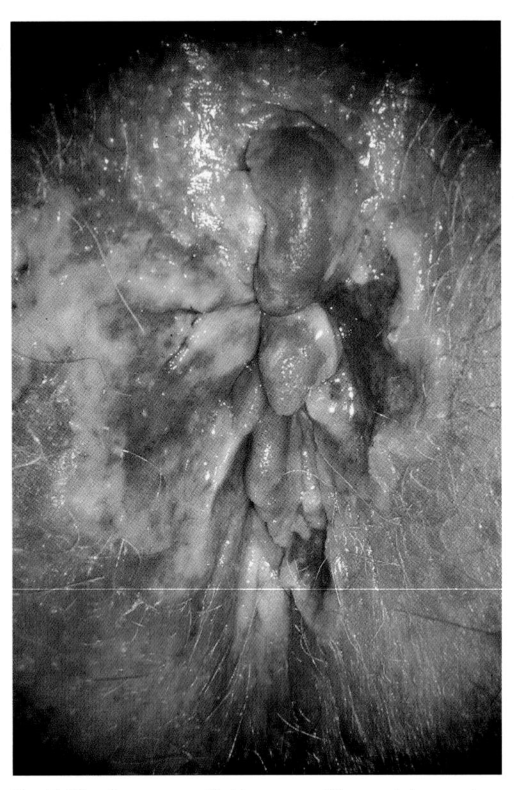

Fig. 7.**48** Severe genital herpes with condylomas in a 21-year-old patient in the terminal stage of AIDS.

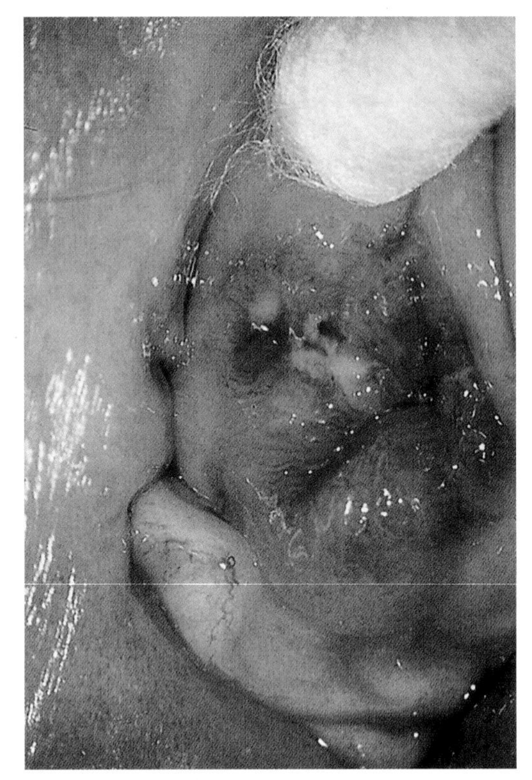

Fig. 7.**49** Recurrent herpes of the external orifice of the urethra in a 45-year-old patient treated for recurrent cystitis for 10 years.

Diagnosis:

- *Medical history of the patient.* Repeated appearance of the symptoms.
- *Clinical picture.* Groups of vesicles, erosions/lesions, crusts.
- *Detection of pathogen.* By means of culture, or by the immunofluorescence test in questionable cases.
- *Serology* hardly plays a role in cases of recurrent herpes because a relapse rarely induces a measurable rise in titer. Serology may be helpful in distinguishing between primary and recurrent herpes and, above all, in determining the patient's immune status in cases of uncertain diagnosis and negative virus detection (exclusion of infection).

Therapy. Treatment with aciclovir is only appropriate during the early phase when the virus is multiplying. At the stage of erosions/lesions and at the crust stage, the treatment cannot be expected to be successful. Because the disease is restricted to certain locations, topical treatment is an option. However, penetration of aciclovir is not satisfactory; foscarnet is slightly more effective.

Oral administration of aciclovir is more effective, for example, 5 × 200 mg per day. In many patients, taking this dose for one to two days is sufficient to stop the spreading of herpes.

In case of frequently recurring genital herpes, continuous medication with aciclovir (suppression therapy) may prevent a relapse for as long as the drug is taken. The required dose varies from patient to patient and should be determined for each patient by slow reduction in the number of tablets. If genital herpes reoccurs regularly—for example, during the period—short-term prophylactic administration of the drug may be indicated at that time.

Special risks:

- risk of infecting the sexual partner
- risk of transmitting the disease to the newborn during childbirth (p. 179).

Differential diagnosis (Table 7.**3**)

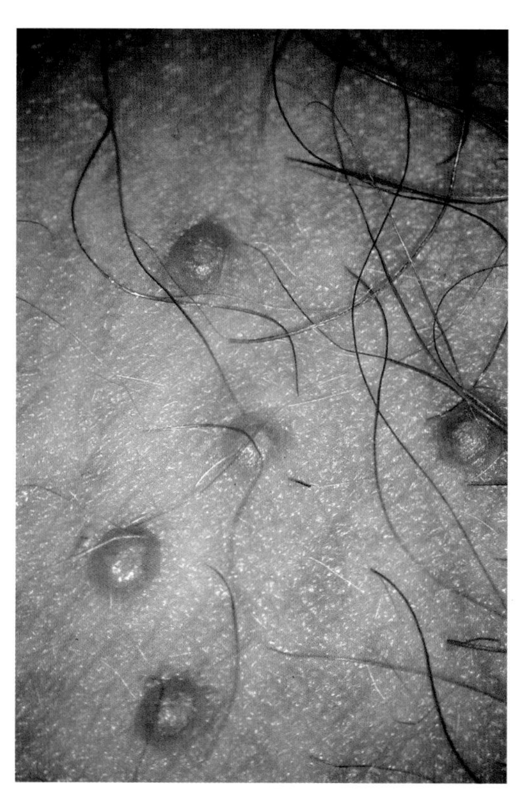

Fig. 7.**50** Molluscum contagiosum of the vulva in a 23-year-old patient.

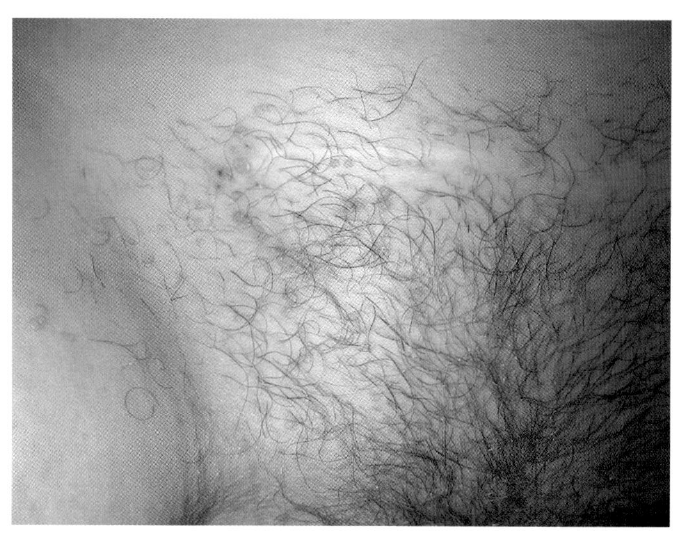

Fig. 7.**51** Molluscum contagiosum in the region of the mons pubis, with mild inflammation due to scratching.

Table 7.**3** Genital herpes: differential diagnosis

Vulvitis pustulosa caused by *Candida albicans* (Figs.7.**4**–7.**6**, pp. 70–71), staphyloderma
Behçet syndrome (Figs. 7.**86**, 7.**87**, pp. 108–109)
Trichomoniasis (Figs. 7.**105**, 7.**106**, pp. 117–118)
Injuries during intercourse, scratching because of itching
Plasma cell vulvitis (Fig. 7.**56**, S. 93)
Varicella or herpes zoster (Fig. 7.**52**, p. 92)
Pemphigus vulgaris, bullous pemphigoid (Fig. 8.**10**, p. 182)
Herpes gestationis (Fig. 8.**9**, p. 181)
Molluscum contagiosum (Fig. 7.**50**, p. 91)
Syphilis (primary lesion, Fig. 7.**72**, p. 101)
Urethritis
Proctitis
Contact dermatitis

Molluscum Contagiosum

Pathogen. Molluscum contagiosum virus.

This infection causes skin lesions consisting of individual small nodules (1–10 mm in diameter). These molluscum bodies are smooth, soft, and waxy and have a depression in their center (Fig. 7.**50**). They are benign tumors caused by a poxvirus. Children are affected more frequently than adults. Transmission occurs through close skin contact, hence, often during sexual intercourse. Occasionally, molluscum bodies become inflamed due to scratching and then cause diagnostic problems (Fig. 7.**51**). Treatment consists of mechanical removal of the nodules, preferably by means of curettage (Stiefel disposable ring curette), but it is also possible by means of electrocoagulation or laser.

Herpes Zoster of the Vulva

Pathogen. Varicella–zoster virus.

This rare disease is easy to diagnose because the vesicles and nodules are restricted to one side of the vulva and to one segment (Fig. 7.**52**). In comparison to genital herpes, the vesicles persist for many days and weeks without therapy (Fig. 7.**53**). High doses of aciclovir (tablets, 5 × 800 mg per day) bring quick relief (see also varicella, p. 184).

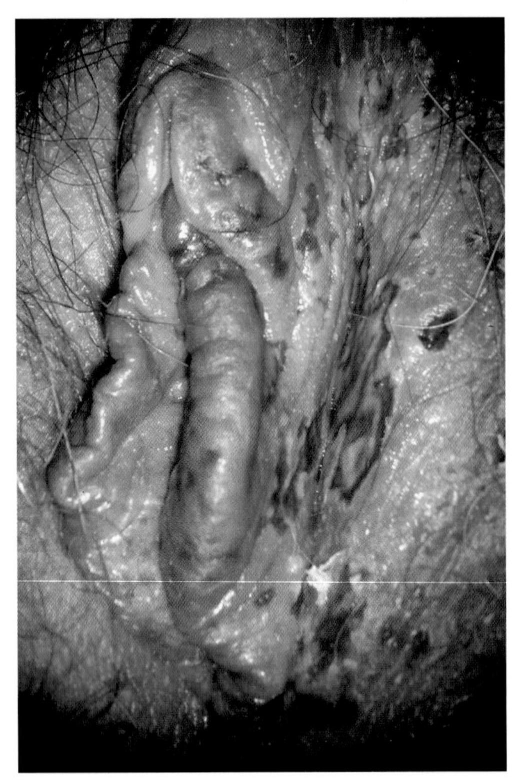

Fig. 7.**52** Herpes zoster of the left vulva in a 64-year-old patient.

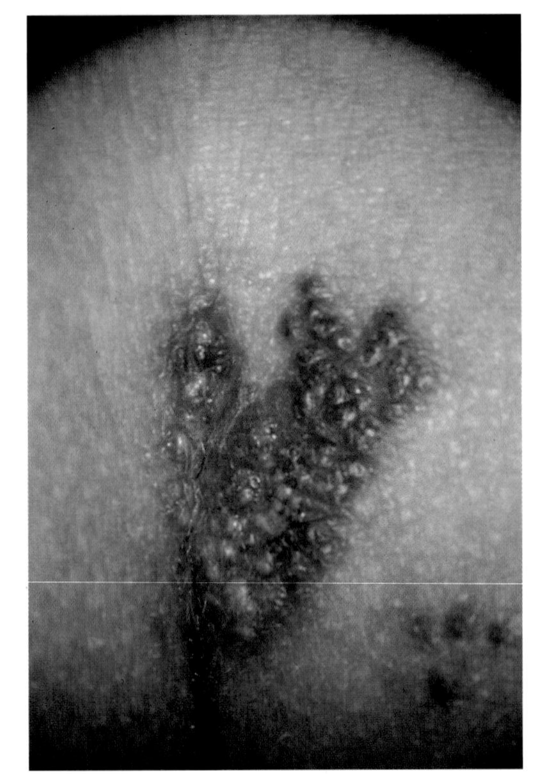

Fig. 7.**53** Herpes zoster reaching from the buttocks to the vulva in a 51-year-old patient with stable vesicles (pustules) for the last 10 days.

Other Forms of Vulvitis

Vestibular Adenitis/Vestibulitis

Pathogen. Unknown.

Clinical picture. This disease occurs especially in young women suffering from dyspareunia. They complain of point tenderness on both sides of the vaginal orifice. Examination reveals an uneven redness around the duct of Bartholin gland (Figs. 7.**54**, 7.**55**). Application of 3% acetic acid sometimes reveals white areas that resemble papillae when viewed with the colposcope, similar to the transformation zone on the portio vaginalis.

This clinical picture probably does not represent an infection or inflammation but is rather because the extremely thin and delicate epithelium in the area around the glandular ducts is sensitive to touch and responds with pain (dyspareunia). An additional inflammatory or infectious component may exist only in rare cases.

Therapy. Treatment attempts to strengthen the delicate epithelium through:

- epithelial denaturation using albothyl (policresolene)
- estrogens (topical application)
- skin care with ointments containing lavender oil.

Plasma Cell Vulvitis (Zoon Vulvitis)

Clinical picture. Painful punctate hemorrhages (Fig. 7.**56**) associated with severe leukorrheal discharge (> 100 leukocytes per field of view at 400× magnification).

Pathogen. Unknown.

Pathogenesis and diagnosis. In contrast to vestibular adenitis, plasma cell vulvitis is an inflammation caused by infection. The pathogen is not yet known. Nevertheless, it is most likely an infection because this type of vulvitis can be cured with an antibiotic (clindamycin, topical or oral application) in more than 90% of patients. So far, all attempts at demonstrating a pathogen through culture or staining methods have been unsuccessful.

Plasma cell vulvitis is the rare vulvar form of plasma cell vaginitis (purulent vaginitis). Patients complain of burning pain because the sensitive vulvar region is affected. Clinically, it can be dis-

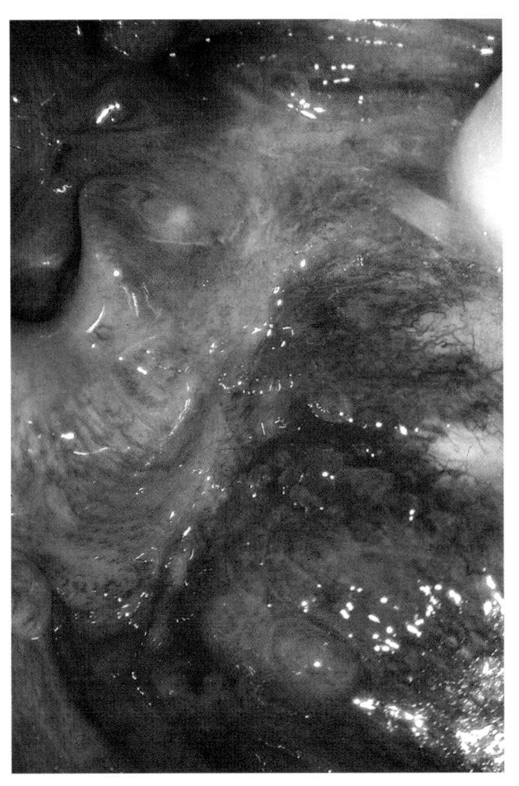

Fig. 7.**54** Vestibulitis in a 25-year-old patient with dyspareunia.

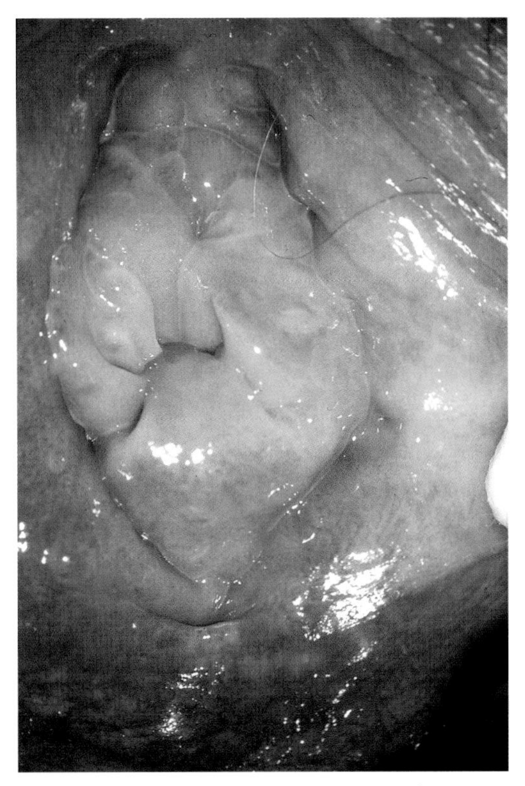

Fig. 7.**55** The same patient as in Fig. 7.**54**, three years later: free of symptoms and with a normal vulva.

tinguished from erosive lichen planus based on the punctate hemorrhage and leukorrheal discharge (see p. 119, plasma cell vaginitis).

Therapy. Topical treatment with clindamycin vaginal cream, two to three times daily for two to three weeks. In case the topical treatment fails—the cream does not stay on the skin long enough—oral treatment may be indicated: clindamycin tablets, 4 × 300 mg per day for two weeks.

Relapses do occur, unfortunately. Hence, a follow-up immediately after the treatment is recommended as only a cure will confirm the diagnosis.

Vulvar Infections without Pain

Pathogen and occurrence. Erythrasma is a bacterial infection of the skin surface (stratum corneum) caused by *Corynebacterium minutissimum.* It is predominantly found in older persons.

Pathogenesis and clinical picture. Onset of the infection is promoted by a warm and humid milieu; in women, this infection is therefore found between the labia majora and the thighs

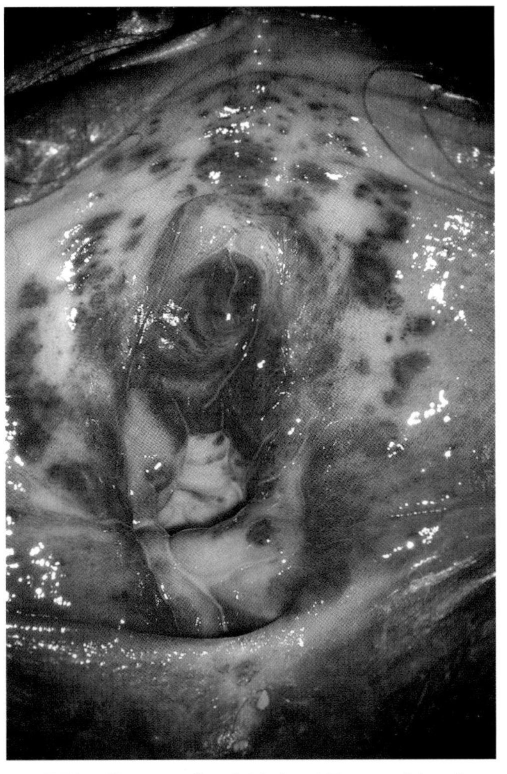

Fig. 7.**56** Plasma cell vulvitis in a 57-year-old patient.

Fig. 7.**57** Erythrasma of the vulva in a 54-year-old patient.

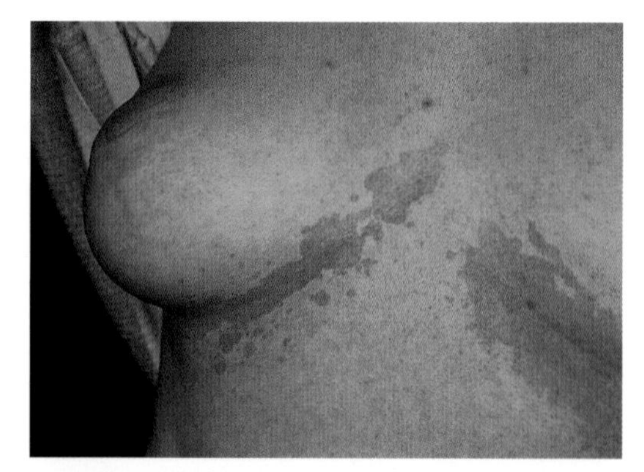

Fig. 7.**58** Submammillary erythrasma in a 36-year-old patient.

(Fig. 7.**57**). The submammary folds (Fig. 7.**58**) or the axillae are less often affected. The infection is further promoted by obesity and diabetes.

The formation of porphyrin by corynebacteria leads to a red–brown, macular skin lesion at the affected site. Usually, there are no subjective complaints.

Diagnosis:

- ▶ clinically typical sites and limited expansion of red–brown spots without scaling
- ▶ examination under Wood light (UV light) results in brick-red fluorescence
- ▶ detection of corynebacteria (this test is rarely performed and also not essential).

Therapy. Topical treatment with imidazole derivatives, such as clotrimazole, miconazole, or econazole.

Differential diagnosis. Tinea inguinalis (infection by dermatophytes), candidiasis (*C. albicans*), psoriasis vulgaris, eczema.

Infections Caused by Human Papillomaviruses (HPV)

Condylomas, Acuminate Condylomas (Genital Warts)

Here, we have to distinguish between the moderately common genital warts (acuminate condylomas) and the much more frequently occurring subclinical HPV infection that probably affects more than 50 % of all adults. Detection of the virus depends on many factors, such as the method, the patient's age, and the collection of samples.

This viral infection is particularly important because certain genotypes are involved in the development of cervical carcinoma and other anogenital carcinomas. Hardly any other infection has given rise to so many publications during recent years. Activities have already advanced to a point at which it is considered that cytological screening for prevention should be replaced by virus screening for high-risk HPV types. However, it has also become evident that only very few persons infected with a high-risk type actually develop a genital carcinoma. Though HPV is an important prerequisite for carcinoma development, additional endogenous factors (immunosuppression, genetic disposition, HLA status) as well as exogenous factors (additional infections, e. g., HIV and chlamydiae, or smoking) also play a role.

Pathogen. Papillomaviruses are small, stable DNA viruses of about 8000 base pairs. So far, they cannot be propagated in tissue culture; they can only be classified into different genotypes by means of DNA analysis. Over 150 genotypes are known today, and about 30 of these have been detected in the genital region. They are now divided into low-risk types—such as HPV-6, which is detected exclusively in benign acuminate condylomas—and high-risk types. The high-risk types have been detected with increasingly sensitive methods in over 95 % of cervical carcinomas.

The most important high-risk types are HPV-16 and HPV-18, which are found in two thirds of all cervical malignancies.

- ▶ Low-risk types (LR types): types 6 and 11 are found almost exclusively in acuminate condylomas.
- ▶ High-risk types (HR types): types 16 and 18 (the most common ones), types 31, 33, 39, 45, 59, and others.
- ▶ HPV-1 and HPV-2 are the pathogens of warts on hands and feet (verruca vulgaris).

Double or multiple infections with various types do occur.

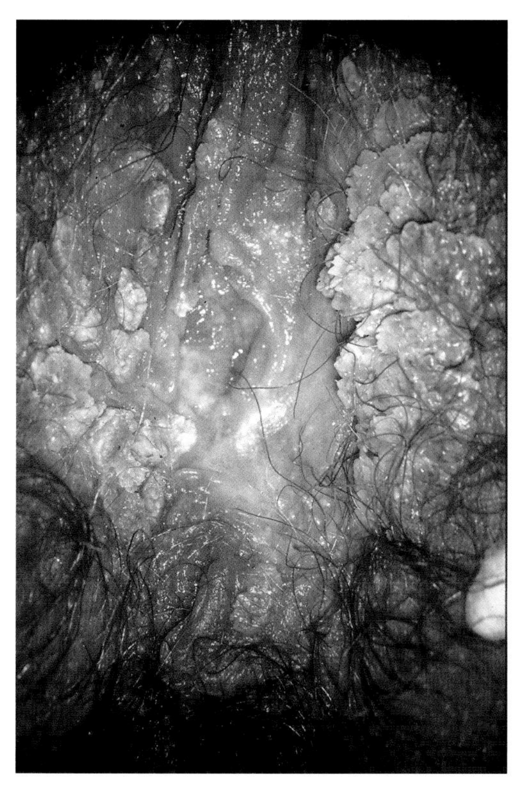

Fig. 7.**59** Acuminate condylomas in a 27-year-old patient.

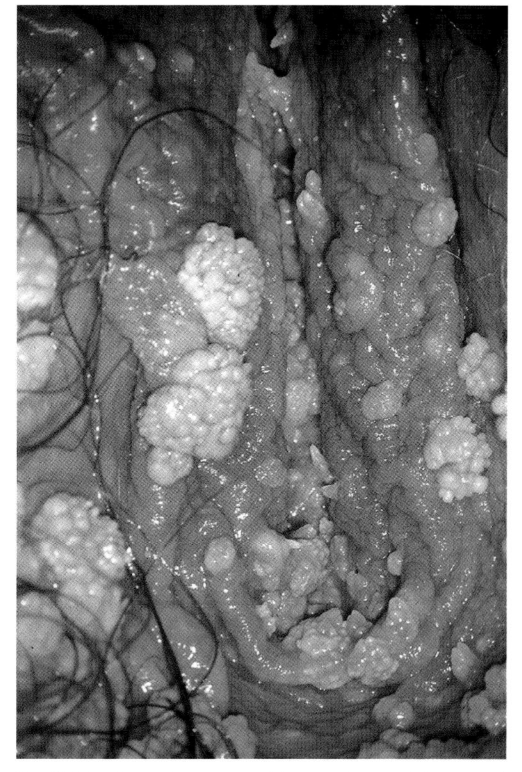

Fig. 7.**60** Acuminate condylomas in a 20-year-old patient.

Frequency:

- *Condylomas.* At least 1 % of young, sexually active persons have acuminate condylomas. During pregnancy, visible condylomas are slightly more common due to mild immunosuppression.
- *HPV infection.* The rate of genital infection with human papillomaviruses in adults is high, though the data vary considerably. Depending on the method and the examiner, values range between 20 % and 80 %.
- *High-risk types.* They have been detected in about 5 % of women over age 30, in about 50 % of women with cervical intraepithelial neoplasia of stage I (CIN I), in about 75 % of those with CIN II, in 95 % of those with CIN III, and in 98 % of women with cervical carcinoma.
- *HPV-specific DNA.* DNA of HPV-16 has been detected in about 50 % of cervical carcinomas, the DNA of HPV-18 in 14 %, and in the rest 20 other types of HPV.

Transmission. Papillomaviruses are mainly transmitted through sexual contact. Due to their resistance to environmental influences, however, they may also be picked up through smear infection and indirect contact through objects. Determining the precise time of transmission is usually not possible because of the slow growth of any visible changes in the skin. Penetration of the pathogen is probably promoted by small skin lesions. Secondary infections may promote the development of condylomas.

Clinical picture. Condylomas do not cause any complaints. Any itching or burning described in the past as being associated with them may be explained today by other infections or skin lesions. At the most, condylomas are disturbing and are rather a nuisance because of their appearance and their size. The virus usually infects large areas.

The clinical picture varies greatly, ranging from individual tiny warts, numerous small acuminate condylomas (Fig. 7.**59**), medium-sized cauliflower-like (Fig. 7.**60**) and fairly large, partly pigmented condylomas (Fig. 7.**61**) to extreme manifestation during pregnancy (Fig. 7.**62**).

The absence of any visible condylomas does not exclude HPV infection (Fig. 7.**63**). Swabbing the vulva with 3 % acetic acid reveals also subclinical HPV infections as white areas with continuous dotting (Fig. 7.**64**). The body can presumably no longer eliminate all papillomaviruses from the genital region. However, the number of virus particles may be reduced to such an extent that they can only be detected with increasingly

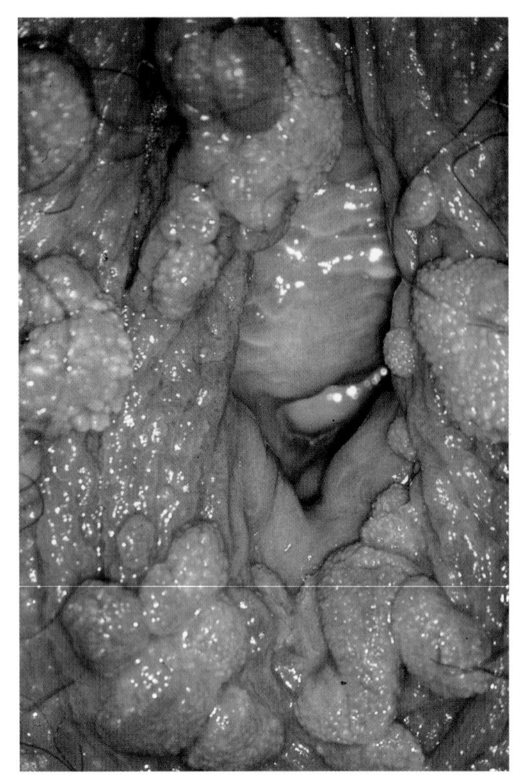

Fig. 7.**61** Large, fairly old condylomas in a 30-year-old patient.

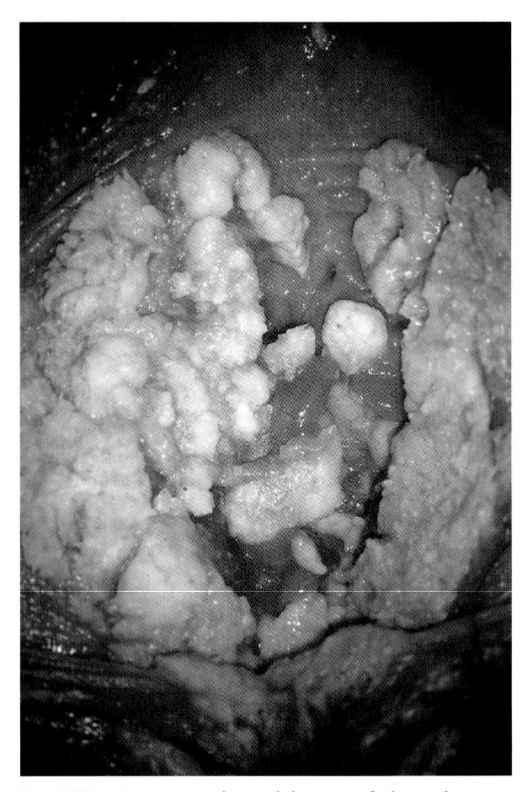

Fig. 7.**62** Pronounced condylomas of the vulva in a 21-year-old patient during the 29 th week of pregnancy.

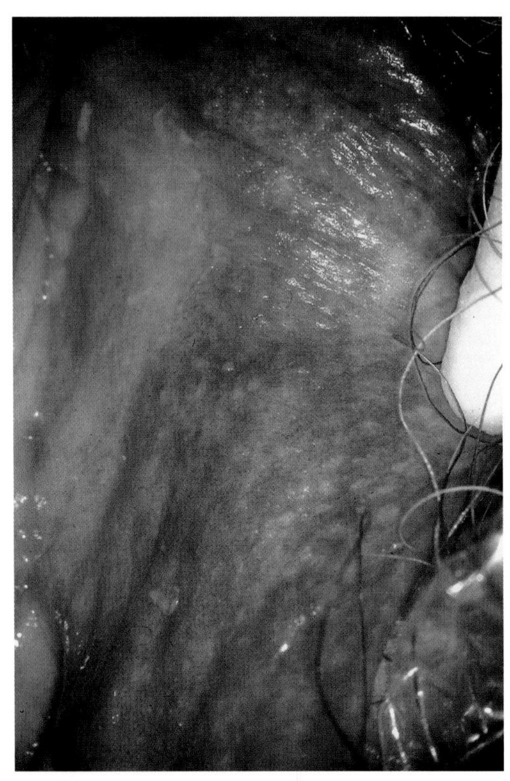

Fig. 7.**63** Subclinical HPV infection in a 45-year-old patient.

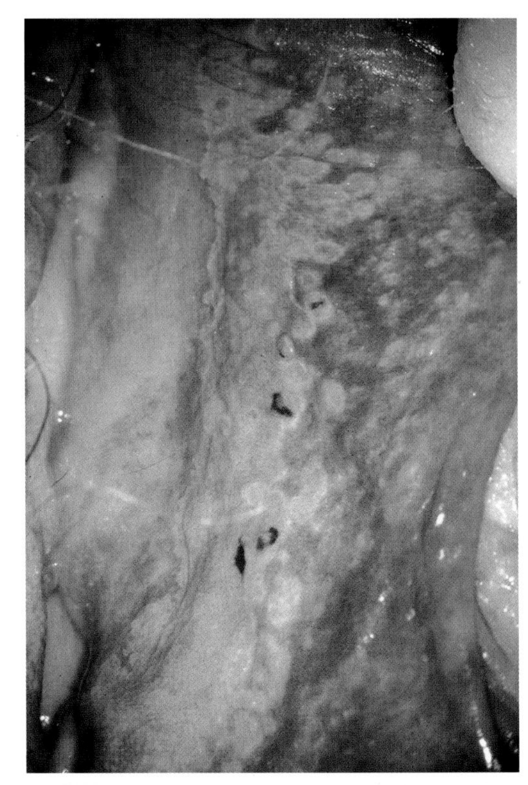

Fig. 7.**64** The same patient as in Fig. 7.**63**. Application of acetic acid revealed white spots with discrete dotting.

sensitive tests—or not at all. This view is supported by the fact that immunodeficiency promotes the appearance of extensive, often very large condylomas that are difficult to remove.

A preferred site for condylomas is the posterior labial commissure, probably because it is subjected to severe mechanical stress. Infection of the perianal region is not necessarily the result of anal intercourse. Here, again, it is more likely the severe mechanical stress during cleaning that causes epithelial lesions and thus promotes penetration of the virus. The risk of transmission can possibly be reduced by following the recommendations for improved skin care with ointments containing lavender oil.

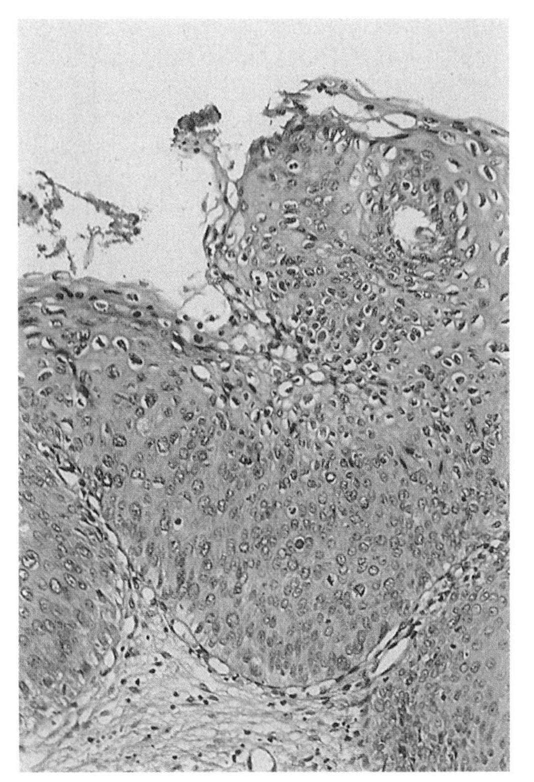

Fig. 7.**65** Histological preparation of a biopsy from the posterior lip of the uterine orifice. The hematoxylin-eosin stained cross-section clearly shows koilocytosis, a sign of papillomavirus infection. Virus typing revealed HPV 18. (Micrograph courtesy of Prof. Dr. Schäfer, Department of Pathology, University of Freiburg, Germany).

Papillomaviruses and Cervical Carcinoma

In the 1970s, zur Hausen postulated that human papillomaviruses might cause cervical carcinoma, and in 1983, HPV-16 was isolated and cloned for the first time from a cervical carcinoma. This triggered a rapid development in tumor virus research. It was soon recognized that the early proteins E6 and E7 of both HPV-16 and HPV-18 are, in fact, tumor promoters and are required for maintaining continued cell division that is so characteristic of tumor growth. Similar proteins with oncogenic properties are produced by other DNA viruses, for example, SV40 and adenoviruses. They are essential for stimulating cell division, for it is only then that the viral DNA replicates together with the cellular DNA.

In normal cells infected with HPV, the viral proteins E6 and E7 are initially synthesized but are then down-regulated by viral control genes as soon as virus particles assemble.

In all HPV-positive cervical carcinoma cell lines studied so far (e. g., HeLa cells), DNA fragments of HPV-16 or HPV-18 have been found integrated in the cellular genome. These fragments always contain the *E6* and *E7* genes but not the viral control genes mentioned above. The site of integration in the cellular genome is at random.

Tumor Development Due to High-risk Types of HPV

Only in 10–30% of women infected with HPV-16 does the infection persist (i. e., the viral DNA can still be detected). Expression of the viral oncogenes *E6* and *E7* increases only in some of the chronically infected women. This causes the cells to enter S phase and subsequently undergo uncontrolled divisions; simultaneously, the cells accumulate changes in the DNA because the p53-dependent systems of DNA repair and apoptosis are inactivated by E6 and E7. In addition, irregular cell divisions may occur because the mitotic spindle apparatus is disturbed. In a few cells, viral DNA fragments are integrated into the cellular genome. This, in turn, causes a deficit in viral replication modulator E2, thus resulting in an increased expression of E6 and E7. This sequence of events takes time and requires additional factors (other infections, smoking, etc.) that promote this rather complex process. It is therefore easy to understand why the development of malignant tumors may take between eight years and several decades and only happens in a few patients.

Diagnosis. When condylomas become disturbing, they are also recognized clinically. Hence, no further diagnostic steps are required. The situation is different in cases of subclinical HPV infection or dysplasia. Here, it is essential to track down the virus. This requires special aids and expensive methods of molecular biology:

- *Clinical picture.*
- *Colposcopy* after swabbing with 3% acetic acid (Fig. 7.**64**).
- *Histology.* Detection of koilocytosis (Fig. 7.**65**), elongated rete ridges, acanthosis, deficient

glycogenesis, para- or hyperkeratosis, and detection of dysplasia (mild, CIN I; moderate, CIN II; severe, CIN III).

- *Virus-specific DNA.* Detection and determination of the type of virus are possible by means of hybridization. The Hybrid Capture II test (DNA in situ hybridization with signal enhancement) is currently the test best suited for routine HPV testing; group tests for the most common HR and LR types are also used.
- *Real-time PCR.* This is used for quantifying the HPV DNA (positive result: 10 copies and more) because a high load of virus increases the risk of dysplasia by a factor of six to eight.
- Possibly also a test involving the amplification of papillomavirus oncogene transcripts (*APOT test*), which detects integrated HPV DNA but is not yet available for routine screening.
- *Cytology*: Pap IIw, Pap III, Pap IIID.

Serology does not yet play a role today. Its significance is still unclear. Commercial tests are not available.

Therapy. Genital HPV infections associated with condyloma formation are found most often in young, sexually active women. In the majority of patients, spontaneous remission occurs without treatment. Adopting a wait-and-see policy is therefore justified. If no spontaneous remission takes place, or if the patient is too much discomforted, the condylomas should be removed. There are a number of methods available for this purpose. However, the virus itself will not be eliminated by these measures.

- *Mechanical ablation* (surgical, electrical, or laser ablation).
- *Mitotic inhibitors.* Treatment with podophyllotoxin, available as a 0.5 % alcoholic solution or as a 0.15 % cream. Podophyllin (which is a mixture of substances) is available as a 5–20 % extract in alcoholic solution but should no longer be used (see p. 48).
- *Denaturation.* Strong acids (trichloroacetic acid, > 50 %; nitric acid), cryoablation, or electrocoagulation. This treatment is permitted during pregnancy.
- *Interferon.* Treatment for several weeks, either by s.c. or i.m. application or as a gel. (So far, there are no additional parameters that allow one to recognize in which patient this method might be successful.)
- *Immunomodulation.* Treatment with imiquimod cream is reserved for stubborn cases (a severe inflammatory reaction may occur if the cream is applied too generously to sensitive skin). The desired result—namely, elimination of the virus—has not yet been demonstrated.
- Possibly, *fluorouracil* (available as a solution or as a cream).

Depending on the examiner, patient cohort, time of observation, and type of treatment, the rates of clinical healing are reported to lie between 50–80 %. There is no true preference of one method. All these methods remove condylomas but do not always eliminate also the virus—which spreads over large areas of the genitals up to the cervix. It therefore depends, first of all, on the immune system whether there will be a visible relapse. Depending on the activity of the virus, the infection may be visible or not. It is largely unknown why one patient develops fairly large condylomas while another patient does not.

Long-term Care of Patients with Dysplasia and High-risk HPV Infection

Strict monitoring is required only for women with an increased risk. Monitoring includes the cytological and histological detection of dysplasia and the detection of HR types of HPV. If dysplasia is detected, HPV typing is justified and necessary. If HR types are not detected through repeated testing, the risk of developing cervical carcinoma later is very low.

Only in 5 % of women over 30 years old can one expect to detect HR types of HPV. If HR types are detected, the risk of developing cervical carcinoma increases by a factor of 70. Even then, only few of these women actually develop cervical carcinoma. Nevertheless, knowing about the presence of HR-HPV in the genitals is helpful. These women should be more tightly monitored by means of colposcopy, cytology, and histology so that precancerous stages and early stages of cervical carcinoma can be recognized and treated in time. Newly developed tests will make it possible to further limit the actual risk also for HR-HPV-positive women. The role of serology in this context is still not clear.

There is no reason, however, to worry these women unnecessarily or even speak about precancerous lesions already at this time.

Prophylaxis:

- *Barrier methods.* Condoms protect only partly from infection with these viruses. Most HPV-infected individuals do not know that they are infected. Transmission is also possible by smear infection. In most patients, the time of inoculation can no longer be determined because condylomas grow slowly. In addition, visible condylomas are caused by LR-types. The use of condoms does not protect from

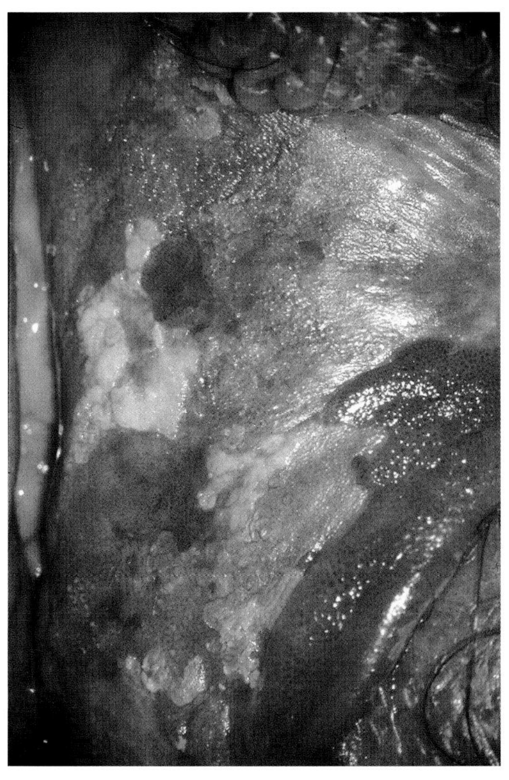

Fig. 7.**66** Bowen disease of the vulva in a 46-year-old patient after long-term treatment for chronic fungal infection.

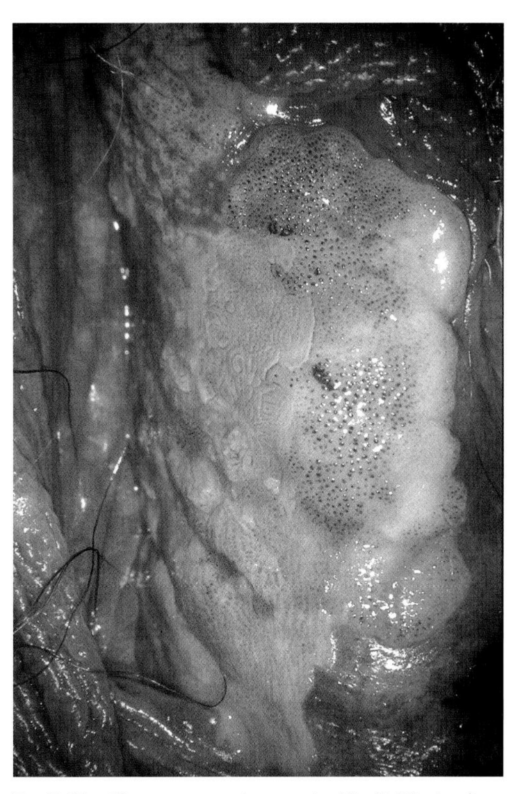

Fig. 7.**67** The same patient as in Fig. 7.**66**. Application of acetic acid revealed severe dysplasia (VIN III).

HR-type infections, which are usually subclinical.

- *Vaccination.* There are promising developments in both prophylactic and therapeutic vaccination. Various vaccines have been successful in animal experiments and are now tested in humans.
- *Immunomodulators.* Expectations that they might help the body to eliminate the virus have not been fulfilled.

Special Forms of HPV Infection

Bowenoid papulosis and **Bowen disease** (vulvar intraepithelial neoplasm of stage III, VIN III) are precancerous dermatoses in which HPV is involved. Diagnosis is established clinically (Fig. 7.**66**), especially after swabbing the vulva with 3 % acetic acid (Fig. 7.**67**), and histologically (Fig. 7.**68**).

Differential diagnosis:

- hyperkeratosis
- papillary vulvar hirsutism (papillomatosis) (Fig. 7.**69**)
- keratoangioma (Fig. 7.**70**).

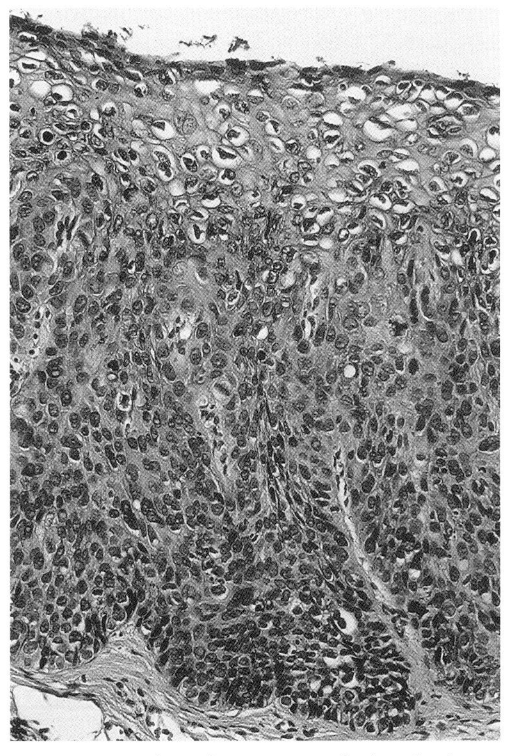

Fig. 7.**68** Histological preparation of vulvar skin from a patient with Bowen disease (VIN III). The hematoxylin-eosin stained cross-section shows a carcinoma in situ.

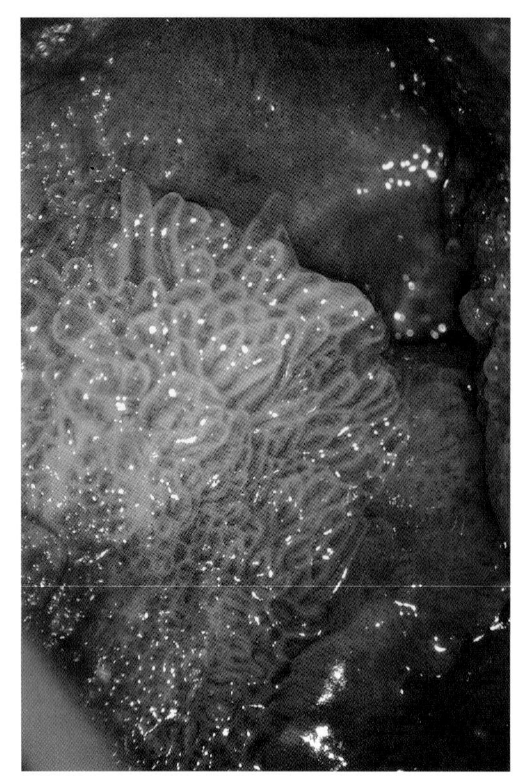

Fig. 7.**69** Harmless papillomatosis (hirsuties) in a 17-year-old patient.

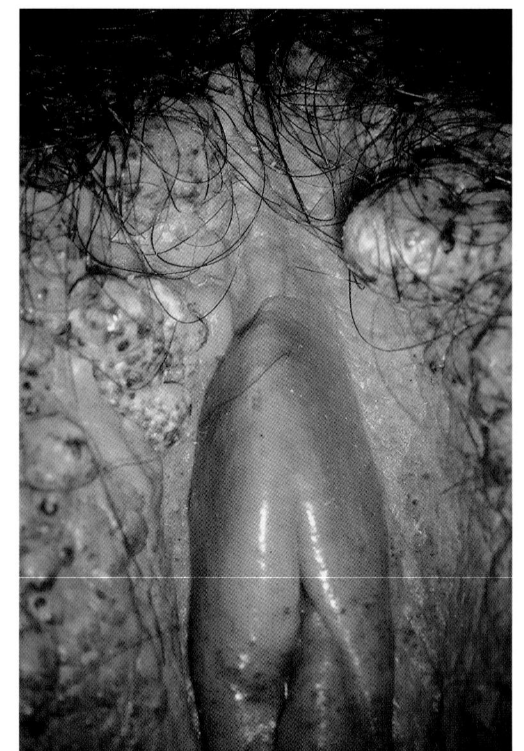

Fig. 7.**70** Keratoangioma (benign) in a 26-year-old patient. (The disease is rarely as prominent as shown here.)

In the presence of extensive acuminate condylomas in the birth canal, the newborn may become infected with papillomaviruses during birth. However, the risk of transmission is low because condylomas contain few virus particles. Hence, cesarean section is justified in rare cases only. Reliable data on the frequency of peripartal transmission of papillomaviruses are not yet available. In addition, the data on recently reported laryngeal papillomas, in which HPV-6 has been detected, are scanty and not convincing. The problem is that the detection methods are costly and that the clinical signs often occur only after months or years.

Syphilis (Lues venera)

Even today, syphilis is still a reportable infection. Formerly called lues, this so-called veneral disease is a sexually transmitted infection that is feared because of its sequelae. It was, and still is, largely limited to certain risk groups and occurs less and less often in the general population. There have been even considerations to abolish obligatory serological screening during pregnancy. This has slightly changed in recent years. In the mid-1990s, there has been a massive spreading of syphilis in Eastern European countries, where the prevalence in some regions increased by a factor of 50. As the infection spread from Eastern to Central Europe, syphilis is now seen slightly more frequently here as well.

Frequency. The prevalence in the general population is three to five infections per 100 000 persons, with only one third of that being women. In risk groups and in heavily populated areas with many immigrants arriving from high-risk countries, the prevalence is up to 10 times higher than in rural areas, where it is far below 1:100 000.

Incubation time. Three to four weeks (in rarer cases one to 13 weeks).

Transmission and pathogenesis. Because the pathogen is unstable, an infection can only occur during intense mucosal contact. The external genitals are usually the port of entrance. Here, the infection causes a painless primary lesion with regional lymphadenopathy (inguinal lymph node swelling) after about three weeks.

Occasionally, the primary lesion may occur on the portio vaginalis (Fig. 7.**141**, p. 140), in which case there is no swelling of the inguinal lymph nodes because the lymphatic drainage is deep seated. Detection of these primary infections is

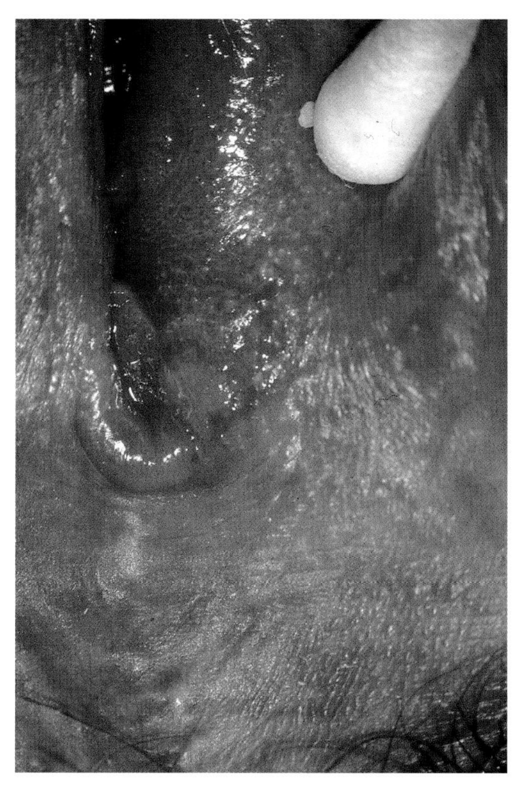

Fig. 7.**71** Fresh syphilis, primary lesion in a 24-year-old patient.

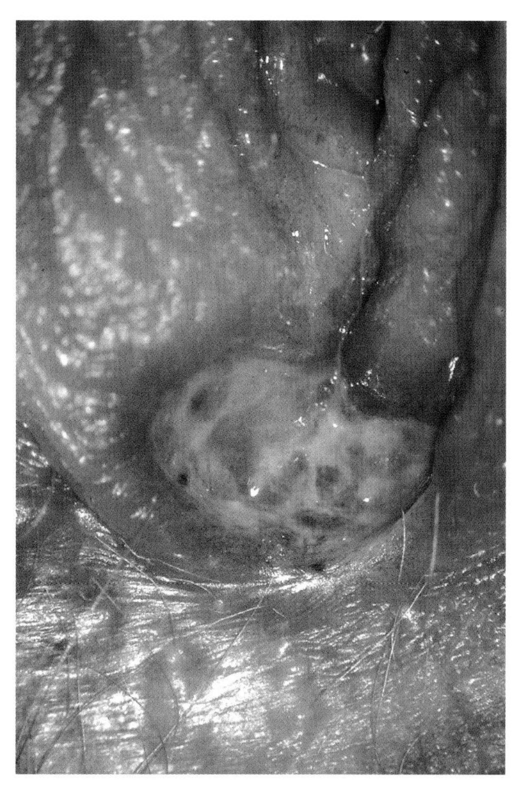

Fig. 7.**72** Primary lesion of syphilis in a 20-year-old patient.

by chance only. Primary lesions may also occur in the oral region due to oral–genital contact, or in the anal region due to anal contact.

Pathogen. The spirochete *Treponema pallidum* is a delicate spiral bacterium (p. 7). It does not grow on artificial media and can only be propagated in rabbit testicles.

Clinical picture:

Primary syphilis. Within three to four weeks, nodules appear which change into a painless ulcer (chancre) with a hardened base (Figs. 7.**71**, 7.**72**). The regional lymph nodes are enlarged, but they are not painful. A secretion containing plenty of *Treponema pallidum* can be squeezed out from the nonbleeding ulcer. The ulcer heals after four to eight weeks, even without treatment.

Secondary syphilis. A skin rash (exanthema) appears six to 12 weeks after infection; it may heal within days or persist for months (Figs. 7.**73**, 7.**74**). Most patients have additional mucocutaneous lesions (syphilids). These changes are accompanied by generalized lymphadenopathy. In addition, the eyes, bones, joints, and internal organs may be affected in some patients.

During this period, also the meninges become affected. Hypertrophic, flat papules may appear in the genital region; they are called flat condylomas (Fig. 7.**75**) and are infectious.

Latent syphilis. This stage may last for years, during which time an infected patient is free of overt symptoms. Two years after the initial infection, the disease is usually no longer infectious.

Late or tertiary syphilis. The clinical course may take various forms. For example, late benign tertiary syphilis appears three to 10 years after the initial infection and is characterized by chronic, granulomatous lesions (gummata). These may occur on the skin but may involve also any other organ or tissue of the body.

Cardiovascular syphilis makes its appearance only after 10 to 25 years. *Neurosyphilis* (meningovascular syphilis) develops in 10–12% of untreated syphilitic individuals. This form of syphilis—which includes general paralysis (resulting in progressive dementia and generalized paralysis) and tabes dorsalis (posterior spinal sclerosis)—is rarely seen today.

Special risks:

- transmission of the infection to the embryo or fetus during pregnancy (p. 193)
- late sequelae of syphilis: cardiovascular syphilis, neurosyphilis.

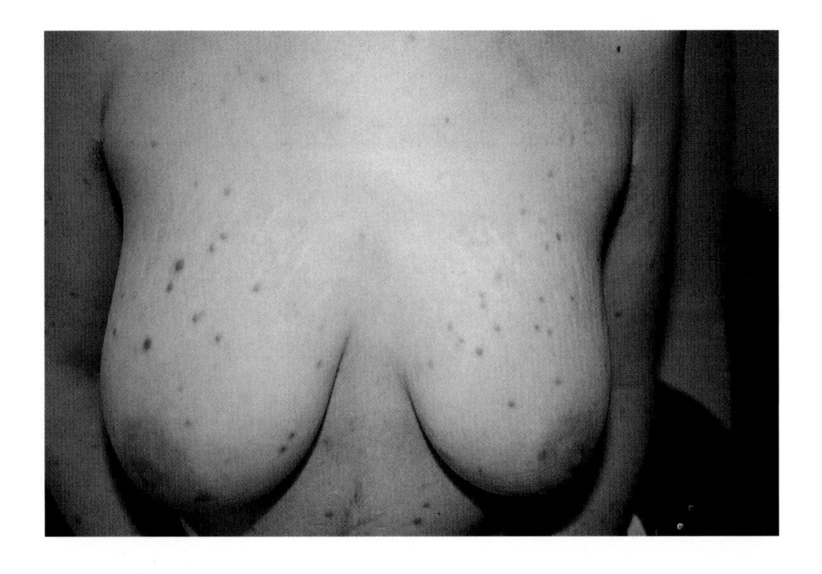

Fig. 7.**73** The same patient as in Fig. 7.**72**, showing exanthema (macular syphilids) due to secondary syphilis four weeks later, in spite of treatment with a macrolide (the patient was allergic to penicillin).

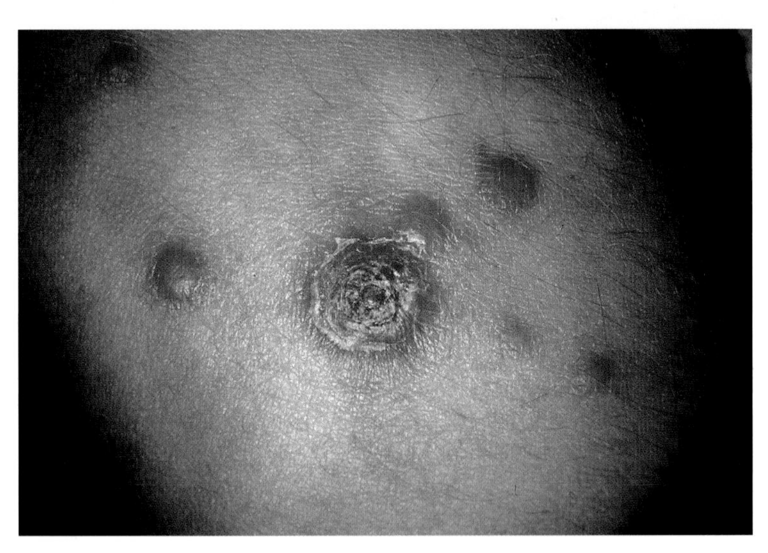

Fig. 7.**74** The same patient as in Fig. 7.**73**. Higher magnification of the syphilitic skin lesions (papules) due to secondary syphilis.

Diagnosis:

- *Direct detection of the pathogen.* In the secretion from primary lesions; occasionally, detection is also possible in secondary lesions, but this is rarely successful:
  - fluorescence test
  - dark field microscopy.
- *Serology:*
  - *Treponema pallidum* hemagglutination test (TPHA test): used as a screening test for detecting previous infection with syphilis. The patient remains positive for life.
  - Venereal Disease Research Laboratory (VDRL) test (a modification of the cardiolipin microflocculation test), or a complement fixation test (CFT) using cardiolipin (or *T. pallidum* antigen). Both tests are nonspecific but are important for obtaining information on the actual infection—and thus the need for treatment—or for monitoring the success of treatment. Cross-reactions with collagenosis and rheumatic diseases occur.
  - IgM antibody detection. Available are the fluorescent treponemal antibody absorption test (FTA–ABS test) and the solid-phase hemadsorption (SPHA) assay.

Therapy:

- Daily intramuscular injection of 1–2 million IU of clemizole penicillin G. This treatment is rarely used today.
- Intramuscular injection of 2.4 million IU of benzathine benzylpenicillin (divided into two doses, one given into each buttock); single treatment in cases of fresh, uncomplicated syphilis, or three treatments at one-week intervals during pregnancy or in complicated cases.

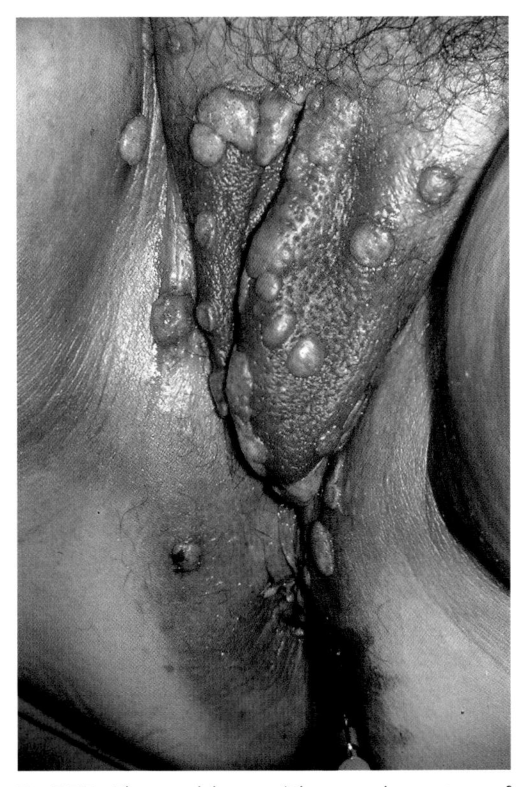

Fig. 7.**75** Flat condylomas. (Photograph courtesy of Prof. Bilek, Leipzig, Germany.)

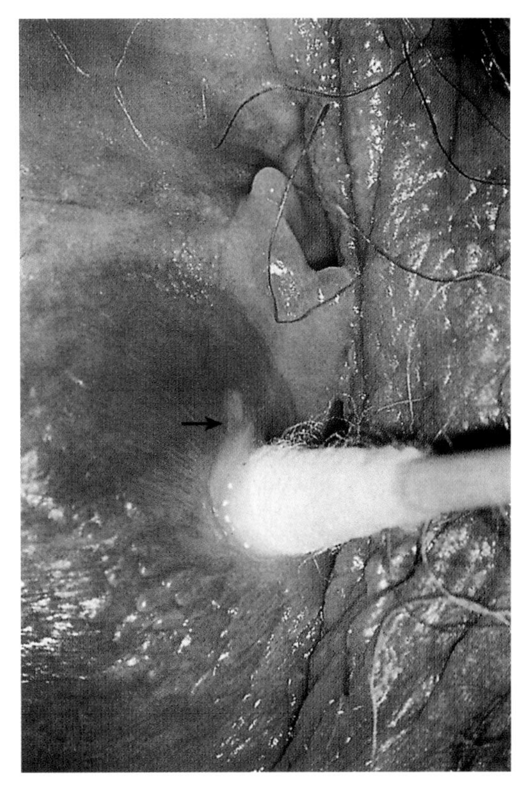

Fig. 7.**76** Bartholinitis in a 31-year-old patient. Swelling of the right vulva and yellow secretion draining from Bartholin duct (arrow).

In case of allergy to penicillin, the following may be used:

- ceftriaxone (2 g per day, i. v.)
- doxycycline (200 mg per day)
- erythromycin (2 g per day).

However, macrolides do not seem to be as effective as first assumed. They are insufficient during pregnancy. Our own experience has confirmed the reservations against macrolides for the treatment of syphilis: a young, petite, nonpregnant patient, who had a penicillin allergy, developed secondary syphilis with maculopapulous exanthema while being treated with roxithromycin.

Duration of therapy. At least two weeks of treatment during the first year of infection, and at least three weeks from the second year on.

Repeated serological monitoring (for two years) is required for recognizing treatment failure. Any decline in the values yielded by VDRL tests and IgM assays will occur slowly over several months.

Note: As we know from the era prior to the use of antibiotics, spontaneous healing occurs in about 50% of patients. Humoral antibodies do not protect from reinfection, although they are always produced—thus making serological detection of syphilis very reliable.

Differential diagnosis. Behçet syndrome, injuries, and carcinoma.

Bartholinitis, Empyema, and Congestion of Bartholin Gland

Bartholinitis is usually caused by obstruction of the excretory duct of the greater vestibular gland (Bartholin gland) and subsequent infection by the local flora (intestinal bacteria) and inflammation. It may develop from the more common congestion of glandular secretion (Bartholin cyst). Inflammation always produces pain and redness. Far less common is the primary infection with pathogens, such as gonococci or *Staphylococcus aureus*.

Pathogens:

- *Neisseria gonorrhoeae*
- *Staphylococcus aureus*
- *Escherichia coli*
- anaerobes (*Bacteroides* species, peptococci, peptostreptococci, etc.).

Pathogenesis. The greater vestibular glands, which open near the vaginal orifice, may become infected, thus leading first to bartholinitis and

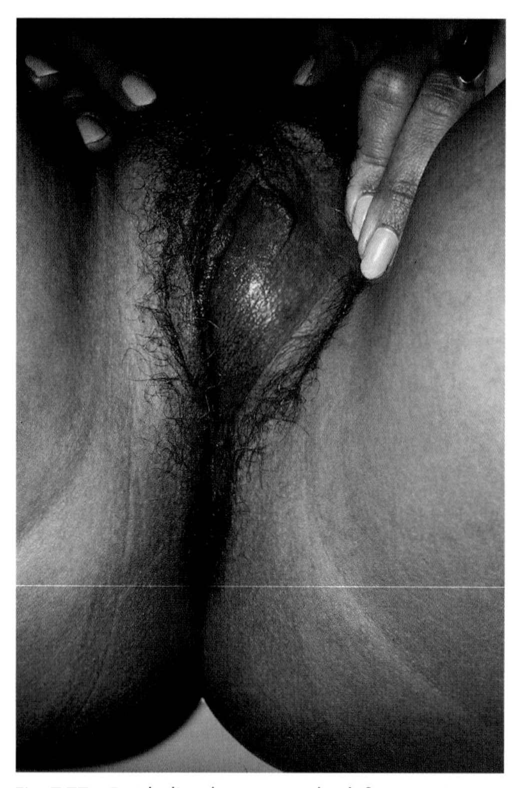

Fig. 7.**77** Bartholin abscess on the left in a 28-year-old patient.

then to Bartholin abscess. This causes a painful swelling of the gland or its duct, usually on one side only. In the presence of pathogens, such as gonococci, the abscess is the result of inflammation, whereas the swelling of Bartholin gland, caused by congestion of the excretory duct, is certainly the prerequisite for an infection with facultative intestinal pathogens.

Clinical picture. Bartholinitis is a painful, red unilateral swelling of the gland in the central region of the vulva (Figs. 7.**76**, 7.**77**). Occasionally, a yellow secretion full of leukocytes can be squeezed out from the duct of Bartholin gland.

The clinical picture is different from that of Bartholin cyst, which is caused by obstruction of the excretory duct without infection and inflammation (Fig. 7.**78**). These cysts are not painful and are only annoying because of their considerable size. They may have existed for years as patients are hardly bothered by them.

Diagnosis:

- *Clinical picture.* The deep location of the hard and painful swelling is characteristic.
- *Ultrasound*
- *Bacteriology* is required only in case of recurrence or when there is a risk for sexually transmitted disease.

Therapy:

- *Marsupialization* (pouch formation by lateral resection of the gland and suture of the cyst's wall to the external skin) is also recommended if the Bartholin cyst is not infected.
- *Antibiotics* are given only if pathogens are detected or when marsupialization is not possible.
- *Spontaneous perforation* is possible; recurrences are common, even after puncture.

Hidradenitis Suppurativa/Pyoderma Fistulans

Hidradenitis suppurativa (so-called apocrine acne) is a rare secondary bacterial infection of the ducts of the apocrine sweat glands following follicular occlusion. In patients with a special disposition, the sweat gland abscesses tend to form fistulas (pyoderma fistulans sinifica, also called fox den disease). Clinically as well as histologically, the condition is often difficult to distinguish from acne conglobata. It is characterized by annoying recurrent purulent discharge and scarring in the paravulvar region.

Hidradenomas are harmless cystic enlargements of sweat glands. Because they are so rare, it is not known whether there is a connection between the two disorders.

Pathogen. Various microbes of the skin flora (*Staphylococcus epidermidis*, streptococci) are found in the culture. One might initially suspect folliculitis, but typical pathogens (*Staphylococcus aureus*) cannot be detected.

Clinical picture. Initially, there is some itching or burning, and there may also be some pain; but often there is hardly any discomfort. The patient may complain that the recurrent purulent nodules and progressive scarring interfere with her sex life. The skin lesions are less extreme than those with acne conglobata.

Hidradenitis suppurativa is more common in the axillae, while pyoderma fistulans appears more often in the vulvar region. Both conditions appear only after puberty. Brown–red, livid, hard nodules develop in the skin (Fig. 7.**79**). They perforate spontaneously or when subjected to pressure, thus draining a turbid leukocyte-containing fluid.

Diagnosis:

- *Clinical picture.*
- *Bacteriology* for differentiation from folliculitis and staphyloderma due to *Staphylococcus aureus.*
- *Biopsy.*

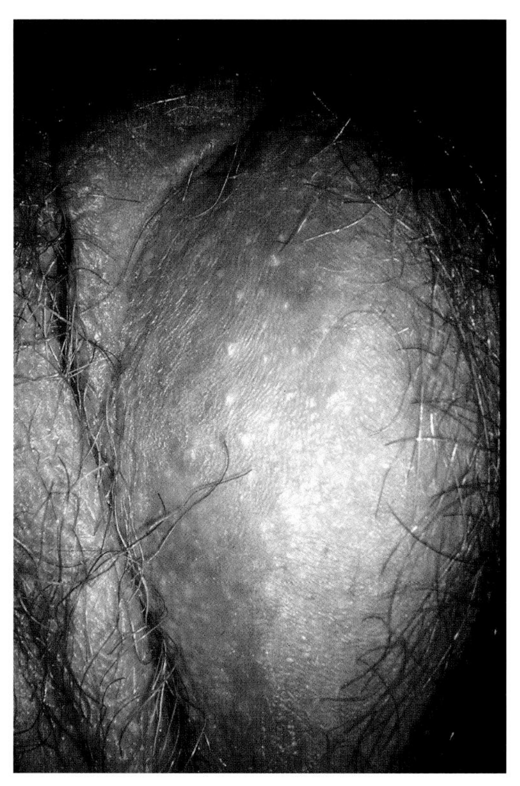

Fig. 7.**78** Bartholin cyst (mild) in a 33-year-old patient.

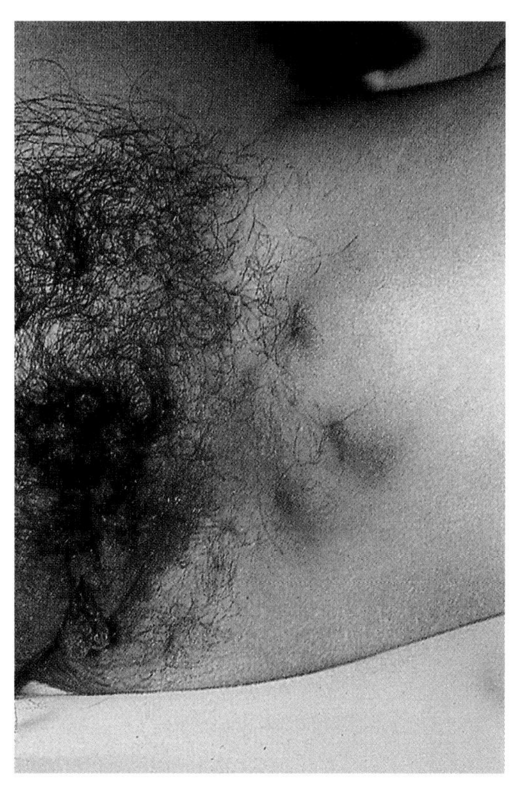

Fig. 7.**79** Pyoderma fistulans existing for five years in a 27-year-old patient.

Therapy:

- Incision of the nodules; subsequent healing may leave distorting scars.
- Excision of the affected area. Systemic antibiotic therapy does not eradicate the infection.

Acne Conglobata

This is an inflammatory disease of sebaceous glands and affects the perivulvar region, in part also the inguinal region. The chronic nodular inflammation of the skin is associated with purulent drainage and disfiguring scarring.

The vaginal orifice and vagina are not affected, and the vaginal flora is mostly normal. Usually, only intestinal or skin bacteria are detected in cultures obtained from the pus of inflamed nodules (Fig. 7.**80**).

The cause is unknown. Treatment with antibiotics does not help. The course of the disease can be alleviated by skin care and local reduction in microbes. In severe cases (Figs. 7.**80**, 7.**81 a**, **b**), only surgical reversion by means of a sliding flap will heal or arrest the inflammation.

Risk factor: smoking.

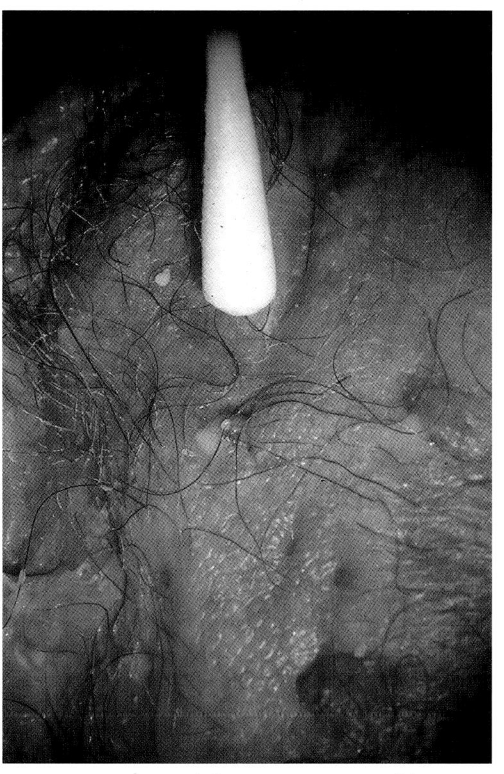

Fig. 7.**80** Acne conglobata in an 18-year-old patient.

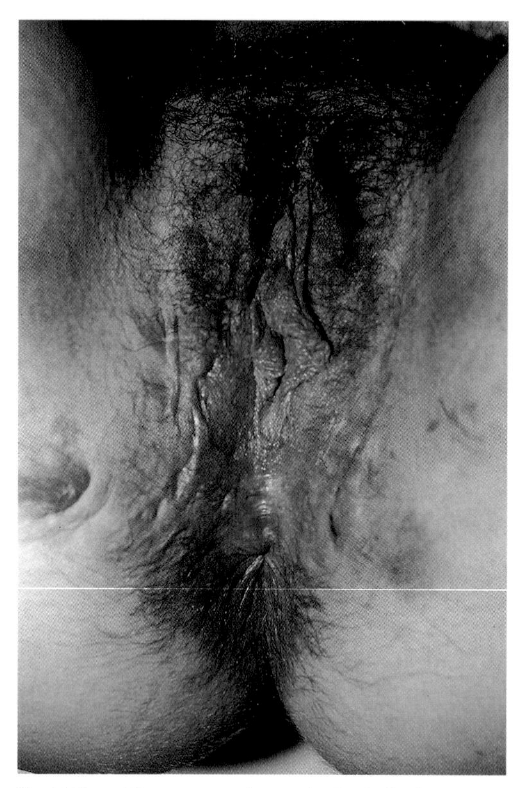

Fig. 7.**81 a** The same patient as in Fig. 7.**80**, four years later.

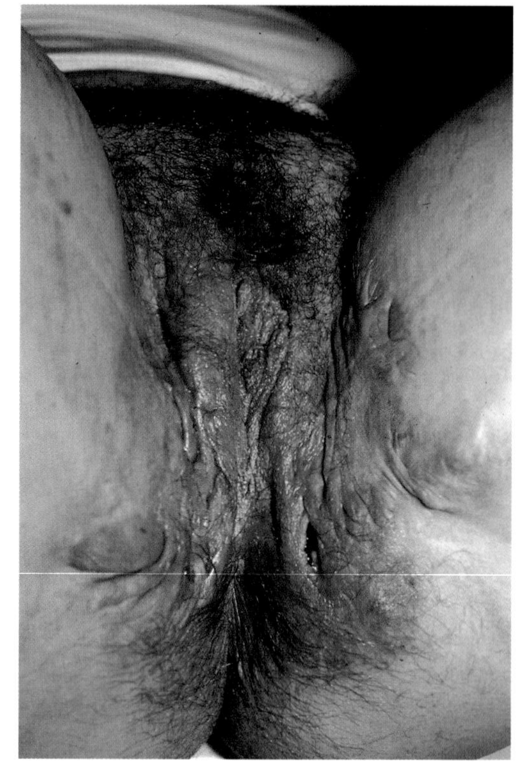

Fig. 7.**81 b** The same patient as in Fig. 7.**81 a**, six years later.

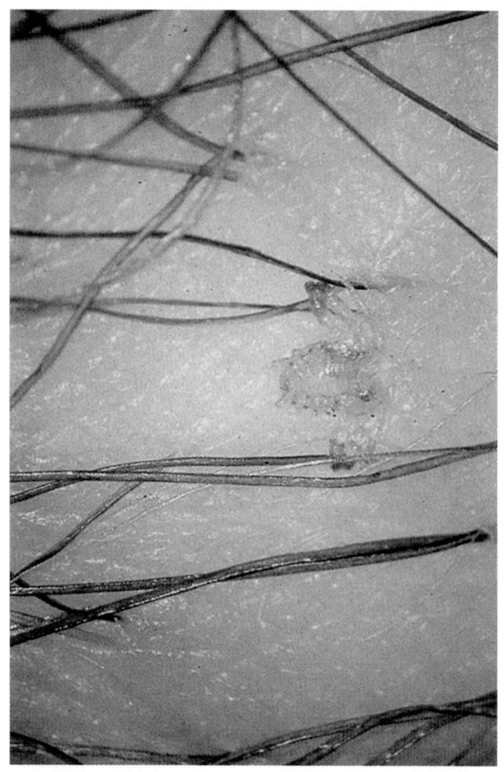

Fig. 7.**82** Infestation of the mons pubis by pubic lice. A pubic louse has anchored itself to two pubic hairs. Nits are not visible here.

Infestation with Pubic Lice (Phthiriasis)

Even nowadays, any itching in the anterior pubic hair region—especially at night in a warm bed—should prompt one to consider also an infestation with pubic lice (pediculosis pubis, pthiriasis inguinalis).

Pathogen. The pubic or crab louse, *Phthirus pubis* (Fig. 7.**82**), reaches a length of about 2 mm. It differs from other louse species by its prominently developed second and third pairs of legs and by the two appendages of the last body segment. The reproduction time is three weeks.

Frequency. Less than 0.1 % of patients.

Transmission:

- sexual contact
- mattresses and blankets (where the survival time is only 24 hours).

Clinical picture and diagnosis:

- scratch marks in the pubic hair region
- colposcopic detection of light-yellowish pubic lice, which are found between the pubic hairs immediately above the skin or buried into hair follicles

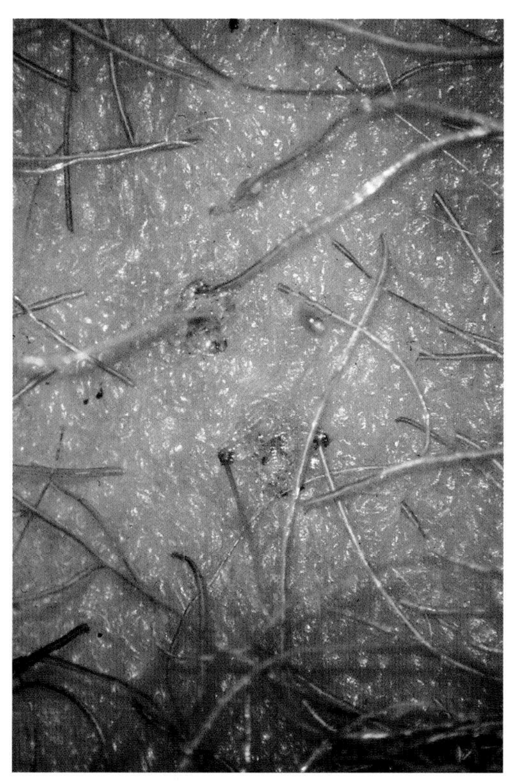

Fig. 7.**83** Pthiriasis pubis with pubic lice and nits in a 24-year-old patient.

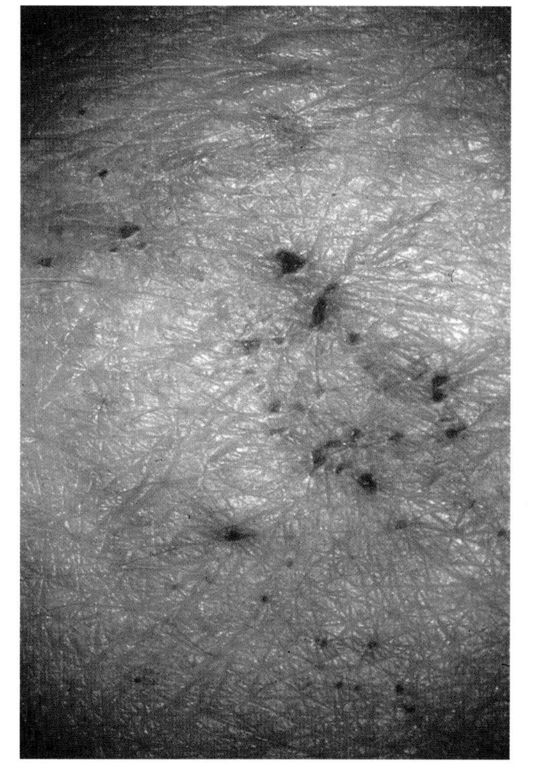

Fig. 7.**84** Scabies in a 41-year-old patient.

- colposcopic detection of nits (the eggs of a louse), which are fixed 2–3 mm above the hair line by means of a waterproof adhesive (Fig. 7.**83**)
- colposcopic detection of crusted blood and fecal balls on the skin between the pubic hairs
- occasionally, so-called maculae ceruleae (blue spots) appear; these are eczematous skin lesions due to substances transmitted through the bite.

Therapy (topical) for pubic lice and head lice:
- permethrin is used preferentially in the United States as a single-dose treatment; it should not be administered during pregnancy
- lindane emulsion, mesulfen; they should not be used during pregnancy, if possible
- pyrethrins: may be used during pregnancy
- malathion.

Duration of therapy. One to three days. Pubic hairs need not be removed.

It is recommended that the treatment be repeated after eight days. After each treatment, the success of the therapy should be monitored.

In case of **treatment failure** (resistances have been reported, but improper application has been more common), the nits have not been killed completely. With the exception of permethrin, none of the preparations has a sufficient ovicidal activity.

Infestation with Mites (Scabies)

Mites are a group of various ectoparasites. Relatively harmless are house dust mites, which occasionally induce allergies, and hair follicle mites (*Demodex folliculorum*).

The itch mite, *Sarcoptes scabiei hominis*, may induce inflammation when the females burrow into the skin to lay their eggs. This is commonly known as scabies.

Clinical picture. Itching nodules and small crusts that spread to other areas (Fig. 7.**84**).

Diagnosis:
- *Clinical picture.*
- *Biopsy* (confirmation of diagnosis is based on the detection of fecal balls; mites are rarely found).

Therapy. The same treatment as for pthiriasis.

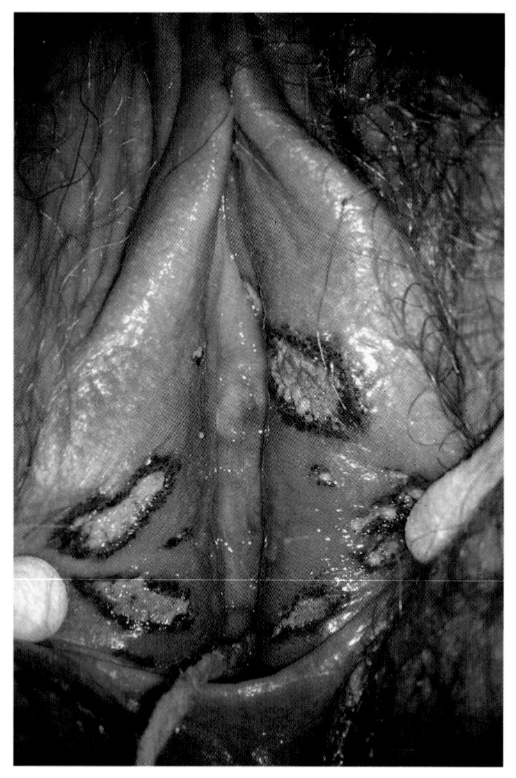

Fig. 7.**85** Behçet syndrome in a 35-year-old patient (very early stage).

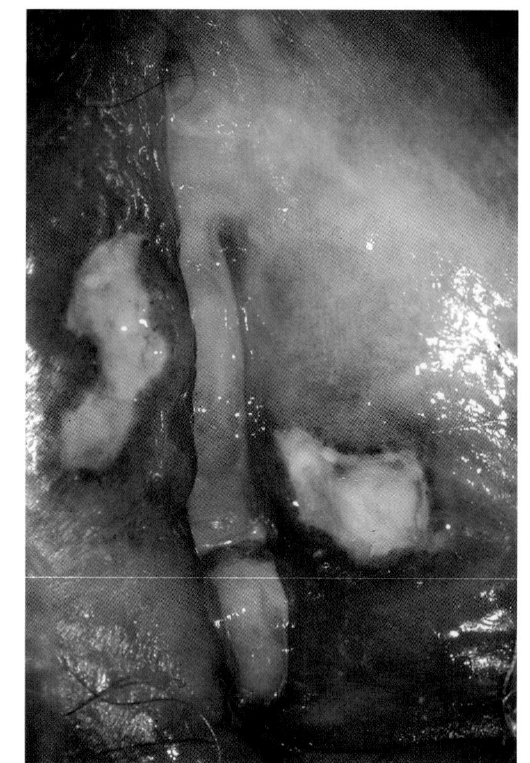

Fig. 7.**86** Behçet syndrome in a 28-year-old patient during the 12 th week of pregnancy.

Differential Diagnosis of Vulvitis Not Caused by Pathogens

Behçet Syndrome

(Differential diagnosis: syphilis, genital herpes, chancroid, carcinoma)

If ulcers are present at several sites of the vulva (Figs. 7.**85**, 7.**86**) and these are particularly painful and deep, one is probably dealing with a form of Behçet syndrome, a recurrent inflammatory disorder involving small blood vessels. Deep necrosis is caused in part by vasculitis of unknown origin. If the condition responds well to topical cortisone, one might suspect an underlying immune disease. If treatment is initiated late, deep necrosis may result in tissue damage that usually takes several weeks to heal. For far too long, Behçet syndrome has frequently been confused with recurrent genital herpes because of its tendency to reoccur.

If a single ulcer occurs for the first time, it is essential to exclude **syphilis** by serology.

Carcinoma of the Vulva

(Differential diagnosis: Behçet syndrome, injury)

If an ulcer does not heal for weeks (Fig. 7.**87**), one should always consider a malignant tumor. Even negative histological findings must not prevent one from taking further biopsies in order to exclude a carcinoma in patients in which the ulcer does not heal or does not become markedly smaller after cortisone treatment. Repeated topical treatment can certainly cause additional problems, as illustrated in Fig. 7.**88**. The figure shows the vulva of the same patient as in Fig. 7.**87** but following anesthesia with ELMA cream prior to biopsy. Here, an irritable dermatitis either developed after application of the cream, or it already existed before that and promoted the malignant growth.

A biopsy should also be performed when a new nodule appears in a chronically inflamed area of the vulva because, as illustrated in Fig. 7.**89**, a small vulvar carcinoma may have developed within the chronically inflamed area. The same applies to other forms of chronic inflammation of the vulva, such as lichen sclerosus or, less often, lichen planus.

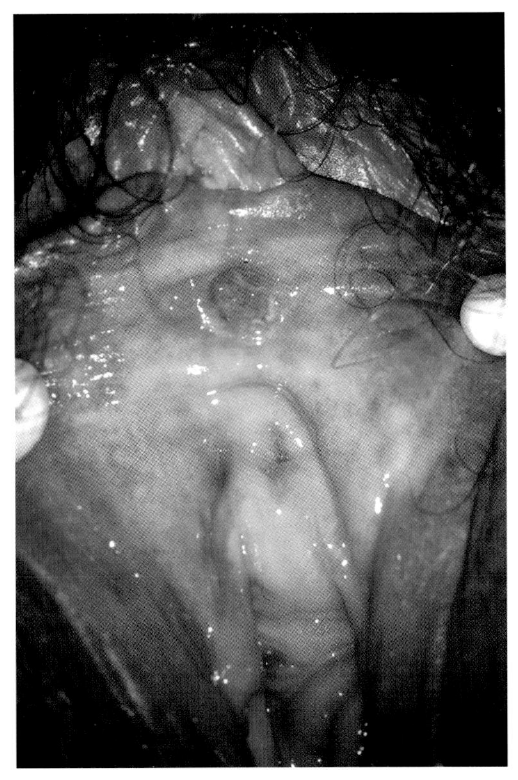

Fig. 7.**87** Small vulvar carcinoma in a 56-year-old patient.

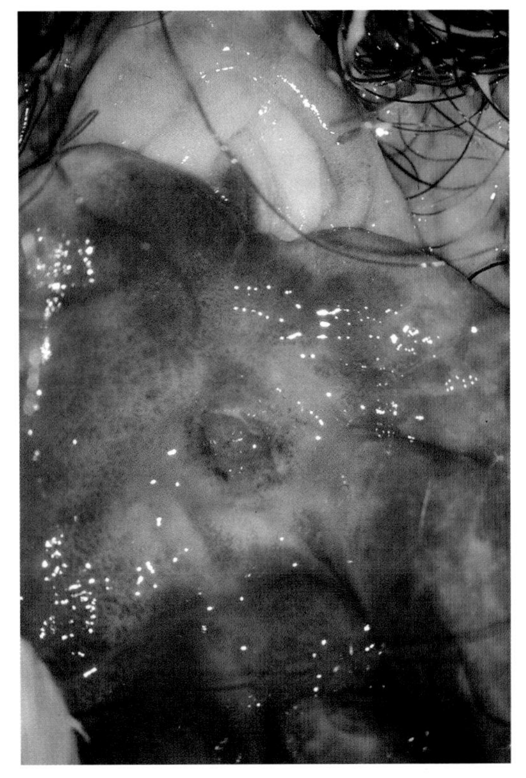

Fig. 7.**88** The same patient as in Fig. 7.**87** after EMLA treatment, revealing irritable dermatitis resulting from numerous topical treatments.

Irritable Vulvitis

(Differential diagnosis: candidiasis, primary genital herpes, plasma cell vulvitis)

This type of vulvitis develops in response to repeated contact with substances applied to the vulva for either treatment or skin care; in the end, this can lead to the development of allergies against these substances (Fig. 7.**90**). Patients usually complain of a burning sensation when applying certain substances, such as the ELMA cream commonly used for anesthesia prior to biopsy.

Local Drug Eruption

(Differential diagnosis: candidiasis, primary genital herpes, plasma cell vulvitis)

The genital region belongs to the preferred predilection sites of this local allergic disorder, which is characterized by keratinocyte damage with vacuole formation and single-cell necrosis.

Initially, the disease is often confused with candidiasis or genital herpes. Diagnosis is established through the clinical picture (redness, swelling, epithelial exfoliation; Fig. 7.**91**), failure to detect a pathogen, no leukocytes in the discharge

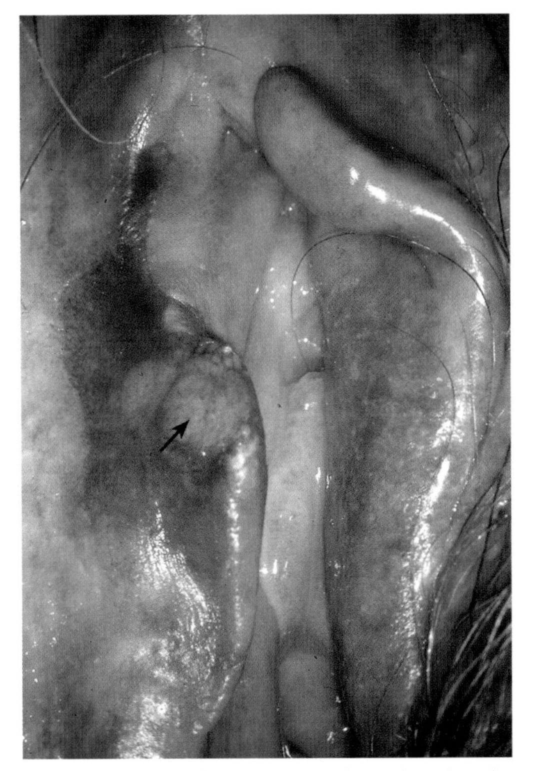

Fig. 7.**89** Small vulvar carcinoma (arrow) within the area of a chronic vulvar inflammation in a 50-year-old patient.

7

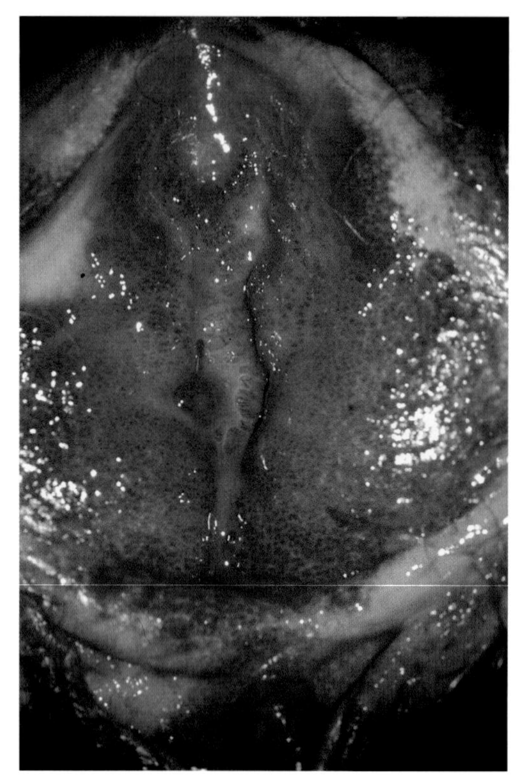

Fig. 7.**90** Irritable dermatitis after numerous topic treatments because of chronic burning and itching.

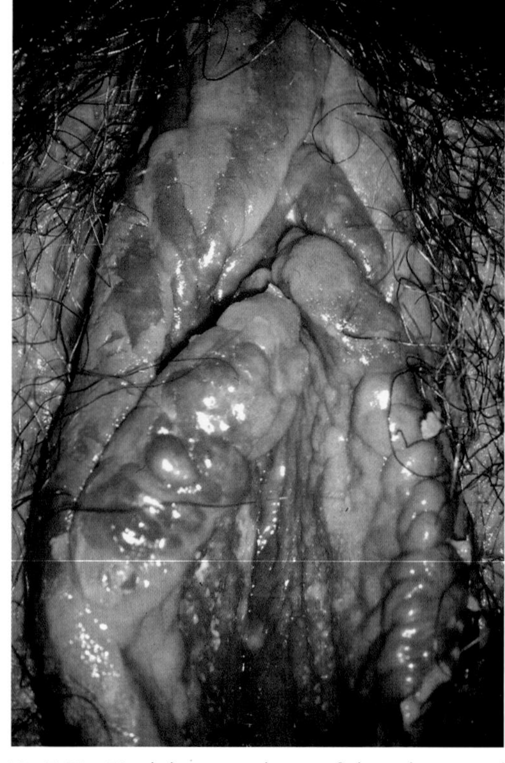

Fig. 7.**91** Fixed drug exanthema of the vulva caused by Co-Trimoxazole in a 41-year-old patient, causing swelling, redness, and exfoliation of the skin.

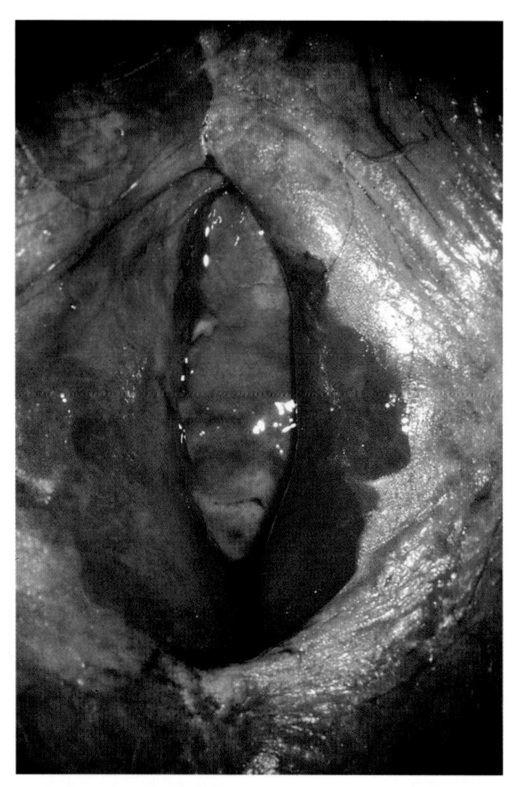

Fig. 7.**92** Erosive lichen planus in a 50-year-old patient, showing a sharp transition between the erosion and the healthy skin.

and, first of all, through a biopsy. Here, too, the discomfort is only alleviated by topical treatment with cortisone.

Unfortunately, the condition cannot be detected through general allergy testing because—as the name "local drug eruption" indicates—it is limited to the site of reaction, for example, the genitals.

Erosive Lichen Planus

(Differential diagnosis: candidiasis, plasma cell vulvitis)

Diagnosis is facilitated by the patient's history: this disease is characterized by its progressive course over many months/years and by the symmetry of the sharp demarcation of the reddened area (erosion) (Fig. 7.**92**).

Affliction of the genital region is particularly uncomfortable as the burning can be very painful in the sensitive region of the vaginal orifice, where contact with urine is always a possibility. As intercourse is often no longer possible with this chronic inflammation, problems with the partner may arise. Diagnosis is established based on the clinical picture, which is characterized by symmetric redness (erosion) with sharp demarcation, the simultaneous affliction of the oral

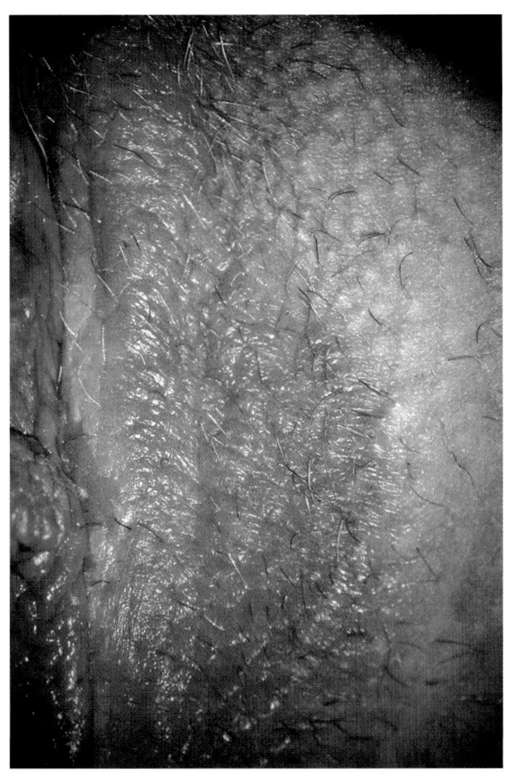

Fig. 7.**93** Psoriasis of the vulva in a 35-year-old patient. Repeated treatment with an antimycotic was unsuccessful.

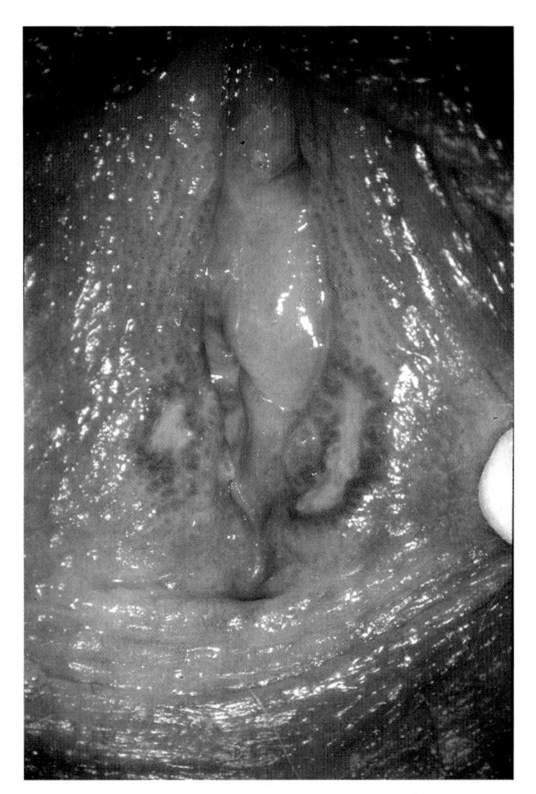

Fig. 7.**94** Injured vulva of a 22-year-old patient, showing symmetric abrasions following intercourse.

cavity, and the biopsy. Here, too, help comes only by sufficient topical cortisone therapy and, if necessary, excision.

Psoriasis Vulgaris of the Vulva

(Differential diagnosis: chronic candidiasis)

For a long time, this disease has been confused with chronic candidiasis due to the clinical picture with chronic redness (Fig. 7.**93**) and itching. In fact, it is reasonable to expect candidiasis to develop on the altered skin in addition to psoriasis. For this reason, monitoring the success of antimycotic therapy is essential in all chronic cases. The suspected diagnosis is based on the clinical picture: the mostly symmetric, flat redness shows a sharp transition to the healthy skin. Diagnosis is confirmed by biopsy, and the biopsy should only be evaluated by an experienced histologist.

Pemphigus Vulgaris

(Differential diagnosis: herpes)

This is a rare, severe immune disease with simultaneous vesicular affliction of the oral region and vulva. It is very painful. Confirmation of the diagnosis is based on the detection of immune complexes. Treatment consists of systemic cortisone administration (starting, for example, with 60 mg of cortisone). A dermatologist should confirm the diagnosis and prescribe the treatment.

Pemphigoid

(Differential diagnosis: genital herpes, candidiasis, folliculitis)

This is a rare, less severe immune disease with vesicles (see Fig. 8.**10**, p. 182). It is not easily recognized. Diagnosis is confirmed by means of biopsy and detection of immune complexes in the biopsy material or serum. Treatment consists of the administration of cortisone or azathioprine.

Injuries/Hematomas

Injuries caused by falls or through abrasion during intercourse can be very painful. Diagnosis is based on the patient's history and the clinical picture of the often-symmetrical lacerations (Fig. 7.**94**) in the absence of pathogens. In case of hematomas, incision is not appropriate; it would only harm and increase the risk of infection. Hematomas regress on their own. The best treatment consists of (initial) cooling and painkillers.

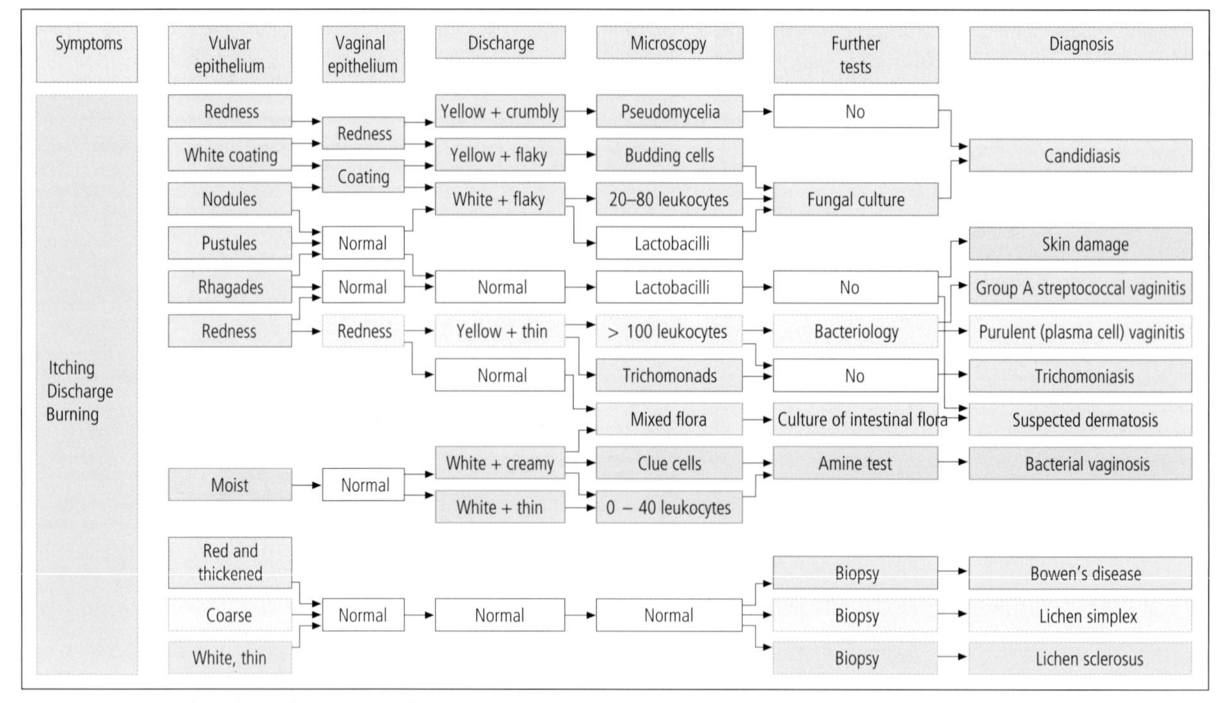

Fig. 7.**95** Practical guide to diagnosing infections.

Infections of the Vagina (Vaginitis)

Almost all pathogens that are able to infect the vulva can also induce infections of the vagina (Fig. 7.**95**). However, they cause less discomfort here because the vagina is poorly supplied with sensory nerves, especially in the proximal region. Frequently, the vulvar and vaginal regions are affected simultaneously.

The main symptom of vaginitis (or colpitis) is discharge. The more of the vulvar region is affected, the more severe the pain associated with it.

Unlike the rather dry milieu of the vulva, the vaginal milieu is moist. This promotes the multiplication of microorganisms and, hence, also the occurrence of vaginal infections, such as trichomoniasis and bacterial vaginosis. Due to the proximity of the vagina to the perianal region and the intestinal flora, bacteria are continuously reintroduced into the vagina. These bacteria are held in check by an intact lactobacillus flora and by the immune system. The lactobacillus flora thus plays a major role in the prevention of bacterial infections.

Vaginitis is characterized by an unusual discharge associated with leukocytes (leukorrhea). Redness of the vagina alone is no evidence of vaginitis; a thin epithelium also lets it appear red.

As an example, one particular patient should be mentioned here. She suffered for years ever since the redness of her vagina had been diagnosed as a chronic, incurable vaginitis. Because of a normal discharge, the vaginal redness in this completely symptomfree patient was finally classified as a harmless vascular display (Fig. 7.**96**).

Dermatosis does not cause leukorrhea if there is no epithelial defect. An increased number of leukocytes (> 40 per field of view at 400× magnification) may therefore originate from cervicitis.

Only few pathogens are able to induce vaginitis. The stratified squamous epithelium of the vagina is very robust. The majority of bacteria detected in case of complaints represent only colonizing microbes from the intestine and the skin and are not necessarily the cause of the complaints but rather a sign of inadequate hygienic conditions.

Vaginitis includes the following forms:

Infections:

- yeast infection (almost exclusively caused by *Candida albicans*)
- trichomoniasis
- vaginitis caused by group A streptococci
- vaginitis caused by *Staphylococcus aureus*
- vaginitis associated with genital herpes
- purulent vaginitis (plasma cell vaginitis).

Other causes:

- atrophic vaginitis
- erosive vaginitis.

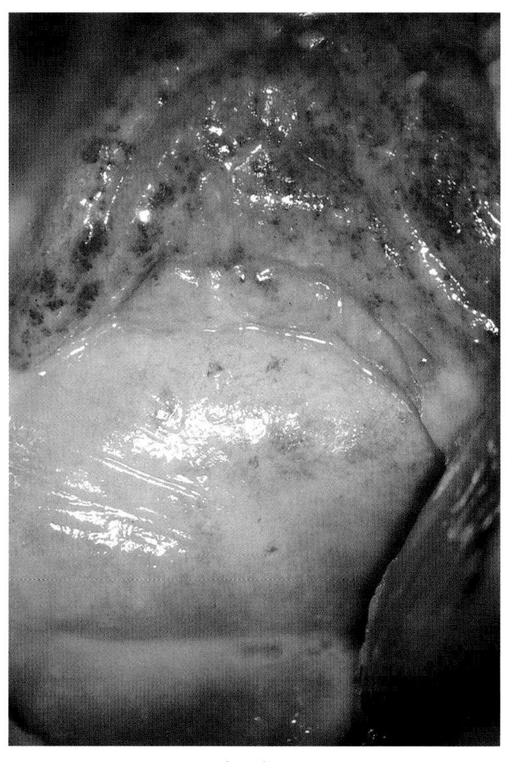

Fig. 7.**96** An apparently therapy-resistant vaginitis existing for 10 years in a 48-year-old patient. However, this is only a harmless vascular display.

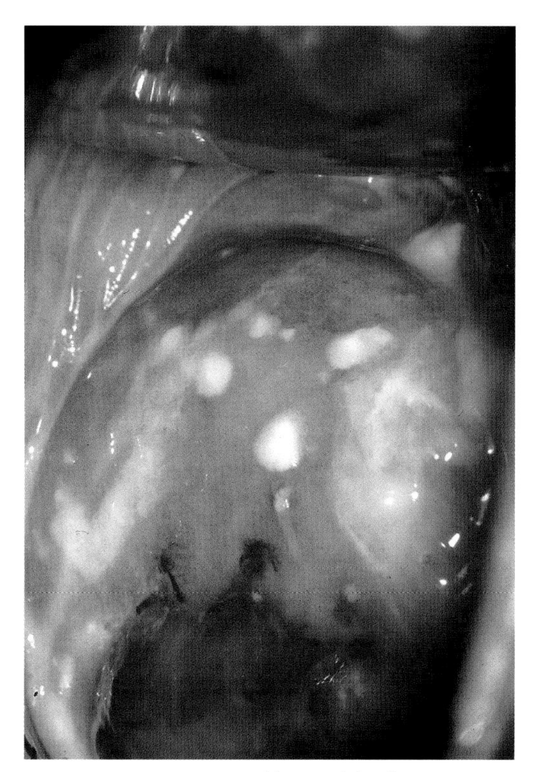

Fig. 7.**97** Vaginitis caused by *Candida albicans* in a 30-year-old patient.

Vaginitis Caused by Fungi

Vaginitis Caused by Candida albicans

It is rather rare that yeasts infect the vagina selectively. Nevertheless, some patients complain of discharge only. In these patients, the vulvar region appears largely normal.

Pathogen. *Candida albicans*, rarely other *Candida* species.

Frequency. Approx. 90 % of fungal infections of the vagina are caused by *Candida albicans*, with 5–8 % of all gynecologic patients being affected. Considering only the patients with distinct signs of inflammation, the former number approaches 100 %.

Clinical picture. The symptoms include itching, burning, pain, and discharge. The clinical picture of vaginitis reaches from discrete redness and single white flakes (Fig. 7.**97**) to massive yellow-crumbly discharge (Fig. 7.**98**). In extreme cases, the entire vagina may be lined with a thick, yellow-white coat. The vaginal wall is then usually reddened. Whereas itching and pain are more pronounced if the vulva is affected as well, no discomfort may be perceived if only the vagina is affected.

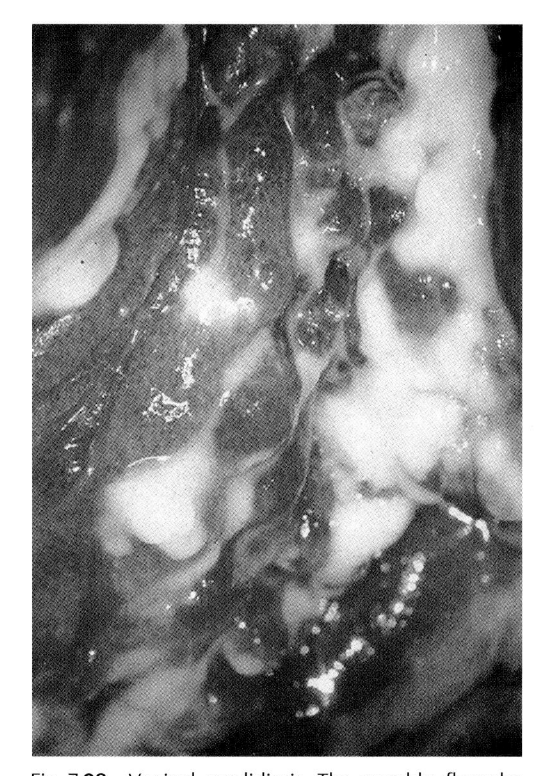

Fig. 7.**98** Vaginal candidiasis. The crumbly, floccular yellowish discharge adhering to the reddened vaginal wall is composed of exfoliated epithelial cells, fungal hyphens, and leukocytes.

7

Fig. 7.**99** Micrograph illustrating symptomatic *Candida albicans* infection. Wet mount of discharge stained with methylene blue, showing pseudomycelia.

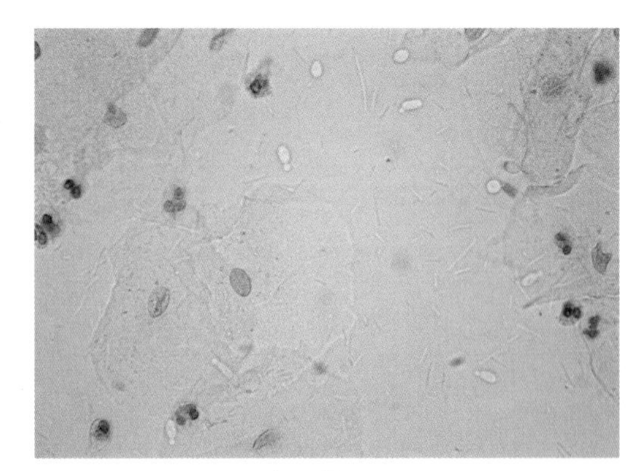

Fig. 7.**100** Micrograph illustrating asymptomatic *Candida* (*Torulopsis*) *glabrata* colonization of the vagina. Wet mount of discharge stained with methylene blue, showing budding cells but no pseudomycelia.

Table 7.**4** Frequency of yeast species in 230 patients, data after culture and differentiation (Women's Hospital at the University of Freiburg, Germany)

Yeast species	Frequency
Candida albicans	205 (89%)
Candida tropicalis	1 (0.4%)
Candida parapsilosis	1 (0.4%)
Candida krusei	0
Candida stellatoidea	0
Candida glabrata	11 (5%)
The genus *Candida*	2 (0.9%)
Saccharomyces cerevisiae	2 (0.9%)
Torulopsis inconspicua	3 (1.3%)
Candida albicans + *Candida lusitaniae*	1 (0.4%)
Candida albicans + *Candida glabrata*	2 (0.9%)
Candida albicans + *Candida parapsilosis*	1 (0.4%)

Diagnosis:

- *Microscopy.* In contrast to the vulva, microscopic detection of fungi in the discharge is much easier here. The detection of pseudomycelia (Fig. 7.**99**) is almost synonymous with the presence of *Candida albicans*, and further diagnostic tests are not required. In case of severe inflammatory reaction, plenty of granulocytes are present (Fig. 7.**10**, p. 72).
- *Culture.* This is only required if no fungal hyphens or only budding cells (Fig. 7.**100**) are found (see also p. 26).

Therapy. Treatment is always necessary in women with symptoms, in case of clinical signs of fungal vaginitis, microscopic detection of pseudomycelia, leukocytes, and budding cells only, and also during pregnancy in case of any detection of *Candida albicans* in culture.

In symptomfree women with a microscopically normal vaginal flora and detection of *Candida albicans* only in culture, treatment is not recommended. In up to 15% of women, *C. albicans* can be grown in liquid culture as a colonizing organism (in very low amounts).

The same drugs and therapeutic approach apply as for candidiasis of the vulva (p. 73).

Harmless Yeast Species in the Vagina

Occasionally, the discharge from a symptomfree patient may show plenty of budding cells under the microscope, but few leukocytes (Fig. 7.**100**). This suggests colonization with harmless yeast species. To be sure that this is the case, these yeasts should always be grown in culture and identified.

Fungal species include (Table 7.**4**, and Table 1.**2**, p. 8):

- *Candida* (formerly *Torulopsis*) *glabrata:* small budding cells that reproduce by budding only and possess no adhesive properties.
- *Saccharomyces cerevisiae:* large, elongated budding cells (brewer or baker yeast).
- *Geotrichum candidum:* a large, harmless imperfect hyphal fungus in feces and dairy products.

Frequency. About 5–10% of isolated yeasts are *Candida glabrata*, and 1–2% are *Saccharomyces cerevisiae*. In women with candidiasis, *C. glabrata* often occurs together with *C. albicans*. After treatment, *C. glabrata* remains because antimycotics do not, or only slightly, inhibit this yeast species.

Clinical picture. Normally, there is no discomfort. The vaginal wall is not reddened, and the discharge is normal. If the patient complains of itching or burning, or if vaginitis with redness and leukocytes exists, one should definitely search for other causes. Yeasts are common microbes of the local anogenital flora and are often associated with skin lesions, excessive washing, irritable dermatitis, dermatosis, or vaginitis of other etiology (see Fig. 7.**95**, p. 112). Other causes should be ruled out—at the latest when fungal treatment does not lead to healing.

Diagnosis:

- *Microscopy.* Only budding cells are present and no, or only very few, granulocytes. If many small budding cells are present, this definitely indicates *C. glabrata;* if many large, elongated budding cells are detected, these could be baker yeast, but *C. albicans* is also a possibility.
- *Culture* is essential for typing these yeasts.

Therapy. If the patient is free of complaints, one should forego treatment. If there are complaints, one should first search for other causes. Fungal therapy does not result in healing because the usual antimycotics are hardly effective. Ciclopirox olamine is said to be more effective. In vitro, itraconazole is slightly more effective than fluconazole. Treatment with high doses of fluconazole (800 mg per day for eight to 10 days) seems to be completely out of proportion for a pathogen that causes no, or hardly any, complaints.

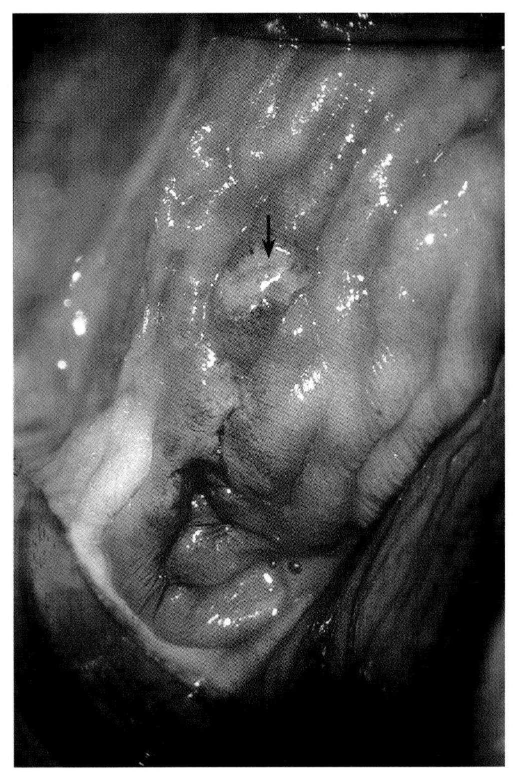

Fig. 7.**101** Primary genital herpes with lesions (arrow) affecting also the vagina.

Vaginitis Caused by Viruses

Herpes Simplex Virus Infection of the Vagina

Primary herpes almost never affects exclusively the vagina; but the vagina and, above all, the portio vaginalis are frequently involved in case of herpes infection.

Recurrent genital herpes may occur exclusively in the vagina, but this is rarely the case. The symptoms may include burning pain, discharge, and moderate increase in leukocytes. To make such a diagnosis, however, herpes-specific lesions (Fig. 7.**101**) must be clearly visible or the virus must have been detected. In case of discharge with increased numbers of granulocytes, therefore, one may consider recurrent genital herpes if other causes have been ruled out. Lesions are only rarely detected, even if the vaginal wall is thoroughly inspected with the colposcope. Another indication of recurrent herpes vaginalis may be the rhythmical appearance of complaints that subside spontaneously after a few days; the presence of such complaints can be shortened with aciclovir.

Serology is not very helpful for making the diagnosis. At the most, it may help exclude herpes if no antibodies can be detected.

For details, please refer to the discussion of vulvar infections caused by herpes simplex virus (see p. 82 ff.).

Papillomavirus Infection of the Vagina

Pathogenesis and clinical picture. In case of extensive acuminate condylomas, the vagina is usually affected in addition to the vulva. However, there are fewer and smaller efflorescences than in the vulvar region.

As already described in case of the vulva, papillomavirus infection of the genitals leads to wide distribution of the virus in the vulvar, vaginal, and cervical regions. However, the extent of lesions may vary considerably (Figs. 7.**102**, 7.**103**). In some women, there are only large or small, flat or acuminate condylomas in the vaginal vault or on the lateral vaginal walls.

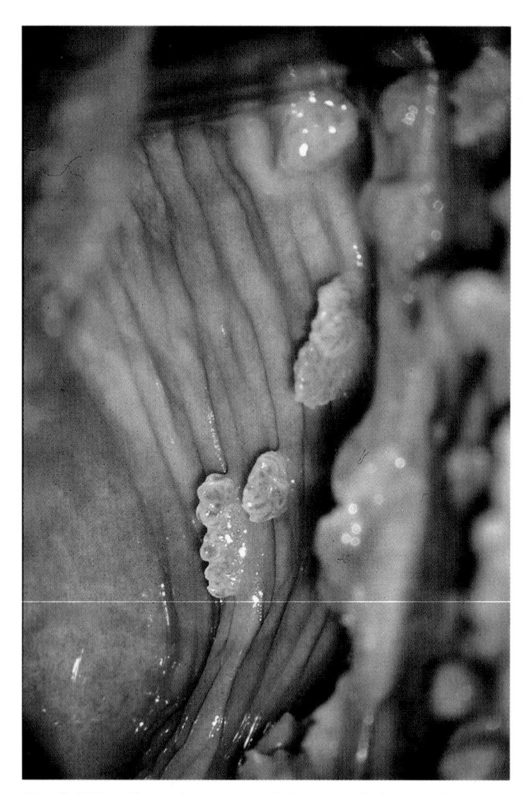

Fig. 7.**102** Acuminate condylomas of the vagina in a 23-year-old patient.

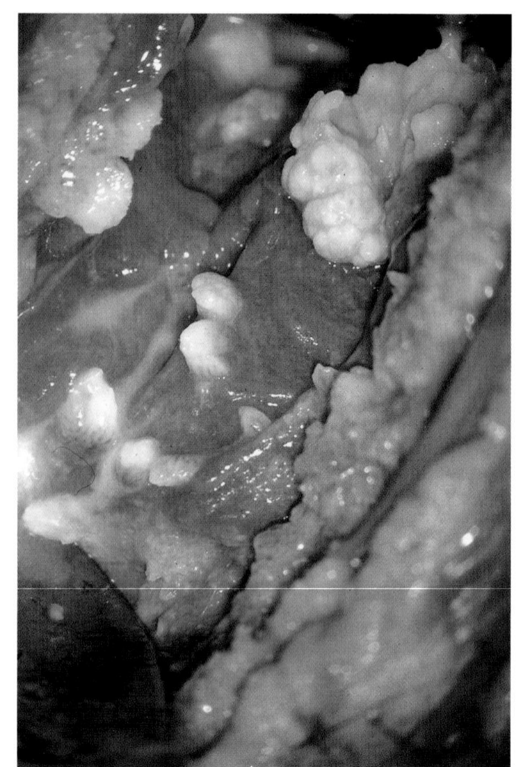

Fig. 7.**103** Pronounced condylomas of the vagina in a 20-year-old patient during the 21st week of pregnancy.

Therapy. Treatment in the vaginal region is rarely necessary. Close monitoring and punch biopsy serve to reassure both physician and patient.

For details, please refer to the discussion of vulvar infections caused by papillomaviruses (see p. 94 ff.).

Differential diagnosis. In case of papillomatosis, the vagina and also the vaginal orifice are strikingly rough. In contrast to condylomas (Fig. 7.**102**), small papillae (hirsuties) completely cover the entire vagina (Fig. 7.**69**, p. 100). In case of doubt, a biopsy will confirm the diagnosis. The detection of HPV-specific DNA by means of highly sensitive tests does not influence the diagnosis of papillomatosis, for subclinical HPV infections are common and may exist at the same time.

Vaginitis Caused by Protozoa

Trichomoniasis

This is a typical vaginal infection. In recent times, however, trichomonads have become rather rare in developed countries, Therefore, they are sometimes no longer considered and thus easily overlooked. They are only detected by gynecologists during microscopic examination. Trichomonads from the usual swab material shipped in transport medium can no longer be stained; hence, they are not detected during routine bacteriology. If the diagnosis is established only by the time the cytologist gets involved—which is often the case—this does not reflect well on the examiner as the sensitivity of cytology is only 50 %, at best.

Pathogen. *Trichomonas vaginalis.*

Frequency. Worldwide, this is one of the most common sexually transmitted infections with > 300 million patients per year. In developed countries , it is now rather rare, with perhaps 0.1–0.3 % of gynecological patients being infected (depending on the patient population).

Clinical picture. The main symptom is discharge, which is green/yellow and foamy in the extreme case. The consistency is usually thin, sometimes sticky. Among the complaints, burning is more severe than itching. The vagina and portio vaginalis are always reddened (Fig. 7.**104**) and often show irregular large, red spots (Fig. 7.**105 a**) or lesions that are reminiscent of those in genital herpes (Fig. 7.**105 b**). The infection causes dysuria if the vulva and the urethra are severely affected.

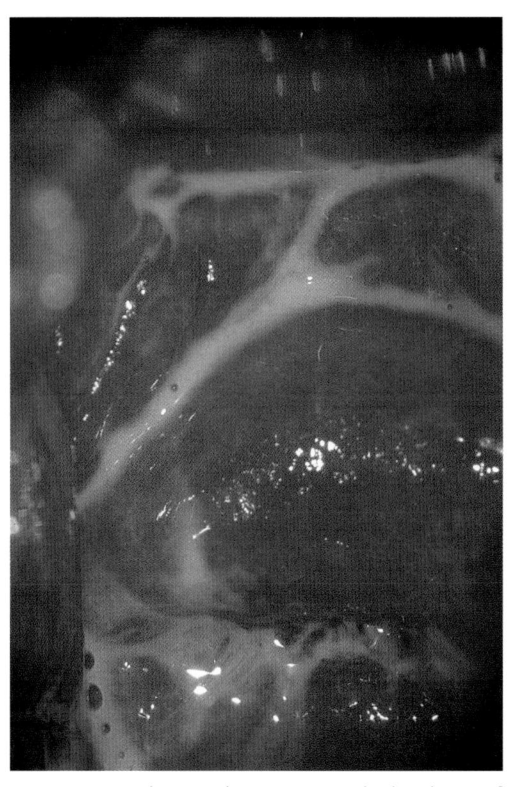

Fig. 7.**104** Trichonomal vaginitis. Marked redness of the vagina and vulva, associated with a yellowish bubbly discharge.

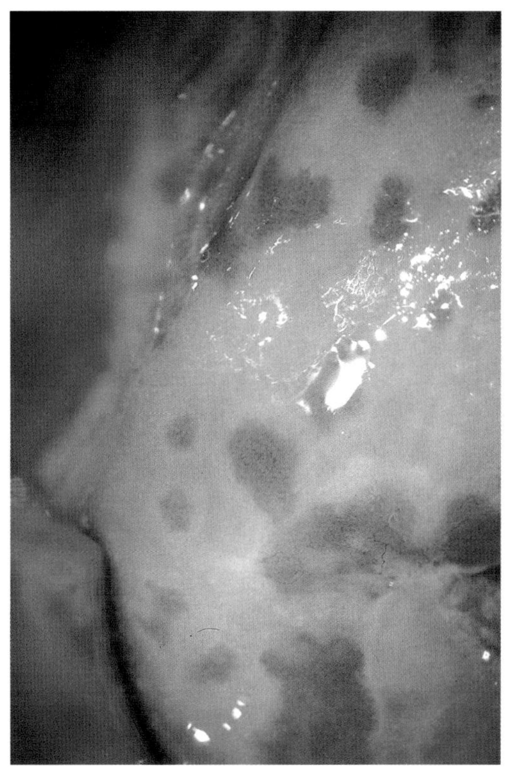

Fig. 7.**105 a** Trichomoniasis with spotlike redness (macular/granular vaginitis).

In men, these complaints are much rarer, and some women do not feel affected at all.

Many patients complain of offensive odor. In the majority of patients, this odor is caused by simultaneously existing bacterial vaginosis. Trichomonads produce a characteristic odor as well, but it is different from that of bacterial vaginosis. Although rarely the case, *Trichomonas* infection is also possible if the lactobacillus flora is normal. Still, trichomoniasis without any increase in the number of leukocytes does not exist.

Trichomoniasis can be very severe and is then associated with considerable discomfort. However, it may also persist over months and years without any symptoms, only to resurface with symptoms when circumstances favor the disease. When there is equilibrium between the body's defenses and the trichomonads' ability to multiply, the number of trichomonads may be so low that they are neither noticed by the patient nor detected by the physician. Any disturbance of the vaginal milieu—through other infections, wound exudation after surgery, or necrotic material derived from a carcinoma of the endocervix or body of uterus—can lead to an increased multiplication of trichomonads and, therefore, to clinical symptoms.

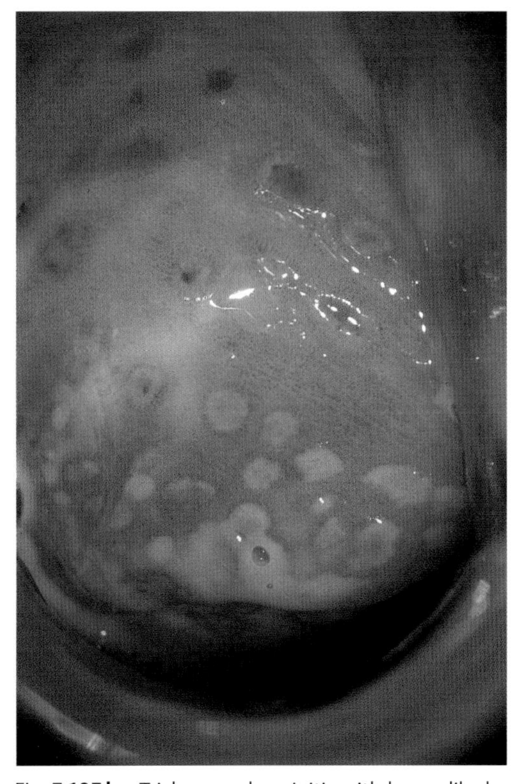

Fig. 7.**105 b** Trichomonal vaginitis with herpeslike lesions. The disease was diagnosed only after 6 months.

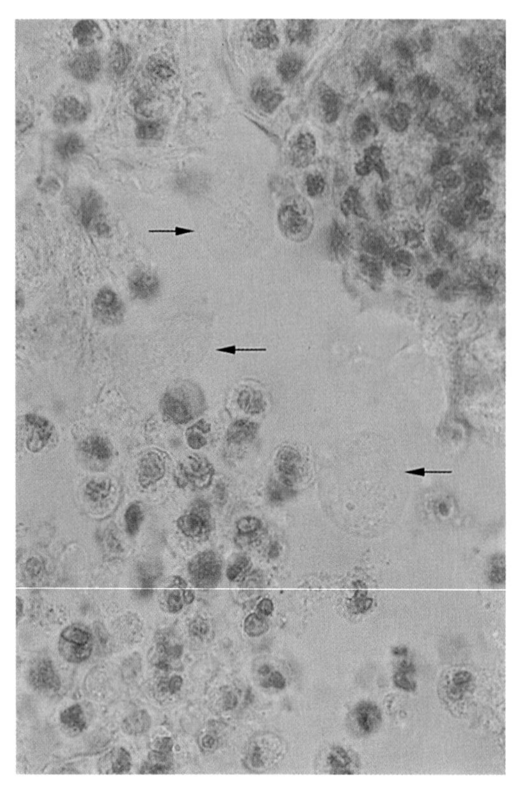

Fig. 7.**106** Micrograph illustrating trichomonal vaginitis. Wet mount of discharge in 0.1 % methylene blue. Apart from numerous leukocytes, three faint trichomonads (arrows) can be identified in middle of the picture.

Diagnosis:

- *Clinical picture.* There is a yellow, sometimes foamy discharge (Fig. 7.**104**) with the pH value usually raised to > 5, and this is often associated with spotlike redness (vaginitis macularis; Fig. 7.**105 a**).
- *Microscopy (sensitivity 50 %).* The wet mount always contains plenty of granulocytes. However, only the presence of jerking trichomonads with their characteristic flagellar movements is proof of an infection. The parasites are slightly larger than a leukocyte (Fig. 7.**106**). In about 80 % of patients, the lactobacillus flora is absent, and small bacteria and clue cells are visible. If trichomoniasis is suspected, the discharge should be diluted with sodium chloride solution because trichomonads are quickly inactivated by 0.1 % methylene blue solution. The preparation should be kept warm, which is achieved by just letting it lie under the microscope with the light switched on. In case of severe vaginitis—which is rather rare—it is recommended that some of the discharge is removed with a syringe to allow for the preparation of a fresh wet mount at the end of the gynecological examination, if necessary, or for further bacteriological examination of the discharge.
- *Phase contrast microscopy* of the unstained wet mount is the best method for recognizing trichomonads. It is superior to examination by normal microscopy and staining with 0.1 % methylene blue solution.
- *Culture (sensitivity 60–85 %).* Cultivation of trichomonads increases the rate of detection almost by a factor of two. However, this requires special culture media and experience.
- *Cytology.* In the cytological smear stained according to Papanicolaou, trichomonads are fairly easy to recognize. They are slightly larger than leukocytes and exhibit 10–20 red dots within their blue cytoplasm (Fig. 7.**107 a**).
- *DNA detection (sensitivity 85–98 %).* This is the most reliable detection method for trichomonads. It is performed by means of a DNA test (Affirm III, available from Becton and Dickens), though this test is offered only by very few physicians and laboratories.
- *Special staining methods (sensitivity 50–65 %).* They allow for good visualization of trichomonads also in smear preparations (Fig. 7.**107 b**). Gram stain (Fig. 7.**107 c**) or methylene blue staining are less suited for the recognition of trichomonads, and even the experienced examiner has occasionally difficulties in finding them in such preparations.

Therapy. The drugs of choice are 5-nitroimidazoles (metronidazole, tinidazole). The majority of these compounds are suited for oral, vaginal, rectal, and intravenous administration.

Oral therapy by a single high dose of 2 g has gained acceptance during recent years, as compared with the original therapy with lower doses over eight to 10 days. Single-dose therapy yields healing rates of far more than 90 %. Topical application often fails because it does not reach all regions that may contain trichomonads. In case of treatment failure, the oral dose may be increased (doubled).

The following preparations are available for single-dose therapy:

- metronidazole, 2 g orally
- tinidazole (also for treating the partner), 2 g orally.

Antiseptics—such as polyvidone iodine, dequalinium chloride, hexetidine, nifutel—also reduce trichomonads, but they lead to moderate healing rates only after prolonged application (more than 10 days). Clotrimazole and vaginal vitamin C are, to a certain extent, also effective against trichomonads.

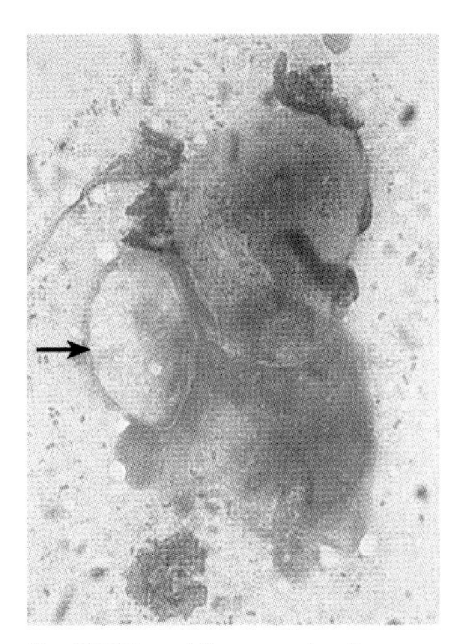

Fig. 7.**107 a** Micrograph of a trichomonad (arrow) in a Papanicolaou-stained smear.

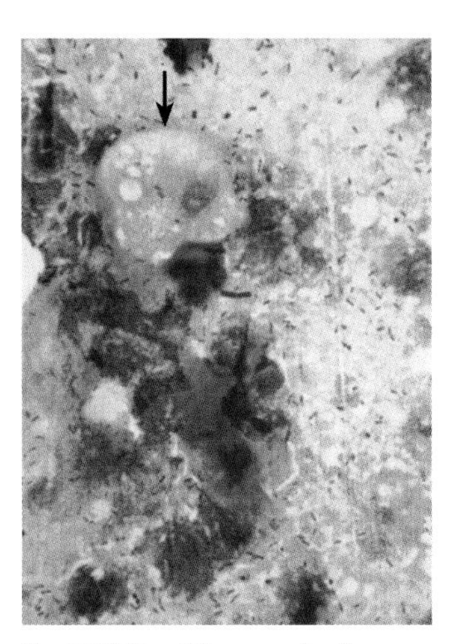

Fig. 7.**107 b** Micrograph of a trichomonad (arrow) in a Giemsa-stained smear. Trichomonads are recognized by their vacuolated cytoplasm.

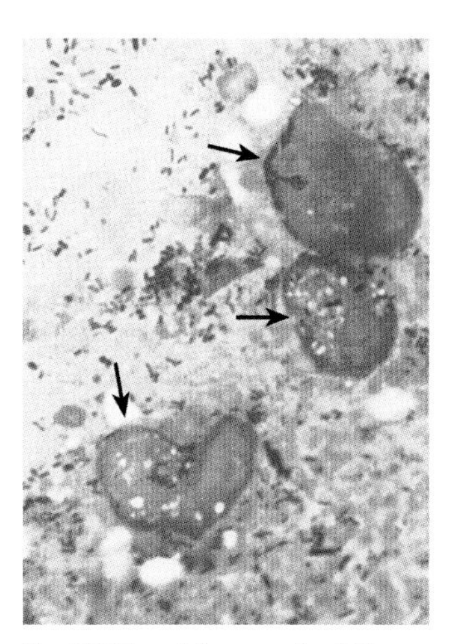

Fig. 7.**107 c** Micrograph of three trichomonads (arrows) in a Gram-stained smear.

Approach to Chronic Recurrent Trichomoniasis

- It is essential to treat the partner as well, even if no trichomonads can be detected (trichomonads are far more difficult to detect in men than in women).
- The dose is doubled and, in particularly stubborn cases, repeated the next day.

Neither intravenous application nor prolonged treatment offer any advantage.

It is assumed that there are no trichomonads that are resistant to 5-nitroimidazoles. Nevertheless, some strains of *Trichomonas* are killed only by high drug concentration. Occasionally, it may be necessary to switch to another compound.

Treatment of the *sexual partner* is always required.

Treatment of Trichomoniasis During Pregnancy

Metronidazole and tinidazole are the drugs of choice also during pregnancy; they can be administered after the 14th week of pregnancy. Topical treatment may be applied, since only about 20% of the substance is resorbed by the body. In case of treatment failure, oral therapy may start from the 20th week of pregnancy onward (see p. 215).

There is no evidence that trichomonads themselves lead to premature births or that trichomonads pose a risk for the child. Still, the vaginal flora in women with trichomoniasis is frequently disturbed, and this most likely explains the increased risk of premature births in these women.

Vaginitis Caused by Bacteria

Plasma Cell Vaginitis (Purulent Vaginitis)

This is mostly a chronic, pronounced vaginitis that is easily confused with trichomoniasis because of the symptoms and the copious amounts of yellow discharge. It is not cured by metronidazole. It is a form of vaginitis that persists after other pathogens have been either excluded or treated. Presumably, it is not a uniform entity. Nevertheless, 90% of the patients can be cured with clindamycin.

Pathogen. No pathogens can be detected. However, because this form of vaginitis can be cured by an antibiotic (administered topically or orally), it is assumed to be a bacterial infection.

Incidence. Unknown, but it is estimated at 0.1%. The disease occurs between age 20 and age 60, with a slight prevalence at premenopause.

Clinical picture. Typically, the patient's history reveals chronic yellow discharge for months or years and many attempts to treat it with various antibiotics or anti-infectives. There is considerable tenderness to touch if the vulva is also affected. The vagina exhibits a diffuse (Fig. 7.**108**) or, more often, spotty redness with flat nodules that are occasionally slightly punctate (Fig. 7.**109**). The pH value of the copious yellow, viscous discharge is between 4.5 and 6.0. The overall picture is reminiscent of trichomoniasis. Microscopy reveals > 100 leukocytes per field of view, and often also an undefined, mixed flora

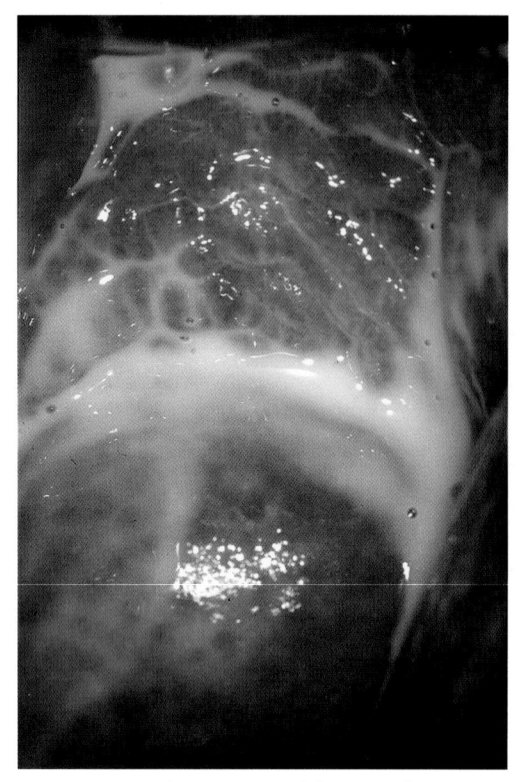

Fig. 7.**108** Purulent vaginitis (plasma cell vaginitis) with marked redness and putrid discharge in a 32-year-old patient.

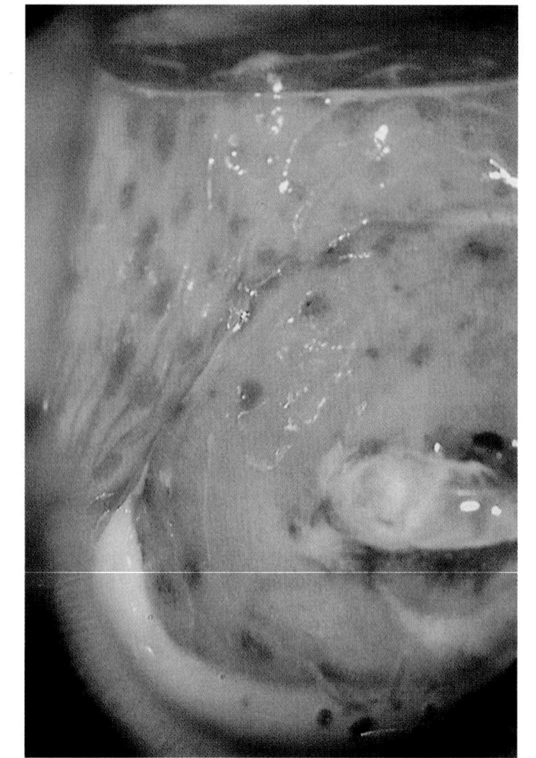

Fig. 7.**109** Purulent vaginitis (plasma cell vaginitis) without pathogen detection in a 24-year-old patient. No improvement after estrogen administration or metronidazole therapy.

and immature epithelial cells (Fig. 7.**110**). Even when examining optimal wet mounts without methylene blue, no motile trichomonads are visible. Treatment attempts with metronidazole do not bring any improvement.

Diagnosis:

- ▶ *Patient's history.* Persistent yellowish discharge, sometimes for months and years.
- ▶ *Clinical picture.* Diffuse or spotty redness (Fig. 7.**109**).
- ▶ *Acetic acid test.* Evidence of mosaic, punctuation, and spotty hyperkeratosis (Fig. 7.**111**).
- ▶ *Microscopy.* Vast numbers of leukocytes (> 100 per visual field at 400× magnification), intermediate cells (Fig. 7.**110**), varying bacterial flora.
- ▶ *Histology.* Possibly plasma cells beneath the rete ridge.

Therapy:

As an initial treatment:

- ▶ clindamycin, topical application as a cream, once daily for one week.

In case of treatment failure or relapse:

- ▶ clindamycin, topical application as a cream once daily for two to three weeks.

Unfortunately, relapses do occur. For this reason, a check-up immediately following the therapy is recommended, for the diagnosis can only be confirmed if the condition is cured by the treatment (i. e., the discharge no longer contains leukocytes). Fading of the redness may take a bit longer.

Supportive measures:

- ▶ estrogen suppositories to strengthen the epithelium
- ▶ vaginal vitamin C tablets to build up the lactobacillus flora (clindamycin inhibits also lactobacilli while it spares *Escherichia coli*)
- ▶ skin care with ointments containing lavender, oil and vitamin E.

Vaginitis Caused by Group A Streptococci

Though this is not a very common form of vaginitis, this infection should be taken very seriously because of the pathogen. Sometimes it cannot be distinguished clinically from trichomoniasis or plasma cell vaginitis, as illustrated by Figs. 7.**112** and 7.**113**.

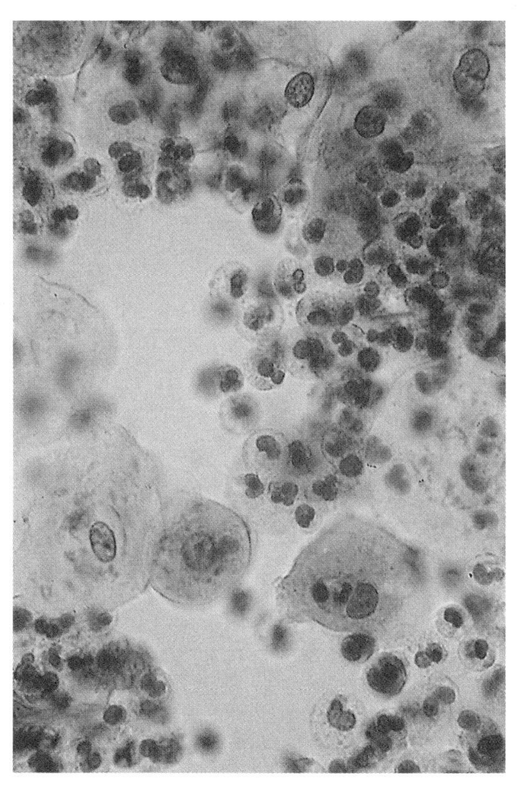

Fig. 7.**110** Micrograph of discharge stained with 0.1 % methylene blue. The abundance of leukocytes and the presence of parabasal cells are characteristic of purulent vaginitis (plasma cell vaginitis) without a known pathogen.

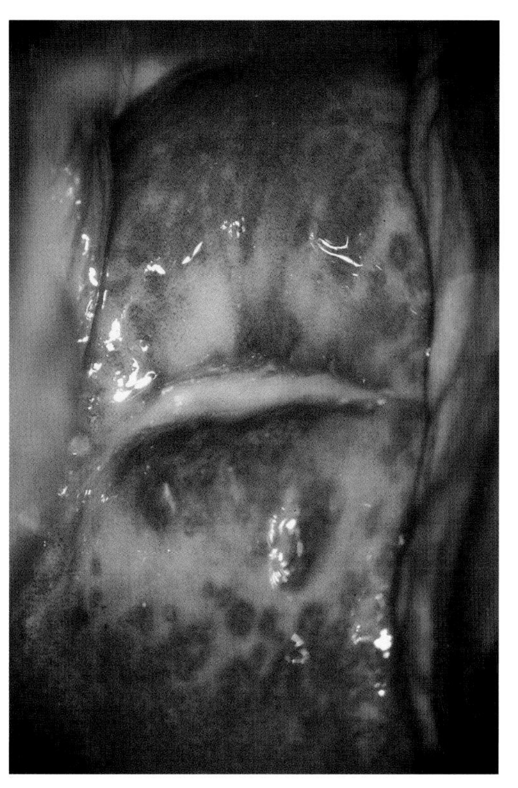

Fig. 7.**111** Purulent vaginitis (plasma cell vaginitis) in a 36-year-old patient, after application of acetic acid.

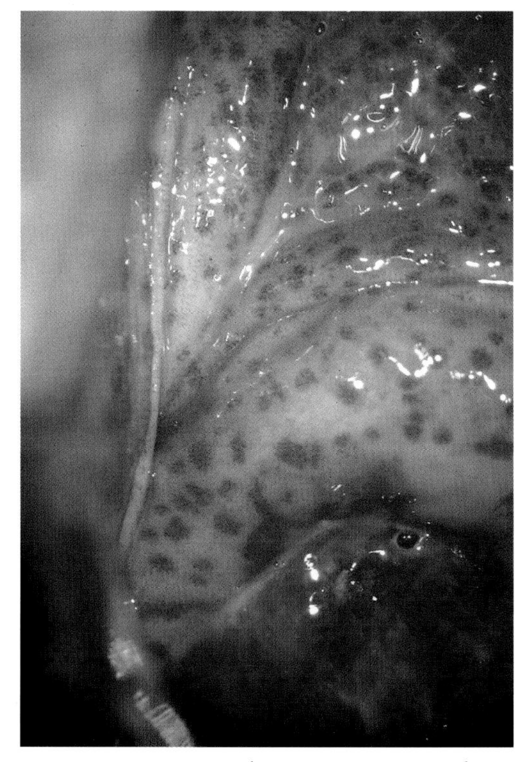

Fig. 7.**112** Vaginitis with intense spotty redness, caused by group A streptococci in a 30-year-old patient.

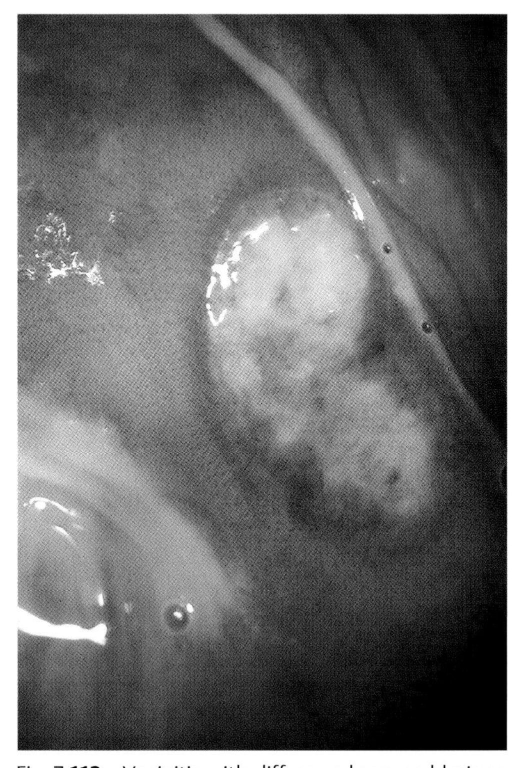

Fig. 7.**113** Vaginitis with diffuse redness and lesions, caused by group A streptococci in a 38-year-old patient.

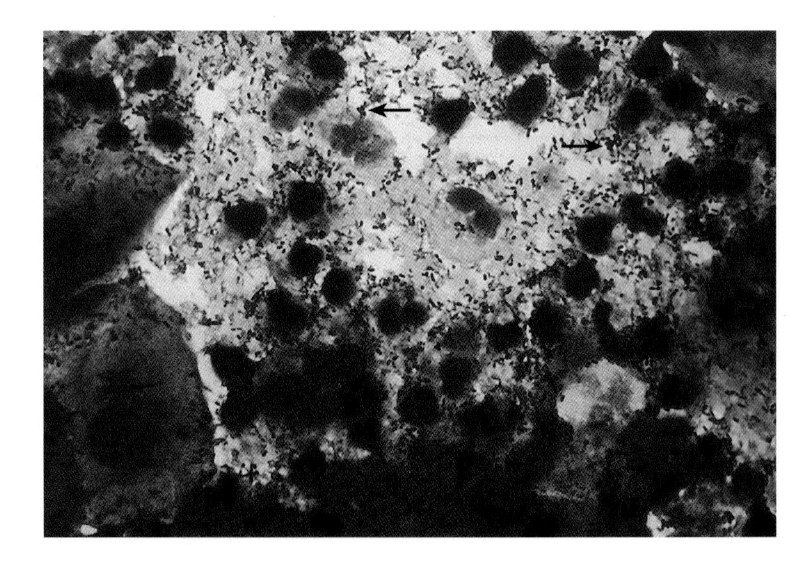

Fig. 7.**114** Micrograph illustrating vaginitis caused by group A streptococci (arrows). The smear shows an abundance of granulocytes and mixed flora (Gram stain).

Pathogen. Group A streptococci.

Incidence. No statistics are available. Depending on the patient population, it is estimated that the incidence might be 0.1–0.3 % of outpatients and thus ranges in the same order of magnitude as that of trichomoniasis and plasma cell vaginitis.

Transmission. Smear infection from oral to genital regions and during sexual contacts. Up to 5 % of children and slightly fewer symptomfree adults carry group A streptococci in the nasopharyngeal space.

Clinical picture. Symptoms in the form of burning and discharge are usually present, and there is always redness of the vagina (Fig. 7.**113**) and, in most patients, also of the vulva. Frequently, the vagina also shows red spots (Abb. 7.**112**). The yellow discharge always contains increased numbers of leukocytes (50–150 per field of view at 400× magnification). Symptoms can be easily confused with those of trichomoniasis (Figs. 7.**104**, 7.**105**, p. 117) and plasma cell vaginitis (Figs. 7.**108**, 7.**109**, p. 120).

Diagnosis. Diagnosis is established exclusively through detection of the pathogen in cultures:

- *Microscopy.* Plenty of granulocytes and cocci (wet mounts in 0.1 % methylene blue solution; Fig. 7.**28**, p. 81) or Gram stain (Fig. 7.**114**).
- *Culture*
- An antibiogram is usually not required because resistance is rare.

Therapy. Antibiotic treatment is indicated whenever group A streptococci are detected in the vagina, for this pathogen may cause the most severe infections.

Penicillin, amoxicillin, or cephalosporin for 10 days.

Bacteriological confirmation of pathogen elimination is recommended. In case of recurrent infections with group A streptococci, one should search for the source, e. g., family members who need to be treated as well.

Vaginitis Caused by Staphylococcus aureus

Staphylococcus aureus belongs to those pathogenic bacteria that are usually not present in the vagina. It may cause vaginitis, but this is not necessarily so. Treatment is advised in case of vaginitis (Fig. 7.**115**) or if the symptoms are associated with the detection of *S. aureus* (Fig. 7.**116**). Because of the limited pathogenicity, one may attempt topical treatment with disinfectants. The pathogen must be eliminated from the vagina prior to surgery or during pregnancy.

Bacterial Vaginosis

Synonyms: aminovaginosis, anaerobic vaginosis, nonspecific vaginitis, *Gardnerella vaginalis* vaginitis.

The term bacterial *vaginitis*, which has been used as a synonym for nonspecific vaginitis (1983), has been changed to bacterial *vaginosis* because this condition is not a true vaginitis but only a bacterial disturbance of the vaginal flora. Because of the characteristic odor of amines produced by many anaerobes, the term "aminovaginosis" is also used in some countries. There are

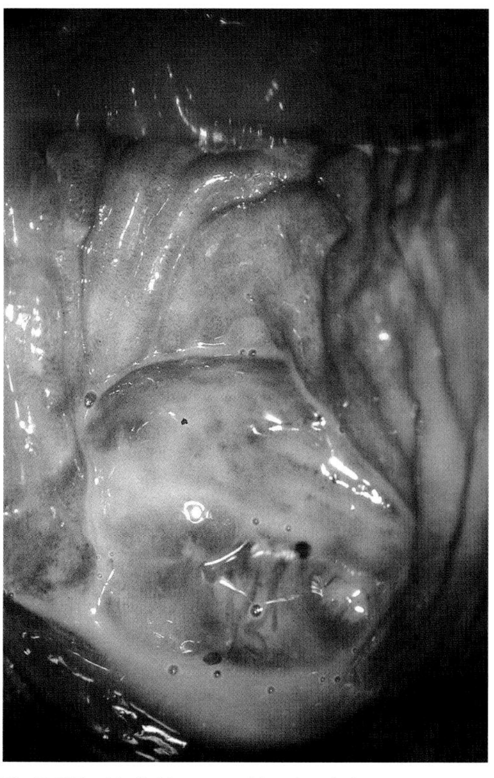

Fig. 7.**115** Vaginitis caused by *Staphylococcus aureus* in a 25-year-old patient.

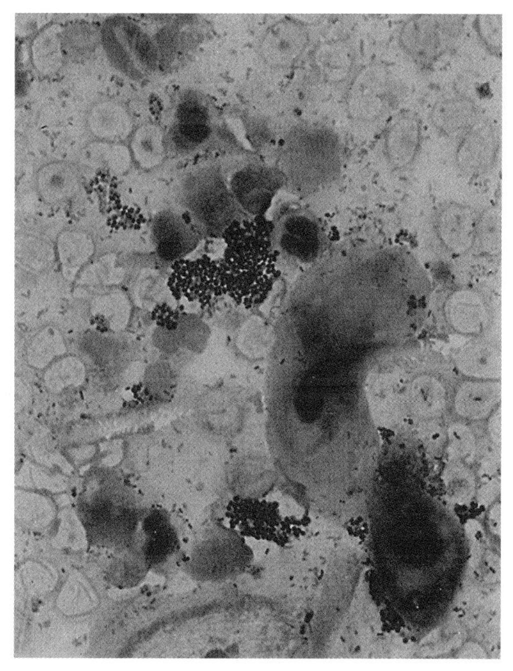

Fig. 7.**116** Micrograph illustrating vaginitis caused by *Staphylococcus aureus* in a 55-year-old patient. Wet mount of discharge, showing numerous staphylococci (Gram stain).

other forms of a disturbed vaginal flora with or without inflammation, but none of them produces enough amines to cause a noticeable odor.

Pathogen. High counts (10^7–10^9/mL) of *Gardnerella vaginalis* and various anaerobes from the intestinal tract. The composition of these bacteria changes; often six or more different bacterial species are found in the culture.

Common anaerobes include species of the family *Bacteroidaceae*:

- *Porphyromonas* (formerly *Bacteroides*) *asaccharolyticus*
- *Prevotella* (formerly *Bacteroides*) *melaninogenicus, bivius, corrodens, disiens*
- Possibly *Bacteroides fragilis* (found only rarely)
- *Peptococcus* species
- *Peptostreptococcus* species
- *Fusobacterium nucleatum* (odor of butyric acid)
- *Mobiluncus* species
- *Veillonella parvula* (family: *Veillonellaceae*).

Aerobic microbes (streptococci of groups B, C, D, F, staphylococci, *Escherichia coli*, *Proteus*) and mycoplasmas (*Mycoplasma hominis*, *Ureaplasma urealyticum*) as well as yeasts are also found more often and in higher numbers when the vaginal flora is disturbed. This reflects the higher risk of exposure as well as better growth conditions.

Transmission and pathogenesis. Bacterial vaginosis is a disturbance of the vaginal flora and comes about by the synergism between *Gardnerella vaginalis* and various anaerobes. While *Gardnerella vaginalis* can be detected in about 40% of all women even at high germ counts (> 10^5/mL), anaerobes without *Gardnerella vaginalis* are hardly ever found in such high numbers in the vagina.

Certain metabolites (e. g., succinate) of *Gardnerella vaginalis* seem to promote the growth of anaerobic bacteria. If the lactobacillus flora is not able to stop the intensified growth of anaerobes, lactobacilli progressively decline in numbers and anaerobes take over until the clinical picture of bacterial vaginosis is complete.

Alkalizing events—such as wound exudation, necrotic tissue, or bleeding—as well as antibiotic therapy, which destroys the protective lactobacillus flora, promote the development of bacterial vaginosis. Bacterial vaginosis does not develop in the absence of estrogens because high concentrations of bacteria cannot build up without the availability of certain nutrients.

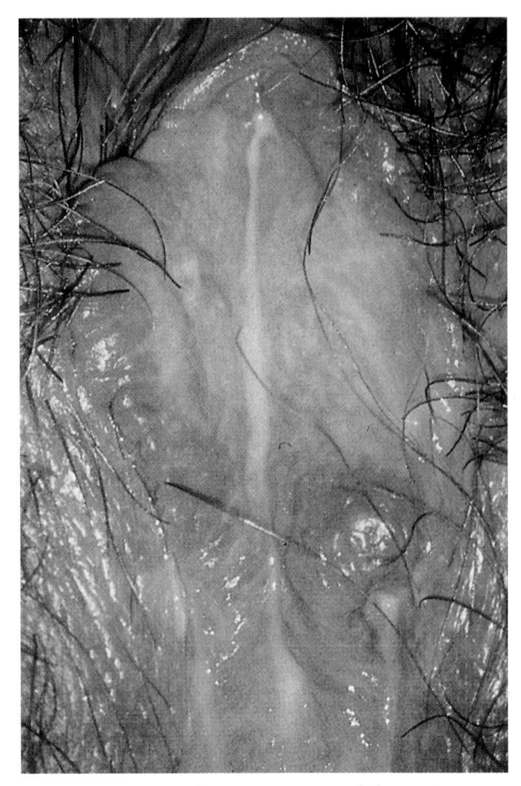

Fig. 7.**117** Bacterial vaginosis. One of the main symptoms is a liquid discharge that gives the patient the sensation of wetness.

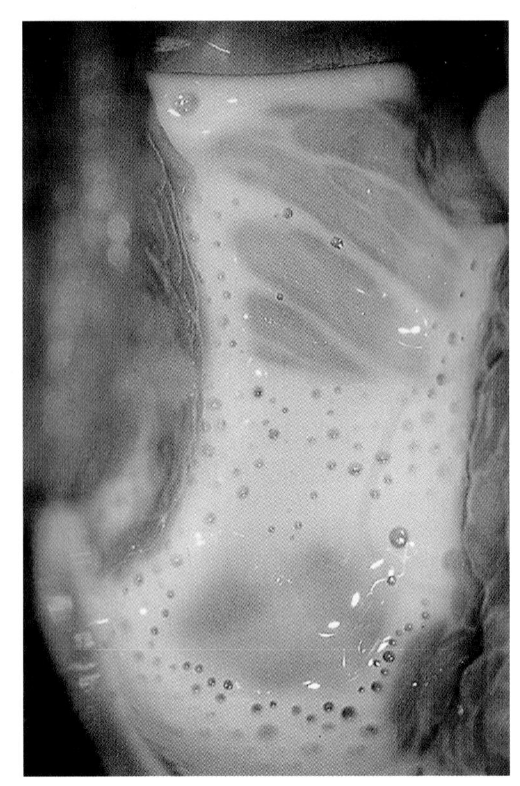

Fig. 7.**118** Bubbly discharge due to bacterial vaginosis in a 28-year-old patient during the 30th week of pregnancy.

Apart from this, the participating bacteria must have been introduced, and sexual contact plays a major role here by transporting the patient's microbes from the perianal region into the vagina, on the one hand, and by introducing the additional flora from the partner, on the other.

Bacterial vaginosis is therefore more common in women who have several sexual partners than in those who have no sexual contact or only one stable partnership. However, even in the latter group, recurrent bacterial vaginosis may develop in individual patients.

One of the main causes of recurrent bacterial vaginosis is colonization of the vagina with atypical lactobacilli. These bacteria look like lactobacilli under the microscope, but they are biochemically different because of their metabolism. Studies have also shown that the affected women are colonized predominantly by lactobacilli that are unable to produce hydrogen peroxide, which is an inhibitor of anaerobes.

Clinical picture. Bacterial vaginosis is the most common bacterial disturbance of the vaginal flora and is found in 5–8% of women. For many women, it represents only an aesthetic problem that is bothersome because of its fishy odor and the sensation of wetness (due to discharge) (Fig. 7.**117**). The wet feeling is usually also present when the amount of discharge is hardly increased. Proteases derived from the anaerobic bacteria degrade the protective mucus, thus making the discharge watery. Degradation of cervical secretion facilitates the intrusion of certain bacteria and their ascent in the internal genitals. If fusobacteria are present, an additional unpleasant odor of butyric acid develops. The intensity of the disturbance may vary significantly, depending on the concentration of undesirable bacteria and on the consistency and amount of the discharge. In an extreme case, the discharge is thin and bubbly (Fig. 7.**118**). In many patients, it is rather creamy; as a result, only its increased pH value lets one suspect bacterial vaginosis.

Risks posed by bacterial vaginosis. Apart from troubling the patient, bacterial vaginosis plays a special role as an increased risk during pregnancy, namely, regarding premature births as well as perinatal and puerperal infections. In addition, the microbes causing bacterial vaginosis may facilitate the ascent of gonococci or chlamydiae and may themselves reach into higher

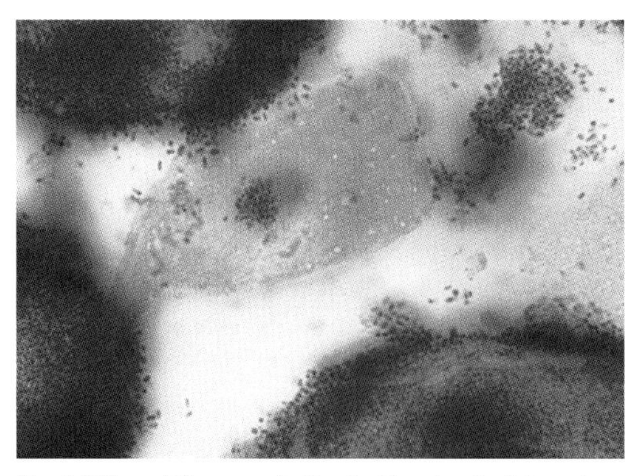

Fig. 7.**119 a** Micrograph illustrating bacterial vaginosis. Wet mount of discharge stained with 0.1 % methylene blue, showing clue-cells covered with *Gardnerella vaginalis*.

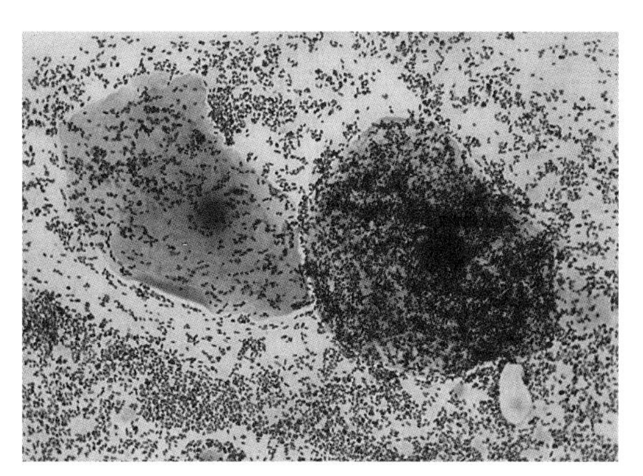

Fig. 7.**119 b** Micrograph of a similar preparation after Gram staining, showing clue cells and masses of small bacteria.

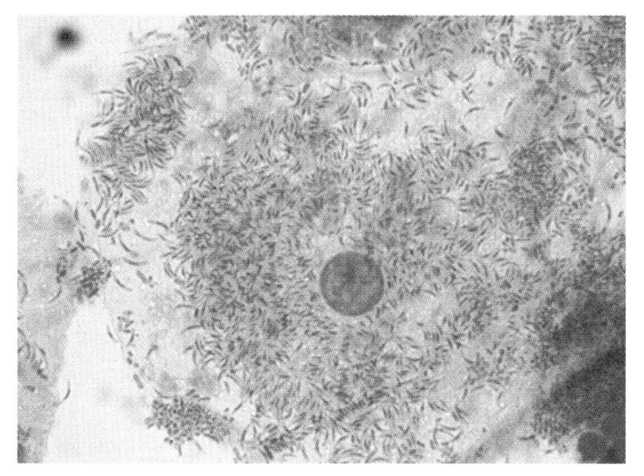

Fig. 7.**120 a** Micrograph illustrating bacterial vaginosis. Wet mount of discharge stained with 0.1 % methylene blue, showing an epithelial cell covered with *Mobiluncus*.

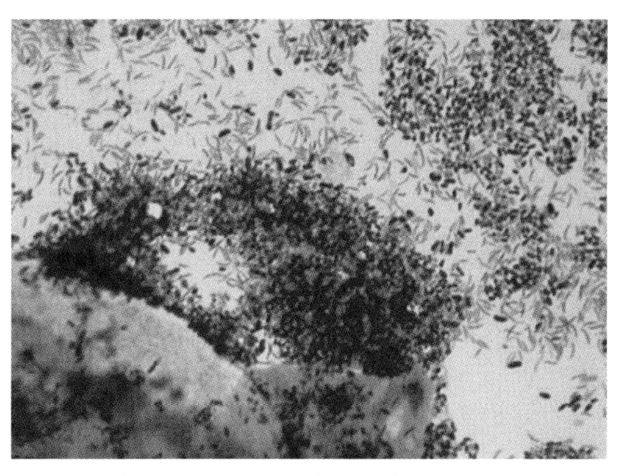

Fig. 7.**120 b** Micrograph of a similar preparation after Gram staining, showing *Mobiluncus, Gardnerella vaginalis,* and other bacteria.

regions where they may induce or support severe, partly abscess-forming infections. Since the pathogenic potential of the microbes causing bacterial vaginosis is low, infectious complications are fortunately far less common than the disturbance itself.

Diagnosis:

- *Clinical picture.* The discharge is white (rarely gray), creamy, bubbly (rarely foamy).
- *pH value.* With bacterial vaginosis, the pH is between 4.8 and 5.5 (pH strips from Merck, product No. 9542), whereas a normal lactobacillus flora is associated with a pH between 3.8 and 4.5, depending on lactobacilli numbers.
- *Amine test.* The fishy odor associated with bacterial vaginosis is caused by amines produced by anaerobic bacteria. The odor is only noticeable when these bacteria are present in high numbers. Addition of one to two drops of 10 % potassium hydroxide solution to the discharge on a cotton swab or microscopic slide intensifies the fishy odor.
- *Microscopy.* Clue cells are visible in wet mounts (Fig. 7.**119 a**) and less clearly in gram-stained preparations (Fig. **119 b**). These are cells from the vaginal epithelium that are covered with a dense layer of small bacteria, most often *Gardnerella vaginalis.* The epithelial cells may also be covered with other bacteria, for example, *Mobiluncus*, fusobacteria, and cocci. They are especially easy to recognize in the wet mount after staining with 0.1 % methylene blue solution. In addition to clue cells, a high count of small, morphologically distinguishable bacteria is also characteristic for bacterial vaginosis; for example, curved gram-negative bacteria like *Mobiluncus* (Fig. 7.**120 a, b**) are easily identified in a wet mount by their spinning movements. Very long, thin, and straight bacteria with pointed ends are also seen occasionally; these are fusobacteria. The methylene blue stain allows only a distinction according to shape and size, whereas it is possible to differentiate between gram-positive and gram-negative bacteria in preparations stained with the Gram method.

- *Culture.* Detection of *Gardnerella vaginalis* and anaerobic bacteria is possible in culture. In normal cases of bacterial vaginosis, culturing bacteria is not very meaningful: because of the multitude of microbes and the costly method, the diagnostic procedures are out of proportion as compared with the simple and problemfree therapy.

Cultures are required only in special cases or when other pathogenic microbes need to be excluded (e. g., gonococci, group A streptococci). A culture may also be helpful if the normal flora is not restored despite treatment with 5-nitroimidazoles.

- *Gas chromatography.* Special detection of typical metabolites of *Gardnerella vaginalis* and anaerobic bacteria.

Therapy. The treatment of choice is with 5-nitroimidazoles. Depending on how severe the disturbance is, what additional promoting factors are present, and to what extent the normal vaginal flora is able to recover, different forms of intensive and long-term therapy may be required.

The following therapeutic options are available:

Oral chemotherapy (used rather rarely):
- *single-dose therapy* (2 g of metronidazole or tinidazole)
- five-day therapy (2 × 400/500 mg of metronidazole per day)
- amoxicillin (3 × 750 mg per day, over five days)
- clindamycin.

Topical/vaginal chemotherapy (preferred today):
- single-dose therapy (500 mg or 1000 mg of metronidazole) is usually sufficient if supportive measures are taken, such as acidification, vulvar and anal care
- five-day therapy (1 × 500 mg of metronidazole per day)
- five-day therapy (2 × 100 mg of metronidazole per day)
- metronidazole gel (2 × 37.5 mg per day, over five days)
- clindamycin cream (over three to seven days).

Other (nonchemotherapeutic) topical treatments:
- vitamin C (vaginal delayed-release tablets)
- antiseptics: dequalinium chloride, hexetidine, nifuratel
- lactic acid preparations (5 %)
- *Lactobacillus* preparations.

The best healing rates (up to 95 %) are observed with 5-nitroimidazoles. The rate with amoxicillin is about 70 %. Nonchemotherapeutic preparations yield a healing rate of 50–80 %.

One problem with treating bacterial vaginosis is the high *relapse rate.* In case of a stable partner relationship, treating also the partner may bring better results—although this is not yet recommended because there is no evidence from studies. A form of treatment is therefore selected that is less burdensome for the patient and is also better accepted, namely, topical treatment. Here, too, the highest healing rates are achieved by high-dose therapy with metronidazole, which is best suited for short-term treatment. Vaginal vitamin C delayed-release tablets are best accepted for permanent treatment.

Approach to Recurrent Bacterial Vaginosis

- Questions regarding sexual habits. The cause is obvious in case of anal intercourse.
- Improvement of anal hygiene, see p. 66.
- Single-dose therapy: vaginal treatment with 500 mg metronidazole. This is followed by repeated acidification of the vagina with vitamin C delayed-release tablets at the end of menstruation for about six days. Acidification accelerates the growth of desirable lactobacilli, thus preventing relapses that usually occur after menstruation.

Detection and Incidence of Other Bacteria in the Vagina

Mycoplasmas

It has been repeatedly suspected that vaginitis may be caused by mycoplasmas. However, mycoplasmas do not seem to be able to induce inflammatory reactions, and mycoplasmas have never been identified as the cause of vaginitis. Mycoplasmas are typical colonizing organisms that are detected most often when the vaginal flora is disturbed. After successful treatment of bacterial vaginosis with metronidazole—which is ineffective against mycoplasmas—mycoplasmas also disappear once the vaginal flora is normal again.

In men, mycoplasmas are assumed to be involved in urethritis and prostatitis, which is why the partners of infected men show up for examination. As mycoplasmas are common colonizing microbes, it is not clear whether any detected mycoplasmas are indeed the cause of disease.

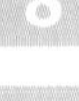

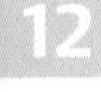
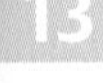

***Mycoplasma* species:**

- ▶ *Mycoplasma hominis*
- ▶ *Mycoplasma genitalium*
- ▶ *Ureaplasma urealyticum* (urea-hydrolyzing mycoplasma)
- ▶ *Mycoplasma pneumoniae.*

Frequency. *Mycoplasma hominis* is found at low counts (10^3/mL) in 5–10% of all women, and *Ureaplasma urealyticum* in about 40% of all women. There are no data available for *Mycoplasma genitalium.*

Clinical picture. Typical symptoms are not known, and there are no clear clinical findings (possibly discharge). In rare cases, mycoplasmas may cause severe infections with inflammatory reactions, or they may be involved in such infections. *Mycoplasma genitalium* is thought to be detected more frequently in connection with inflammatory processes.

Diagnosis:

- ▶ *Culture.* Mycoplasmas can only be detected by culturing. They grow particularly well on special agar media, especially during anaerobic incubation, and form typical colonies within two to four days (daisy-head colonies in case of *Mycoplasma hominis*). So far, only very few specialized laboratories are able to identify *Mycoplasma genitalium.*
- ▶ *Serology* is not important for infection of the genital region, but rather for pulmonary diseases.

Therapy. Treatment is only justified if there are complaints and mycoplasmas are the only microbes found at high counts (10^5/mL). Another reason for treatment is the repeated detection of mycoplasmas in the vagina of women without symptoms if their partners show symptoms (e. g., prostatitis):

- ▶ doxycycline (tetracyclines)
- ▶ erythromycin (effective only against *Ureaplasma urealyticum*)
- ▶ azithromycin (particularly effective against *Mycoplasma genitalium*)
- ▶ clindamycin (very effective against *Mycoplasma hominis* but not against *Ureaplasma urealyticum*)
- ▶ fluoroquinolones.

The duration of treatment should be 10–14 days.

The role of mycoplasmas during pregnancy—for example, as a cause of premature birth—has not yet been clearly established. As mycoplasmas are frequently present in the vagina, their detection in the discharge does not help with the recognition of an impending premature birth. On the other hand, increased counts of mycoplasmas have been detected by some examiners in the amniotic fluid and in the fetal membranes of premature births.

Intestinal Bacteria and Skin Bacteria in the Vagina

Due to the resistance of the vaginal epithelium, intestinal bacteria do not play a role as a cause of vaginitis. Bacteria of various kinds are frequently found in the vagina, at low or even high concentration, due to the close proximity to the anus. However, they do not normally lead to any signs of inflammation. Skin bacteria, such as propionibacteria or *Staphylococcus epidermidis*, are often also found in the vagina, but they are harmless. In recurrent urinary tract infections, intestinal bacteria are frequently detected at high counts on the vulva and in the vaginal orifice. However, antibiotics do not persistently eliminate these bladder-derived microbes from the external genitals. Proper skin care in the anal and vulvar regions is more effective (see p. 66) in reducing the number of bacteria and, thus, the incidence of infections.

During childhood, in childbed, and at old age, intestinal and skin bacteria are more frequently, or exclusively, detected because of the absence of lactobacilli (which only grow to protective concentrations in the presence of estrogen). At low concentration, they should be regarded as normal flora.

If there are signs of inflammation or discharge, a swab should be taken for bacteriological culture. If pathogens like streptococci of group A or even *Staphylococcus aureus* can be detected, treatment is advised even in the absence of major complaints. These bacteria may lead to clinical manifestation of vaginitis in individual patients. The sole detection of other bacteria, such as *Proteus* species, *Escherichia coli*, enterococci, or streptococci of group B, has no clinical significance.

Vaginitis Not Caused by Pathogens

In addition to infections and a disturbed bacterial flora, there are forms of vaginitis in which pathogens cannot be detected and antibiotics are ineffective. Apart from atrophic vaginitis, these are heterogeneous forms of vaginitis, some of which are probably immune diseases as they improve only upon topical cortisone treatment (e.g., clobetasol ointment) and may occasionally even be improved this way.

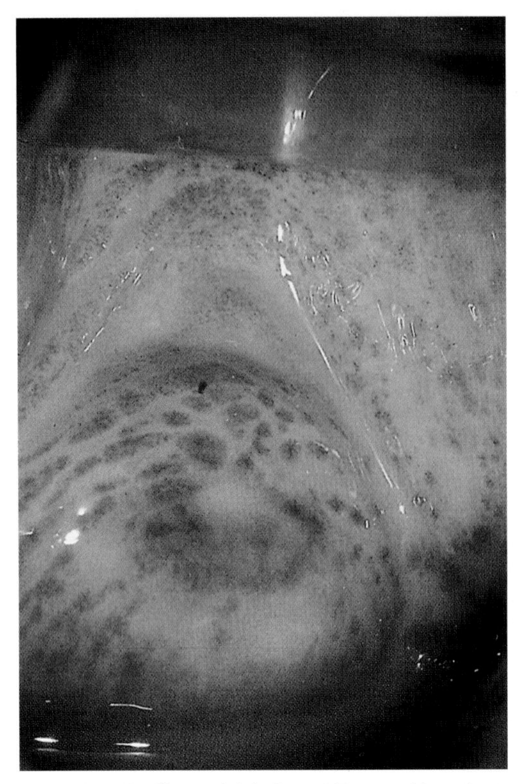

Fig. 7.**121** Senile vaginitis in a 57-year-old patient. The condition improved after topical application of estrogen.

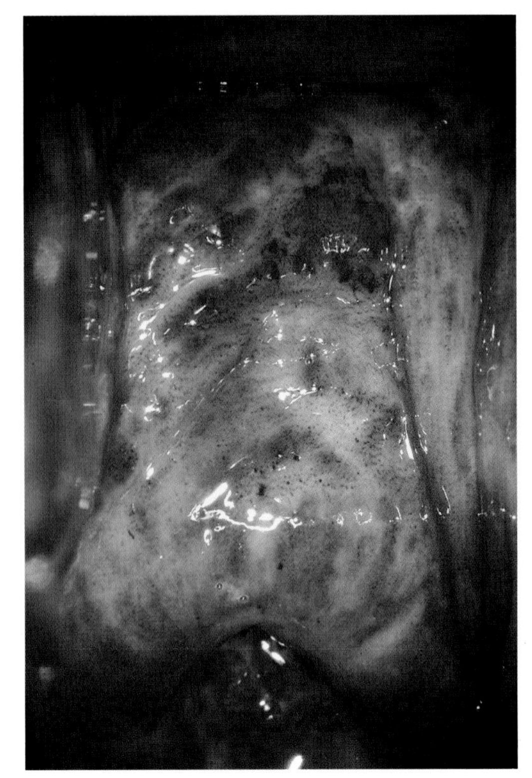

Fig. 7.**122** Atrophic vaginitis in a 47-year-old patient with petechial bleeding.

Atrophic Vaginitis/Senile Vaginitis

Pathogenesis. Estrogen deficiency causes the vaginal epithelium to become very thin and more susceptible even to harmless microbes. This leads to redness and vulnerability of the epithelium (Fig. 7.**121**).

Clinical picture. Atrophic vaginitis can easily be mistaken for trichomoniasis, vaginitis caused by group A streptococci, or plasma cell vaginitis (purulent vaginitis) (see Fig. 7.**108**, p. 120). The redness and yellow discharge are very similar in these conditions. However, the response of the epithelium to pressure is different. For example, rubbing with the cotton swab causes small to large petechial hemorrhages only in cases of atrophic vaginitis (Fig. 7.**122**).

Diagnosis:

- *Clinical picture.* Appearance of petechial bleeding, with the discharge having a pH of > 6.0.
- *Microscopy.* Plenty of granulocytes and mostly intermediate and parabasal cells (Fig. 7.**123**), absence of lactobacilli, and usually many small bacteria (intestinal flora).
- Normalization upon topical estrogen application.

Therapy:

- Topical estrogen application by means of ovules or cream; initially daily, then once or twice a week.
- Antibiotics only in the presence of pathogenic bacteria.

Erosive Vaginitis

This is a form of vaginitis that leads to cracks in a very strong vaginal epithelium (Fig. 7.**124**). The patients complain of pain and mild bleedings that intensify if intercourse is still possible at all. Special pathogens cannot be detected. So far, even biopsy has been of little help for the diagnosis. Antibiotics do not improve the clinical picture. The most effective treatment is by means of clobetasol cream applied inside the vagina, together with estrogen ovules. It is not yet clear if vaginal vitamin C delayed-release tablets result in stabilization of the epithelial condition.

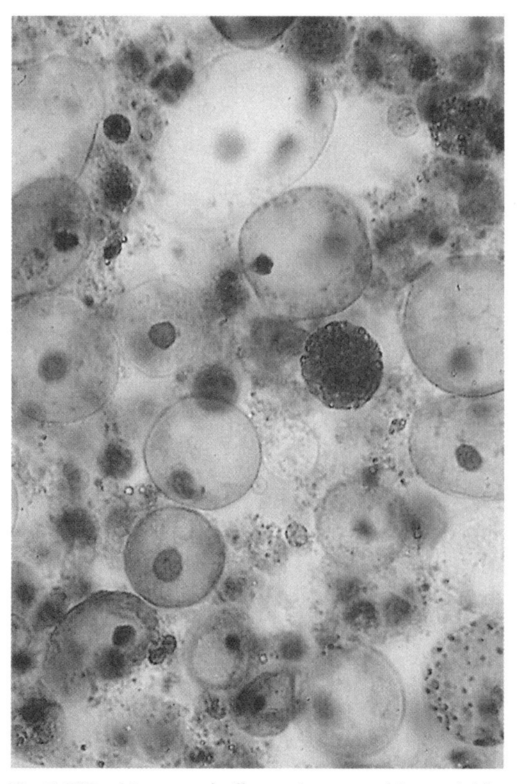

Fig. 7.**123** Micrograph illustrating atrophic vaginitis. Wet mount of discharge stained with 0.1 % methylene blue, showing granulocytes and intermediate and parabasal cells.

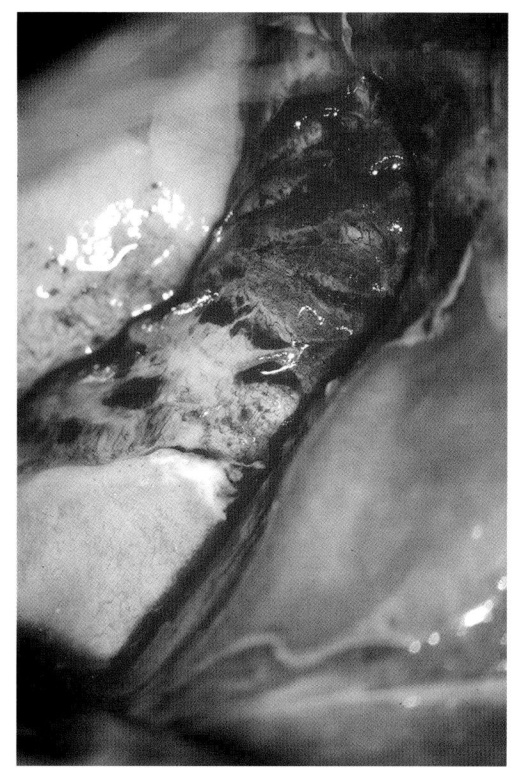

Fig. 7.**124** Erosive vaginitis with exfoliating epithelium in a 49-year-old patient.

Ulceration of the Vagina (Behçet Syndrome)

Deep ulceration of the vagina (Fig. 7.**125**) causes only little discomfort, due to the low sensitivity of the vagina. Frequently, the patients are known to have experienced previous vulvar and oral ulceration, thus letting one suspect Behçet syndrome. Vaginal carcinoma is extremely rare in young women and should be excluded by biopsy. Personally, I have never seen a vaginal carcinoma and, hence, cannot present an example.

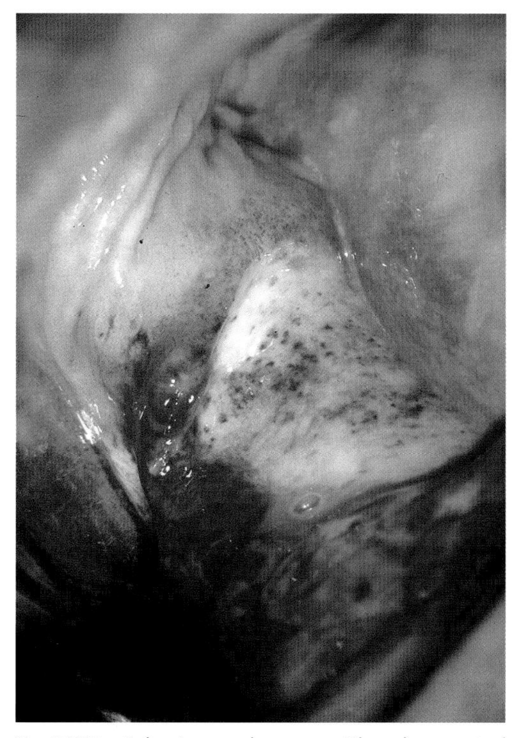

Fig. 7.**125** Behçet syndrome with deep-seated ulceration in a 30-year-old patient during the 20th week of pregnancy.

Granular Vaginitis

In contrast to Behçet syndrome, which heals after a few weeks, there are also ulcerating and granulating forms of vaginitis that persist over months and years and, in part, look like a malignancy. They have been cured with cortisone in cases where the histology has repeatedly been negative.

In one such case of vaginitis (Fig. 7.**126**), after 10 years, only topical treatment with clobetasol could temporarily bring complete healing.

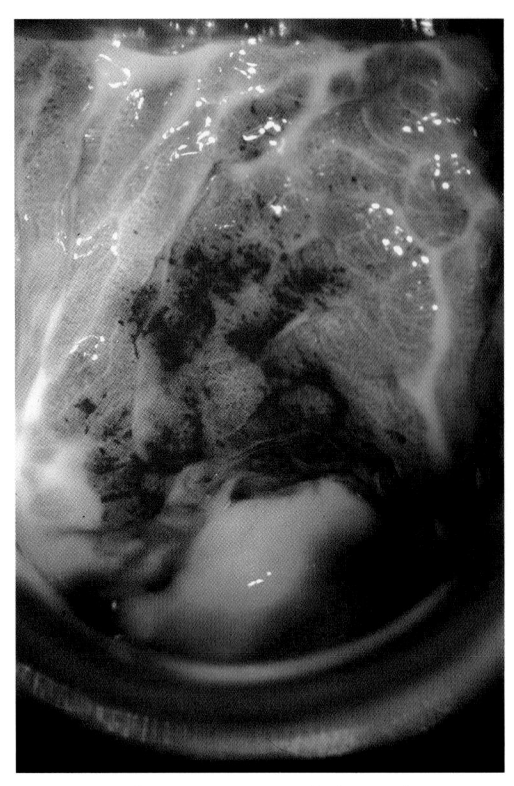

Fig. 7.**126** Chronic vaginitis with hemorrhages in a 48-year-old patient (possibly an immune disease).

Caution. There are also forms of vaginitis that result from combinations of known infections, plasma cell vaginitis, and immunological diseases. These have been improved or cured only after several treatments or combined treatments. In all severe cases of vaginitis, therapy should be followed up by regular checks.

Infections of the Cervix (Cervicitis)

The cervix with its numerous glands and their secretions—particularly the viscous, gestagen-rich cervical secretion—is an important barrier against microorganisms. Only few pathogens are able to pass it or even cause inflammation.

For sexually transmitted viruses (HBV, HIV, CMV), the cervix is only a portal of entry, or transit station, and serves as an asymptomatic site of pathogen elimination. Viral passage and also infections are helped along by a large ectopia of the portio, which is physiological after puberty and is often further enhanced by ovulation inhibitors. Besides, young women are more susceptible to pathogens due to their delicate genital epithelium, which explains why sexually transmitted infections are more common in younger and sexually active women. Foreign bodies (such as an intrauterine device, IUD), bleeding, estrogen deficiency, and surgery promote ascending infections as well.

Only a few pathogens cause cervicitis. We have to distinguish between infections of the single-layered columnar epithelium of the cervical canal and infections of the external stratified squamous epithelium of the portio vaginalis (Table 7.**5**).

Infections of the stratified squamous epithelium tend to occur always together with infections of the vaginal orifice and the vagina. By contrast, infections of the single-layered columnar epithelium are specific cases in which only a few pathogens are detected exclusively. First, there is *Chlamydia trachomatis*. If there is no uterus, chlamydial infections in the vaginal region are no longer possible.

The cervix is also the initial site of ascending bacterial infections due to chlamydiae or gonococci. Vaginal microbes originating from the intestine do not cause cervicitis, but they can easily reach the upper abdomen together with an ascending infection and may cause additional inflammation in the peritoneal region.

Clinical picture. In cases of cervicitis, patients complain only of discharge and contact bleeding. Cervicitis is often accompanied by a disturbed vaginal flora and sometimes even by vaginitis.

After inserting a speculum, typical cervicitis reveals a reddened, slightly thickened cervical opening that is covered by a yellow sticky secre-

Table 7.**5** Infections of the cervix

Site of cervicitis	Pathogens	Other causes
Single-layered columnar epithelium	Gonococci *Chlamydia trachomatis*	Adenocarcinoma
Stratified squamous epithelium	Gonococci Herpes simplex viruses Papillomaviruses* Trichomonads Group A streptococci Syphilis, primary lesion (very rare)	Squamous cell carcinoma Behçet syndrome

* Infection with very little inflammatory reaction.

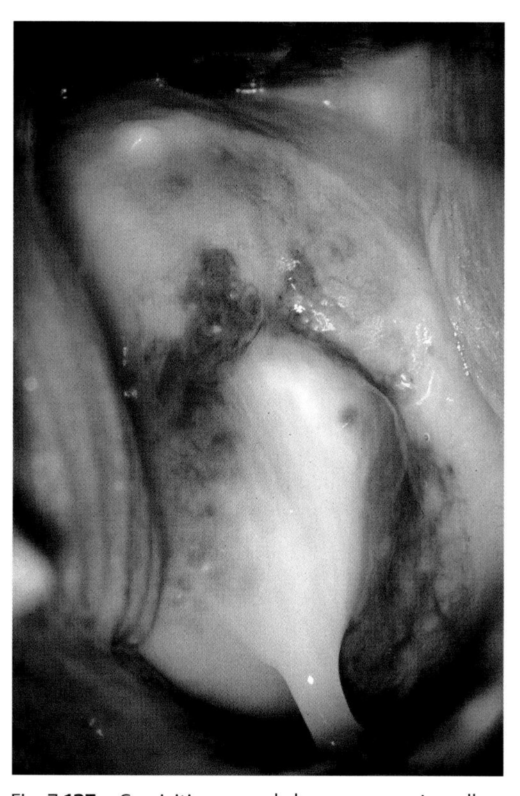

Fig. 7.**127** Cervicitis caused by gonococci: yellow secretion in a 20-year-old patient.

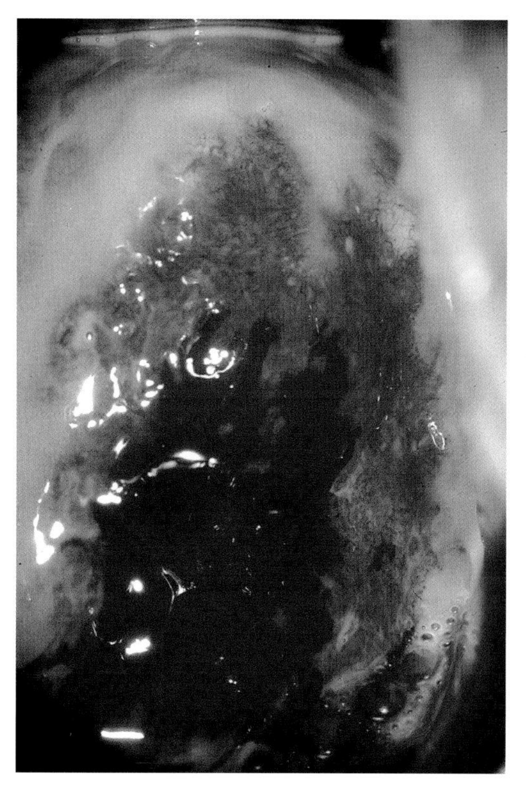

Fig. 7.**128** Cervicitis caused by *Chlamydia trachomatis:* hemorrhage in a 22-year-old patient.

tion (Fig. 7.**127**). The cervix is easily injured, and contact causes bleeding (Fig. 7.**128**). Contact bleeding and dysfunctional bleeding are therefore another characteristic symptom of cervicitis.

The clinical picture of cervicitis is very impressive when there is a large ectopia of the portio (Fig. 7.**129**). Nevertheless, there are individual patients where cervicitis is strictly endocervical and hardly anything suspicious can be found by colposcopy (Fig. 7.**130**). In these patients, however, a possible indicator is discharge containing plenty of leukocytes, without any pathogen being detected as a cause.

Chlamydia Infections

Chlamydiae are the smallest bacteria (0.3 µm). They can only reproduce within cells because they do not produce ATP as a source of energy. They have adapted extremely well to the human body during millions of years. Chlamydial cells come in two forms: elementary bodies and reticulate bodies. Elementary bodies (0.3 µm) are the infectious form that is visible in inclusion bodies of the infected cells (Fig. 7.**131 a, b**). They hardly metabolize and, hence, cannot be attacked by antibiotics.

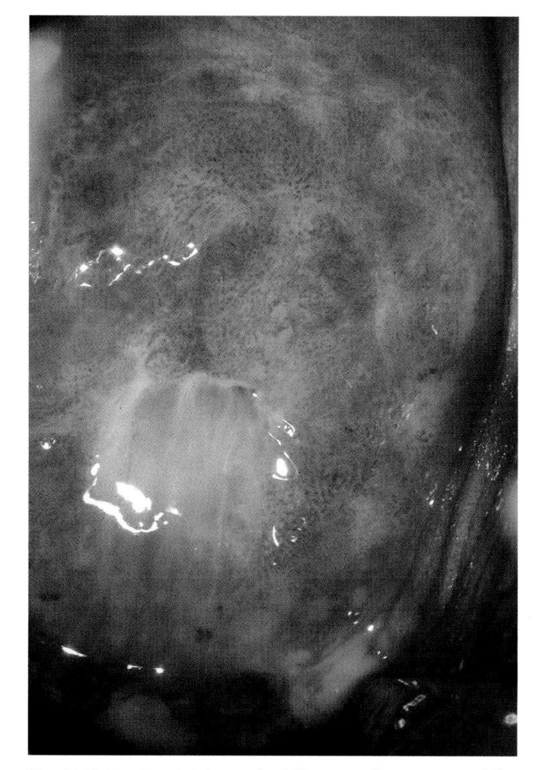

Fig. 7.**129** Cervicitis with diffuse redness caused by *Chlamydia* after menstruation in a 22-year-old patient with a large ectopia of the portio.

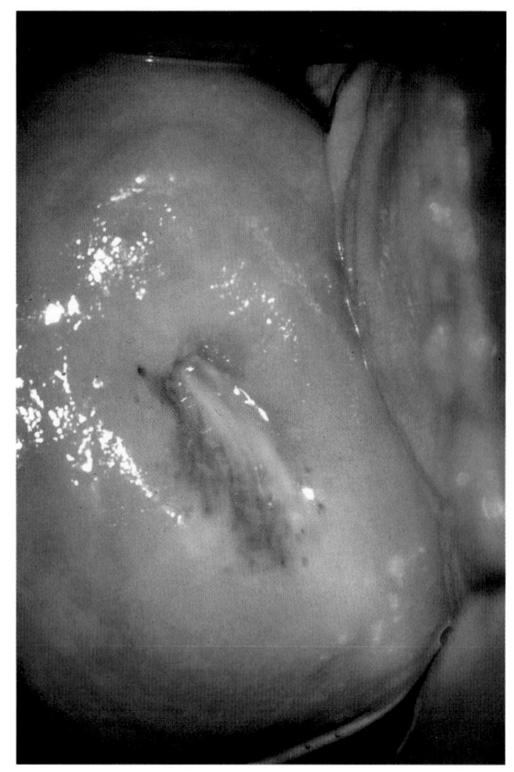

Fig. 7.**130** Discrete cervicitis caused by *Chlamydia* in a 24-year-old patient.

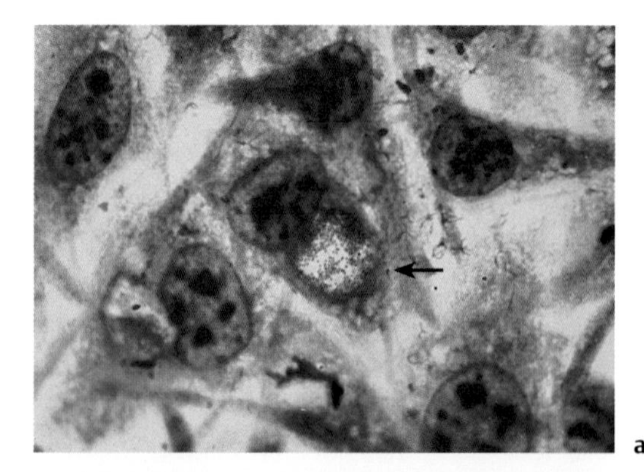

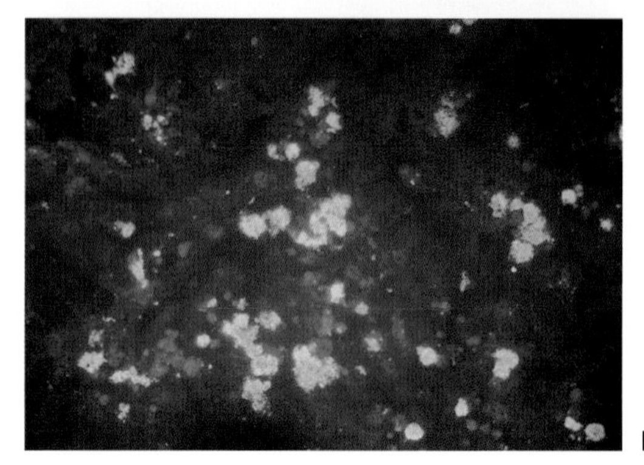

Fig. 7.**131** Micrographs illustrating *Chlamydia* infection. **a** Infected cell culture (Giemsa staining) with inclusion body (arrow) filled with elementary bodies of *Chlamydia*. **b** Detection of *Chlamydia* infection by immunofluorescence microscopy. The large yellow spots are inclusion bodies, and the small spots are elementary bodies.

During the phase of reproduction within the cell, the elementary bodies change into reticulate bodies, which divide by fission. Now, antibiotics can be used to inhibit multiplication of the pathogen. A complete cure of chlamydial infection can be best achieved at an early stage and in cooperation with an uncompromised immune system. Whereas chlamydiae actively divide in all infected cells at the start of an infection and can therefore be attacked by antibiotics, more and more chlamydiae are in the resting phase during chronic infections so that antibiotics are ineffective. There are three groups of chlamydiae. So far, only *C. trachomatis* is known to have various serotypes with quite different pathogenic properties (Table 7.**6**).

Table 7.**6** Classification of *Chlamydia*

Chlamydia trachomatis	***Chlamydia pneumoniae***	***Chlamydia psittaci***
Serotypes **A–C:** – trachoma **L1–L3:** – lymphogranuloma venerum (LGV) **D–K:** – urogenital infections – arthritis – conjunctivitis	No serotypes – mostly mild, respiratory infections – pneumonia – reactive arthritis – suspected role in atherosclerosis, myocardial infarct, emphysema, bronchial asthma, multiple sclerosis, sarcoidosis, Alzheimer disease	No serotypes – widespread in animals – atypical pneumonia

Chlamydia trachomatis, Serotypes A–C (Trachoma)

These bacteria spread through smear infection. They are the pathogen of trachoma, a chronic inflammation of the eye (Table 7.**6**). If left untreated, the infection causes scarring of the external eye and leads to blindness after 10–30 years.

Chlamydia trachomatis, Serotypes L1–L3 (Lymphogranuloma Venereum)

Lymphogranuloma venereum is a sexually transmitted genital infection usually seen only in warm climates (see p. 232).

Chlamydia pneumoniae

This is the most common *Chlamydia* species in humans. In 50–70% of adults, antibodies against this species can be detected with species-specific tests. They spread by means of airborne infection and cause mild respiratory infections.

This chlamydial species is particularly important because of the sequelae of infection after years and decades. The blood vessels seem to be affected in particular, thus promoting atherosclerosis as a result of chronic inflammation.

C. pneumoniae, like *C. trachomatis*, may cause arthritis by affecting the cartilage of joints. It is not yet clear whether or not, and to what extent, this species is involved in degenerative diseases.

Diagnosis is established by means of serological methods. Treatment is similar to that of *C. trachomatis.*

Chlamydia psittaci

Here, humans are only rarely the terminal host of an infection that leads to atypical pneumonia. This pathogen plays a role in animals—for example, birds and koala bears—and, above all, in poultry farming.

There are still other species of *Chlamydia* causing infections in the animal kingdom, for example, in cattle. As far as we know, they do not pose a thread to humans.

Table 7.**7** Special features of genital infections caused by *Chlamydia trachomatis*

Over 90% of the infections take an asymptomatic course in men and women
– recognition only through screening of asymptomatic persons
– chronic course over many years
– the most common sexually transmitted bacterial infection
– considerable consequences, such as extrauterine pregnancy, sterility, arthritis, particularly when the course is asymptomatic
– one of the most common infections transmitted during childbirth
– intracellular multiplication produces only few progeny, thus making pathogen detection difficult
– increase in prevalence in most populations
– increase in the detection and understanding of essentially asymptomatic infections
– antibodies do not protect from reinfections
– transmission is also possible during petting

Genital Chlamydial Infections (*C. trachomatis*, Serotypes D–K)

Infections caused by *C. trachomatis* are among the most important causes of inflammation in the genital region because of the frequency of infections and their sequelae (Table 7.**7**). They are among those bacterial infections that are most often transmitted sexually. They do not directly cause severe inflammation and life-threatening diseases. Nevertheless, the sequelae—such as rupture of a tubal pregnancy—may become life threatening. In addition, these infections cause considerable expenses due to chronic pain, with or without inflammation of the joints, and because the methods of in vitro fertilization (IVF) in case of tubal occlusion are very costly.

Pathogen. *Chlamydia trachomatis*, serotypes D–K.

Frequency. We distinguish between two types of infection:

- ▶ Florid infections with detection of the pathogen in 2–5% of young, sexually active men and women (Fig. 7.**132**).
- ▶ Subacute chronic infections in the upper genital region or in other parts of the body (e.g., joints), where detection of the pathogen is not possible and where an ongoing florid infection is only suspected because antibodies are present. Antibodies against genital chlamydiae are found in 15–20% of adults.

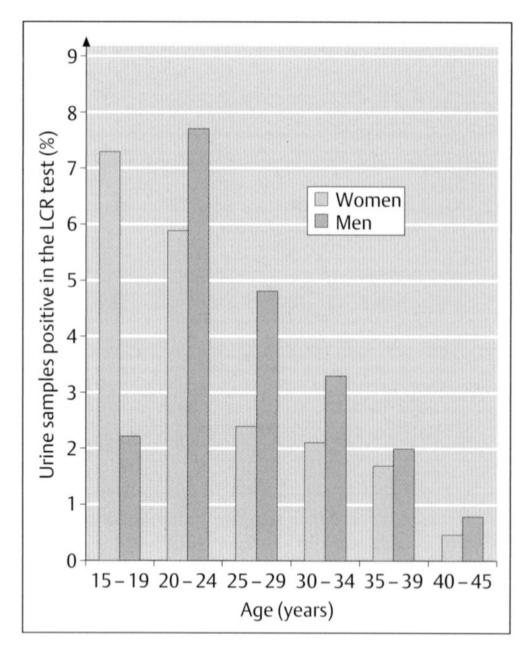

Fig. 7.**132** Prevalence of genital *Chlamydia* infection in Germany, based on the examination of 4381 asymptomatic men and women in 1996. Of 1652 couples, at least one partner was positive in 4.5 %.
LCR = ligase chain reaction

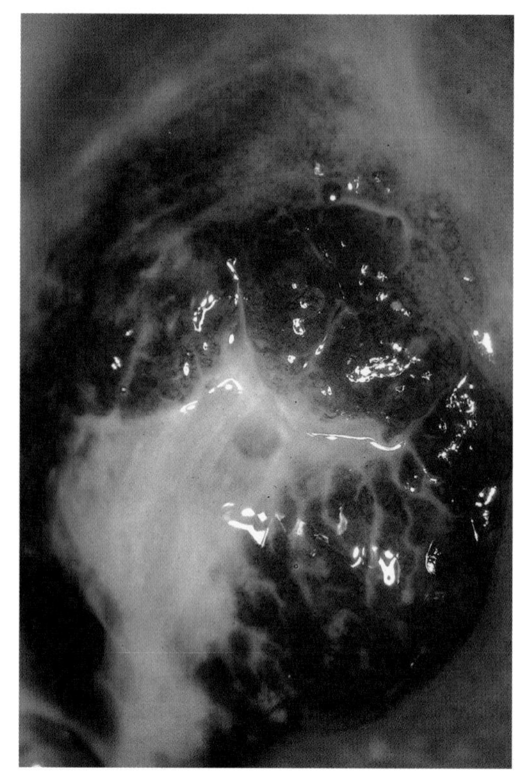

Fig. 7.**133** Hyperplastic cervicitis caused by *Chlamydia* in a 20-year-old patient with arthritis.

Transmission and pathogenesis. *Chlamydia trachomatis* is predominantly transmitted by sexual contact and thus primarily found in the genital region. In individual patients, chlamydiae may be transferred into the eyes by smear infection, where they cause conjunctivitis. The typical mode of infection in humans is by ascending in the genitals, causing far greater damage in women than in men.

Due to the high turnover of cervical cells, chlamydiae can last only for a few months in the cervix as they are eventually shed together with the cells. By contrast, they can survive for many years in the fallopian tubes. Consequently, it is here where they do the greatest harm. Chronic inflammation of the tubal epithelium develops, thus leading to loss of function, adhesion, and finally occlusion of the tubes. Since tubal occlusion does not slow down the infection, it may develop into pyosalpinx or hydrosalpinx.

Chlamydiae then reach the peritoneal cavity through the orifice of the fallopian tube and are transported by the blood into the joints.

They spread slowly and cause only a moderate inflammatory response because of the slow cycle of intracellular reproduction. The resulting symptoms of a persistent or advancing infection are often hardly noticeable—if there are any symptoms at all.

This explains why the majority of genital chlamydial infections occurring inside the genitals are either not recognized or only when irreversible secondary damages have already occurred.

Unlike in women, the main portal of entrance in men is the urethra. From here, the chlamydiae ascend and cause epididymitis and, after years, infertility (azoospermia and oligospermia) (Table 7.**8**).

Chlamydial persistence and chlamydial reinfection are both possible and often difficult to distinguish from each other. Not much is known about the resistance of specific *Chlamydia* strains.

Clinical signs. In 90 % of patients, there are no symptoms or only mild ones, such as a yellow sticky discharge (Fig. 7.**133**), contact bleeding, mid-cycle bleeding (endometritis). There are no systemic symptoms, and local findings vary widely. There may be edematous, polypiform swelling of the cervix with mucopurulent secretion, or intense vascular display (Fig. 7.**134**) where the dilation of blood vessels may persist for months. Spontaneous healing does occur, or the infection moves upward and is then no longer detectable in the cervix. In addition, in men, chlamydial infections are asymptomatic in 90% of patients. Recent polymerase chain reaction (PCR) studies using first-stream urine have shown that, in couples, the man is as frequently infected with chlamydiae as the woman, if not even more often, without showing any symptoms (Fig. 7.**132**).

Specific risk factors:
- ascending infection (> 40%) associated with infestation of the fallopian tubes (see salpingitis, p. 151)
- infection of the newborn during delivery
- late puerperal endometritis (four to six weeks post partum)
- unnecessary appendectomy due to undiagnosed chlamydial salpingitis
- contributing factor in other infections of the cervix
- increased infectiosity in case of leukocyte-mediated infections (e. g., HIV).

The most common cause of tubal sterility is a previous chlamydial salpingitis. The infection usually progresses subacutely and, hence, remains often undiagnosed. It is not uncommon that appendectomy is then performed because of lower abdominal pain. The incidence of transmission of chlamydiae to the newborn during delivery is high. In case of exposure, 40% of the newborns contract conjunctivitis and up to 20% contract chlamydial pneumonia. Late pulmonary damage in children is also possible.

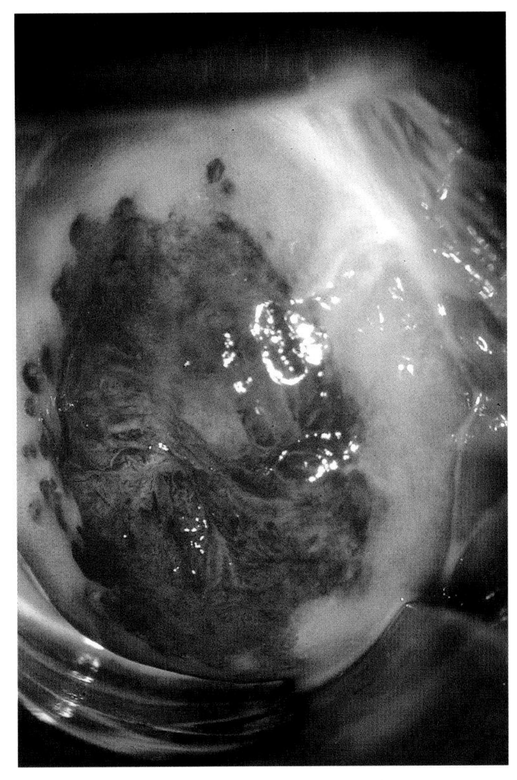

Fig. 7.**134** Chlamydial cervicitis with prominent vascular display in a 21-year-old patient.

Diagnosis:
- Typical complaints: yellow sticky discharge, contact bleeding.
- *Clinical picture.* Insertion of a speculum reveals a yellow *cervical secretion* with unremarkable vaginal flora (Fig. 7.**135**).
- *Colposcopy.* Vasodilatation (Fig. 7.**136**; this may be only a cause of suspicion, since it persists for a long time even after successful treatment and—in rare cases—may have other, largely unknown, causes.
- *Microscopy.* The *vaginal discharge* usually contains plenty of leukocytes (granulocytes and lymphocytes), and the vaginal flora consists of normal lactobacilli in the majority of patients.
- *Cytology* is unsuitable, yielding only accidental findings.
- *Laboratory diagnostics.* Detection of the pathogen confirms the infection (Table 7.**9**).

Table 7.**8** Diseases caused by serotypes D–K of *Chlamydia trachomatis*

In women	In men	During pregnancy and childbirth
Urethritis	Urethritis	Premature delivery
Cervicitis	Prostatitis	Bleeding during pregnancy (subchorionic hematoma)
Endometritis	Epididymitis	Puerperal endometritis
Salpingitis (subacute)		Infection of the newborn
Peritonitis		– conjunctivitis
Perihepatitis		– pneumonia
Conjunctivitis	Conjunctivitis	– genital infection
Arthritis	Arthritis	– possibly primary sterility
Exanthem	Exanthem	
Reiter syndrome	Reiter syndrome	

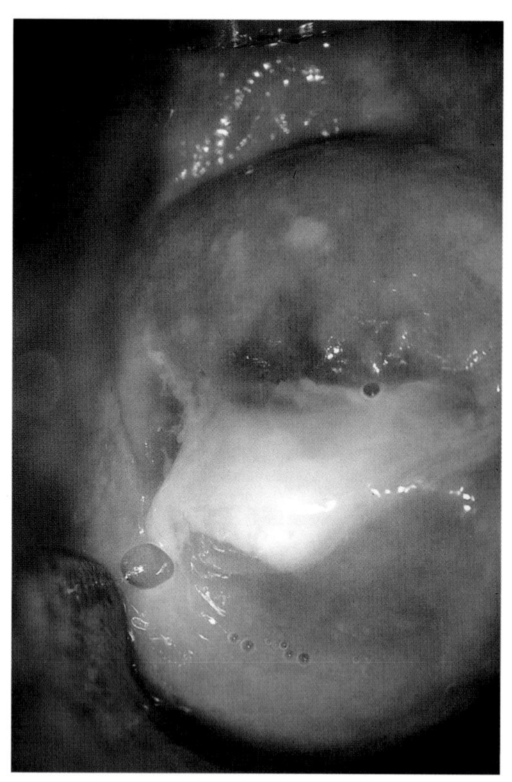

Fig. 7.**135** Chlamydial cervicitis with unremarkable vaginal flora but yellow cervical secretion in an 18-year-old patient.

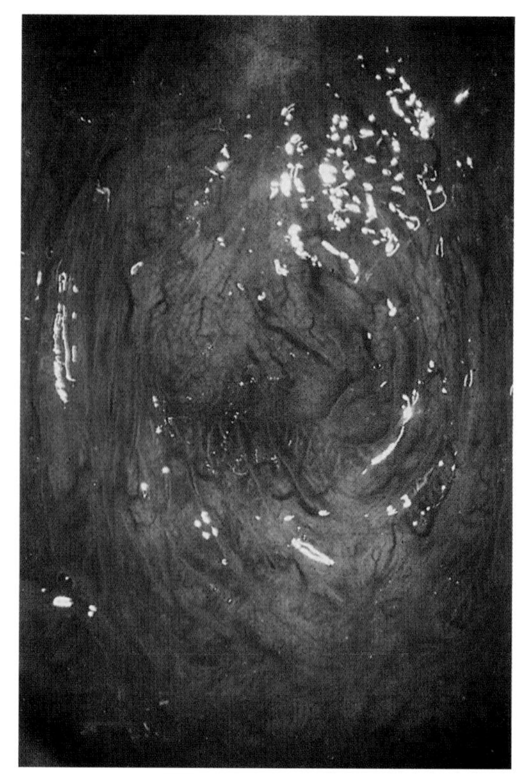

Fig. 7.**136** Cervicitis in a 19-year-old patient. The portio vaginalis exhibits plenty of dilated blood vessels as a sign of an inflammation that has already existed for several weeks.

Table 7.**9** Diagnostic procedures in case of *Chlamydia* infections

Primary diagnosis **Detection of pathogen, antigen, or DNA**	**Sensitivity**
Cell culture (e. g., on McCoy cells): although this method has the highest specificity, it is seldom offered by laboratories because it is laborious, time-consuming, and expensive	60–70 % (old gold standard)
Fluorescence test (FT) of a few samples	70–90 %
Enzyme tests (ELISA)	50–90 %
– rapid tests/individual tests (e. g., ClearView): partly with poor specificity and low sensitivity, therefore unsuitable	50–60 %
– laboratory tests (EIA, IDEIA, etc.): less frequently used today; sensitivity is too low, although specificity is good	80–90 %
DNA probe tests (e. g., gene probe): not better than enzyme tests	80–90 %
Amplification tests (PCR,): high specificity and sensitivity; also suitable for **urine diagnostics** (first-stream urine) and other test materials	95–98 % (new gold standard)
Secondary/additional diagnosis	
Serology: Detection of antibodies indicates that the body reacted against the pathogen. Whether or not the infection is still florid may be suspected from certain values, but this does not prove it. – CFT (only group-specific) – LPS test (group-specific), e. g., rELISA, is only used as an early test for all *Chlamydia* species – microimmunofluorescence test: species specific, though expensive and subjective – ELISA/ImmunoComb: species specific (has been one of the first tests of its kind) – synthetic peptide tests: species specific, highly sensitive, though it does not include all types – detection of antibodies against heat shock proteins (HSP 60)	

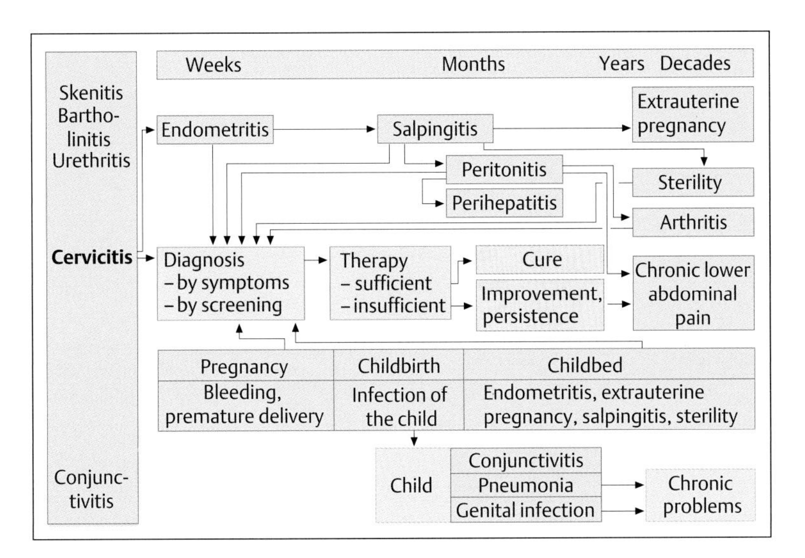

Fig. 7.**137** *Chlamydia* infection. Clinical course and sequelae.

Development of pathogen detection tests for *Chlamydia:*

- 1975–1985, era of cell culture
- 1985–1995, era of antibody tests (no cultures involved), e. g., enzyme immunoassay (EIA), enzyme-linked immunosorbent assay (ELISA)
- 1995–present, nucleic acid amplification test (polymerase chain reaction, PCR).

The only convincing tests are those for species-specific antibodies against *Chlamydia trachomatis.* To a great extent, negative titers exclude chlamydial infection of the inner genitals. However, cervicitis may be so superficial that no antibodies are formed. Persistent titers even after therapy indicate an already existing infection that is not restricted to the cervix. In case of a fresh infection (up to several weeks) and adequate antibiotic therapy (> two weeks), antibody titers actually turn negative. If the pathogen is detected, serology can help with distinguishing a fresh infection from a chronic one due to persistence or reinfection. In addition to eliminating the pathogen from sites where specimens can be taken for confirmation, a shift to negative antibody titers is the best evidence for a complete cure (Fig. 7.**137**).

Sampling of material for pathogen detection. Because chlamydiae reproduce only within cells, a smear containing many cervical cells is essential for the diagnosis. For this purpose, a cotton swab or brush is introduced deep into the cervix and rubbed intensely over the tissue. The cells are then carefully transferred onto a special microscopic slide or into a solution; the swab may remain in the solution. In case of urine sampling, only the first 10–30 mL are collected (first-stream urine) because the chlamydiae are primarily present in the epithelial cells swept along with the urine.

A special transport medium is required for cell cultures. Smear samples for fluorescence microscopy, enzyme test, or PCR may be stored for some time (days) and may also be shipped; the same is true for urine if it is cooled.

The right moment for taking a cervical smear is immediately after the period or during childbed. The wrong moment is in the middle of the cycle when there is plenty of cervical secretion; only few cells can be picked up, and the excessive cervical secretion may interfere with the PCR tests (Table 7.**9**).

Table 7.**10** Treatment of *Chlamydia* infection

Medication	Dosage
First choice:	
– doxycycline	200 mg per day
– tetracyclines	4 × 500 mg per day
Second choice (macrolides):	
– erythromycin	4 × 500 mg per day
– roxithromycin	300 mg per day
– azithromycin	1 × 1.5 g or, better, 2 × 1.5 g per day
Third choice (fluoroquinolones):	
– ofloxacin	2 × 200 mg per day
– moxifloxacin	1 × 400 mg per day
Fourth choice:	
– amoxicillin	3 × 750 mg per day
– clindamycin	
– sulfonamides, Co-Trimoxazole	
Cephalosporins are ineffective against *Chlamydia.*	

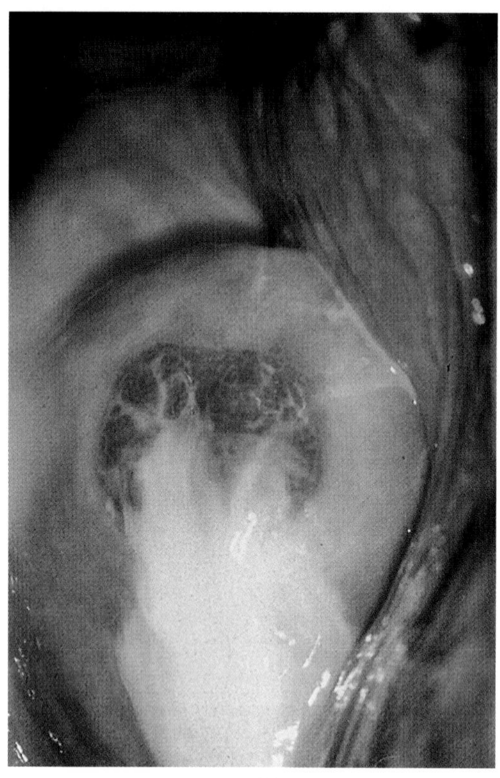

Fig. 7.**138** Cervicitis caused by *Neisseria gonorrhoeae*. A yellowish secretion containing leukocytes flows from the reddened cervix.

Therapy. Many antibiotics are effective against chlamydiae, with doxycycline being the standard medication (Table 7.**10**).

The recommended duration of therapy is:

- 10 days for cervicitis
- 20 days for salpingitis
- 30–90 days for arthritis.

Chlamydial infection should be considered in the following cases:

- discharge without vaginitis
- dysfunctional bleeding
- contact bleeding
- reddened cervix
- yellow cervical secretion
- increase in leukocytes in the discharge, while the lactobacillus flora is normal and no other pathogens are present
- varying discomfort in the lower abdomen
- pain in the right shoulder
- change of the sexual partner.

Gonococcal Cervicitis

Gonococci are rarely detected today even in women with exposure, though they are found occasionally together with chlamydiae. Here, too, the symptoms are mild or absent, and the detection of gonococci is often just by chance.

Pathogen. *Neisseria gonorrhoeae* with several known subtypes.

Frequency. About 0.02–0.2% of gynecological patients.

Incubation time. Two to six days (or even weeks).

Transmission and pathogenesis. Gonococci belong to the pathogenic microbes of the genital region. Nevertheless, asymptomatic infections of the cervix are common. Transmission takes place almost exclusively through sexual contact. In women, it is the cervix that is most frequently affected. However, infections of the urethra, rectum, Bartholin gland, and the nasopharyngeal region may also occur.

Certain factors (bleeding, insertion of an IUD, abrasion) promote ascending infections. Once the infection has reached the uterus, endometritis will develop, followed by acute salpingitis with pain, fever, and leukocytosis.

Especially women may occasionally develop a disseminated gonococcal infection with bacteremia (generalized dissemination of gonococci). Fever, malaise, pain in the limbs, and pustular or petechial skin eruptions are the result. This stage may run a mild course, and only subsequent arthritis may cause severe discomfort.

Gonococcal infection of a newborn during delivery is now a rare event. Nevertheless, gonorrheal conjunctivitis is still a feared sequela because it may lead to blindness (see also Ocular Prophylaxis in Newborns, p. 242).

Clinical picture. There are no systemic symptoms; the local symptoms include increased yellow discharge and a reddened, swollen cervix (Fig. 7.**138**).

Special risks:

- ascending infection affecting the endometrium and the tubes, often associated with severe symptoms and subsequent sterility (see salpingitis, p. 149)
- disseminated infection (in 1–3% of untreated patients) associated with intermittent febrile attacks, migrating joint pain, and skin lesions (vasculitis, hemorrhaging pustules)
- during pregnancy: premature amniorrhexis with infection of the newborn
- postpartal endometritis and disturbed wound healing after cesarean section
- risk of infecting the sexual partner.

Diagnosis:

- *Clinical picture/colposcopy.* Putrid discharge, suspected cervicitis (Fig. 7.**139**).

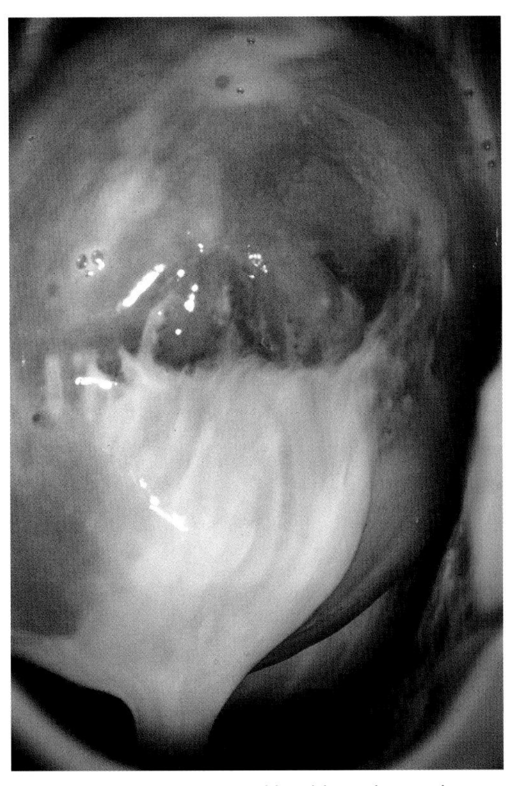

Fig. 7.**139** Cervicitis caused by chlamydiae and gonococci in an 18-year-old patient.

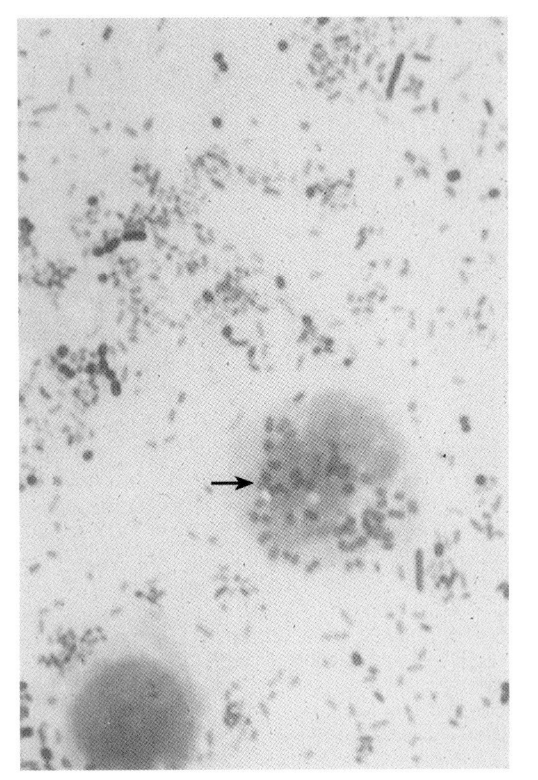

Fig. 7.**140** Micrograph illustrating gonorrhea. The cervical smear (Gram stain) shows scattered leukocytes covered with gram-negative diplococci (arrow). Other bacteria are also visible in large numbers because these patients frequently also suffer from bacterial vaginosis.

- *Microscopy.* Plenty of leukocytes in the cervical swab (more granulocytes as compared with chlamydial cervicitis). Because high numbers of various bacteria are often present at the same time, the typical gram-negative, intracellular diplococci are hardly recognizable in preparations stained with methylene blue or Gram stain (Fig. 7.**140**). The diagnosis should never be based on microscopic findings, for there are also apathogenic *Neisseria* species.
- *Culture.* Transport medium is required as neisserial cells are not stable. When using a transport medium, culture is still possible after two to three days if enough neisserial cells are present. Selective media (Thayer–Martin medium) and oxidase reaction are essential if there are gram-negative diplococci. Antibiogram is required.
- *Serology* does not play a role in cervicitis as there is no measurable immune response.

Therapy. Treatment is essential. With the exception of β-lactamase-producing strains (which are still rare), gonococci are very sensitive to almost all antibiotics (except for clindamycin and lincomycin).

Suggested antibiotics include:

- penicillin, 2.4 million IU, i.m. or orally
- amoxicillin, 3 × 750 mg per day
- tetracyclines, 2 g per day
- spectinomycin, 1 × 2 g, i.m. (suitable also for β-lactamase-producing strains),
- cephalosporins (effective also against β-lactamase-producing strains), for example, 250 mg of ceftriaxone, i.m.
- fluoroquinolones.

Duration of therapy. Treatment may be short in cases of uncomplicated gonococcal cervicitis: one to three days; in cases of complicated or disseminated cervicitis, it should last five to 10 days.

Treatment of the partner is essential.

Primary Lesion of Syphilis on the Cervix

Although this is rarely seen, one should nevertheless take it into consideration. A case is illustrated in Fig. 7.**141**. The patient was free of symptoms, and the inguinal region was not swollen because

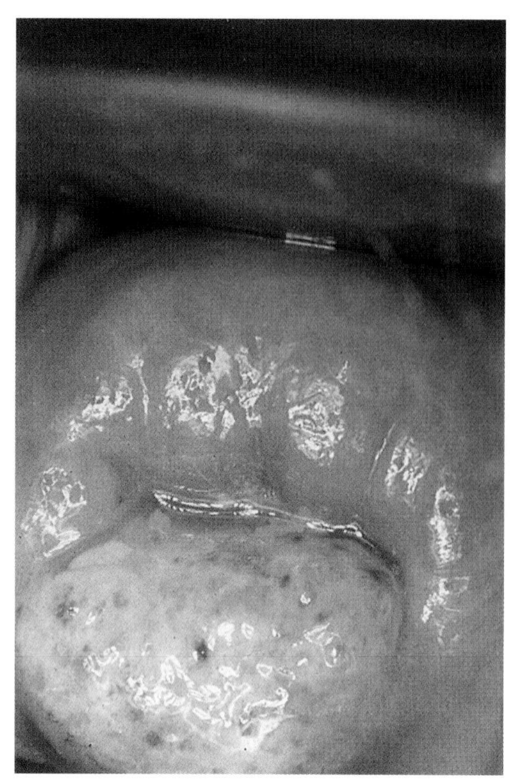

Fig. 7.**141** Primary syphilitic lesion on the portio vaginalis. In the region of the posterior lip of the cervix, a soft tumor (histologically rich in granulocytes) can be recognized.

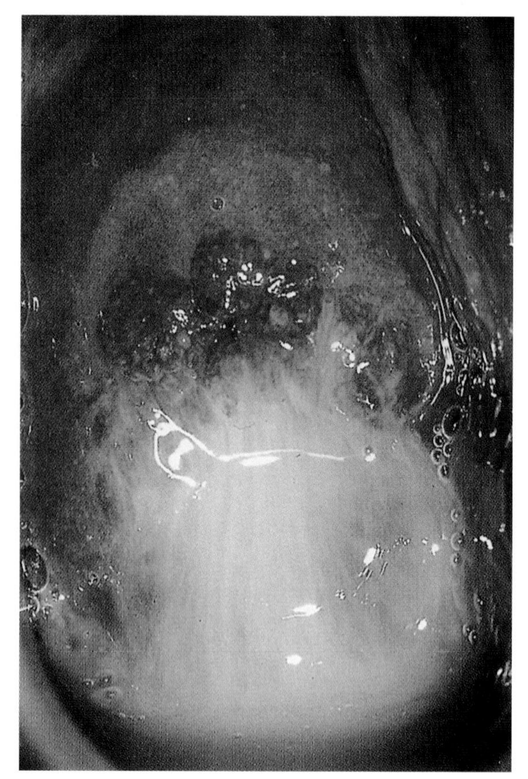

Fig. 7.**142** Cervicitis caused by group A streptococci in a 21-year-old patient.

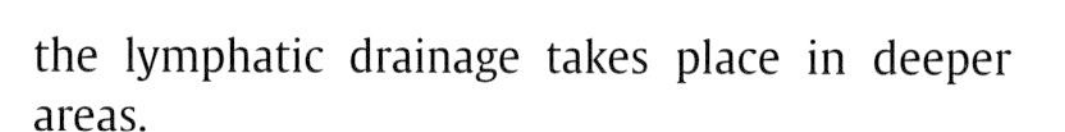

the lymphatic drainage takes place in deeper areas.

Diagnosis:

- ▶ *Detection of pathogen* by immunofluorescence microscopy or dark field microscopy (rarely successful).
- ▶ *Histology* of sample excision (nonspecific).
- ▶ *Serology* (confirmatory together with the clinical picture).

Therapy:
See Syphilis, p. 102.

Cervicitis Caused by Other Bacteria

The cervix may also be colonized by staphylococci, group A streptococci (Fig. 7.**142**), *Enterobacteriaceae* (*Escherichia coli* and others), anaerobes, or mycoplasmas. However, solitary cervicitis caused by one of these microbes is rare. Frequently, one is dealing also with an infection or colonization of the vagina, or with coinfection of the cervix in case of endometritis, for example, after delivery or surgery.

Genital Herpes of the Cervix

Solitary cervicitis caused by HSV is to be expected only in cases of recurrent genital herpes. Due to the lack of symptoms at this site, detection of such an infection occurs rather by chance.

In cases of primary genital herpes, however, the portio vaginalis is often affected as well. Insertion of a speculum is usually rightly foregone because of severe pain in the vulvar region. As a result, the considerable inflammatory response on the portio vaginalis is little known.

Clinical picture. Cervicitis associated with primary genital herpes may, in fact, resemble chlamydial or gonococcal cervicitis in the short term (Figs. 7.**143**, 7.**144**). Unlike chlamydial cervicitis, this is nevertheless a very transient picture, the more so as herpetic skin eruptions change rapidly. Upon first examination, the portio vaginalis is still covered with yellow, adhesive necrotic material (Fig. 7.**145**) and shows the typical undulating demarcation, while the clinical picture has completely changed five days later (Fig. 7.**146**) as the erosion is healing under aciclovir treatment.

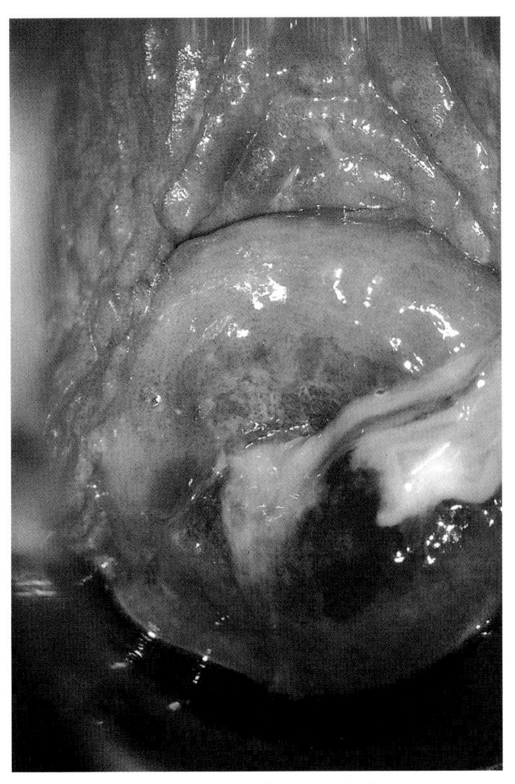

Fig. 7.**143** Primary genital herpes of the portio vaginalis with diffuse redness in a 19-year-old patient.

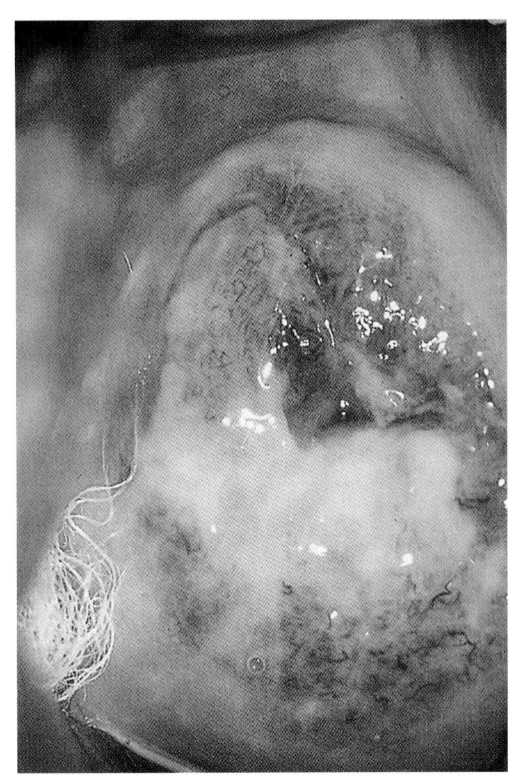

Fig. 7.**144** Primary genital herpes of the portio vaginalis in a 17-year-old patient. The initial tentative diagnosis was malignant growth.

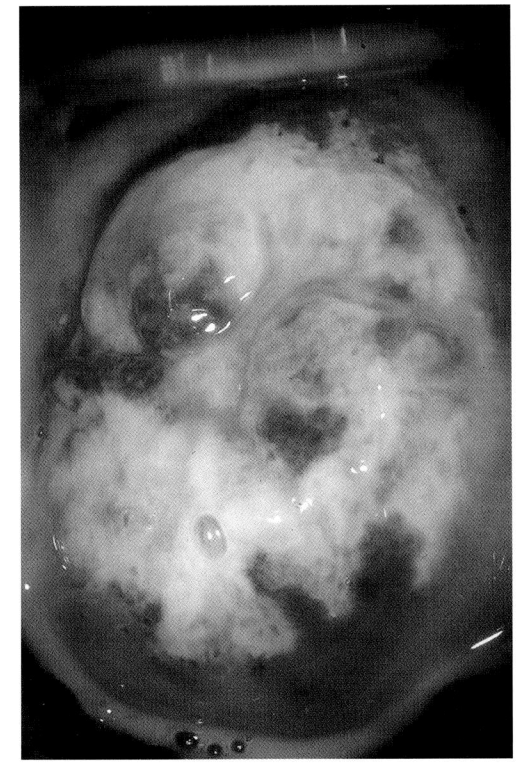

Fig. 7.**145** Primary genital herpes of the portio vaginalis in a 26-year-old patient, showing necrosis with infiltrating leukocytes and undulating demarcation.

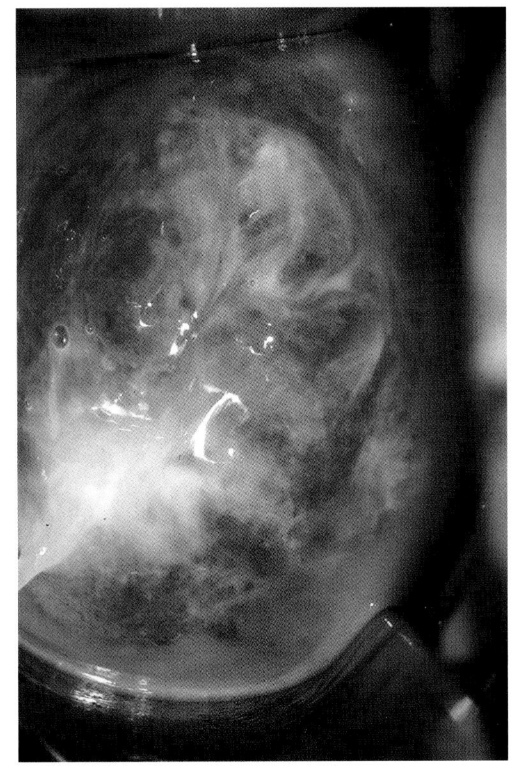

Fig. 7.**146** The same patient as in Fig. 7.**145** five days later, showing hardly any typical findings after acyclovir treatment.

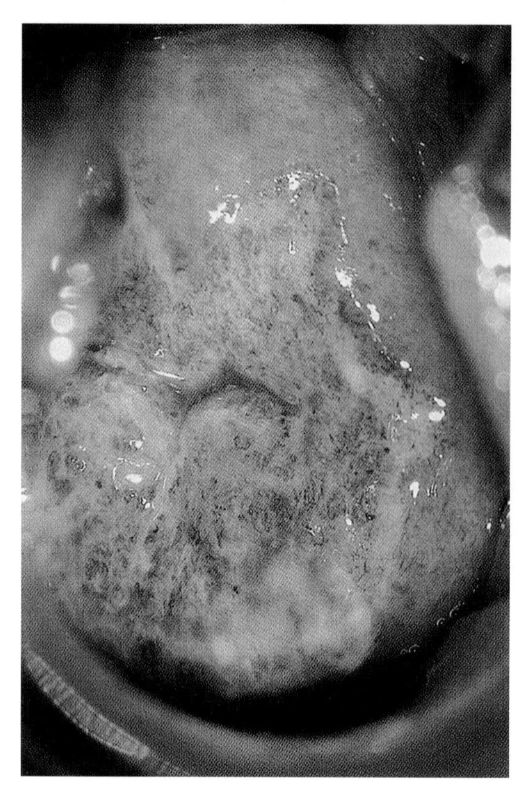

Fig. 7.**147** Primary genital herpes in a 26-year-old patient. The infected portio vaginalis exhibits an undulating erosion resulting from confluent lesions.

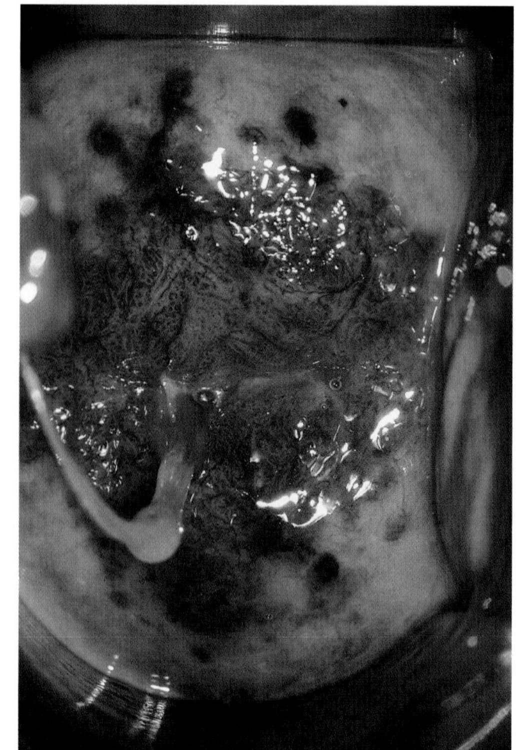

Fig. 7.**148** Recurrent genital herpes of the portio vaginalis in a 26-year-old patient.

Erosion by necrosis is characteristic for genital herpes (Fig. 7.**147**), whereas the cervix is rather thickened in cases of chlamydial cervicitis.

Occasionally, a malignant tumor rather than genital herpes is suspected (Fig. 7.**144**).

The detection of cervicitis in cases of recurrent genital herpes occurs more by chance, namely, when there are vesicles on the portio vaginalis or when a swab has been taken for viral culture in questionable cases of cervicitis (Fig. 7.**148**).

Special risks:

- risk of transmission to the newborn during delivery
- risk of infecting the sexual partner
- possibly a cofactor in the development of cervical carcinoma.

Diagnosis:

- *Clinical picture.* Often sufficient for establishing a diagnosis.
- *Detection of pathogen.* Isolation of the virus from the vesicular content or from the lesion; fluorescence microscopy of a swab preparation, PCR.
- *Serology.* No measurable amounts of IgM antibodies are produced in cases of recurrent genital herpes.
- *Cytology.* Only possible under favorable circumstances and therefore unsuitable.

Therapy. Treatment of solitary recurrent herpes of the cervix is usually not necessary because there is no pain. The situation is different during pregnancy (p. 179).

Caution. HSV is excreted in the cervix even if there are no lesions visible by colposcopy.

Papillomavirus Infection of the Cervix

As is the case with the vulva, we have to distinguish between condylomas on the portio vaginalis and a papillomavirus infection that has been identified by means of virus detection (e. g., in cases of dysplasia). Special forms and intermediate forms are described as flat condylomas.

In addition, we have to differentiate between low-risk and high-risk types of HPV (see p. 94).

Solitary infection of the cervix with papillomaviruses is probably a rare event. By contrast, coinfections are fairly common in the genital region.

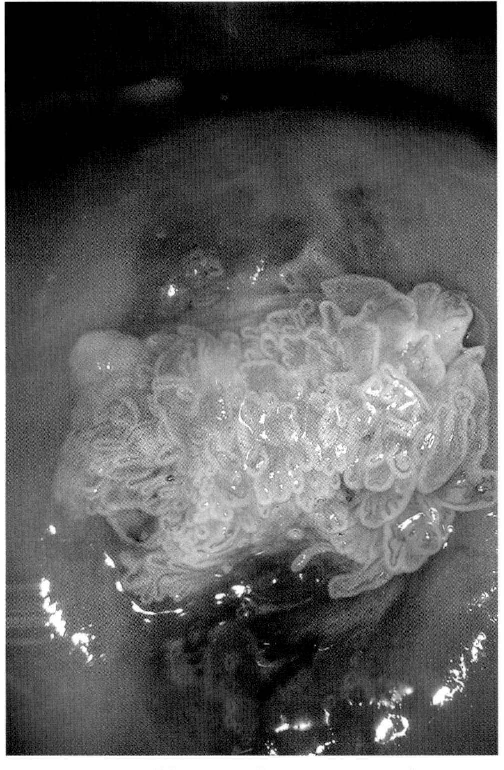

Fig. 7.**149** Condyloma on the portio vaginalis in a 24-year-old patient.

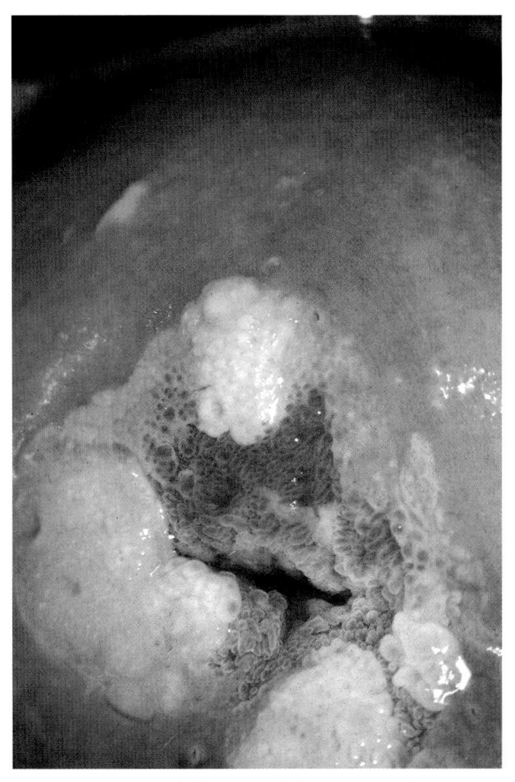

Fig. 7.**150** Several flat condylomas on the portio vaginalis in a 23-year-old patient, after application of 3% acetic acid.

Clinical picture. No complaints.

Condylomas caused by HPV-6 are easily visible by the naked eye (Fig. 7.**149**), whereas flat condylomas are better recognized with the help of a colposcope (Fig. 7.**150**). Infections caused by high-risk types of HPV are associated with severe dysplasia (CIN III) and usually become clearly visible only after swabbing with 3% acetic acid (Figs. 7.**151** and 7.**152**).

Pathogens. High-risk types (HPV-16 and HPV-18) as well as low-risk types (HPV-6 and HPV-11). The former are found more frequently, since viral detection and typing are performed if dysplasia is present (i.e., the frequent detection may be a selective effect).

Frequency. High-risk HPV types are detected in about 3% of 30-year-old women; the frequency of low-risk HPV types is not known.

Pathogenesis and pathological anatomy. Typical acuminate condylomas similar to those in the vulvar region and caused by HPV-6 and HPV-11 are found only occasionally. In most patients, the lesions are flat condylomas (Fig. 7.**153**) that become visible only after swabbing the portio vaginalis with 3% acetic acid. In a large majority of patients, these changes are found on the

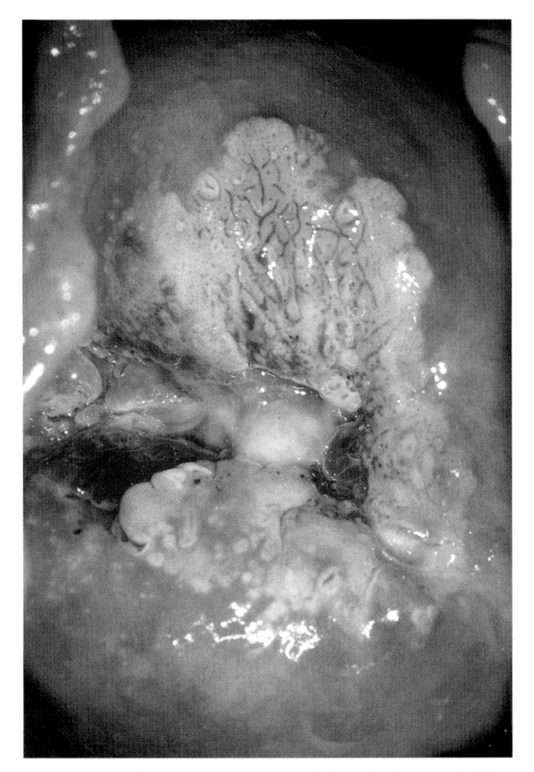

Fig. 7.**151** Flat condylomas and dysplasia (Pap IVa) in a 27-year-old patient during the 12th week of pregnancy, after application of 3% acetic acid.

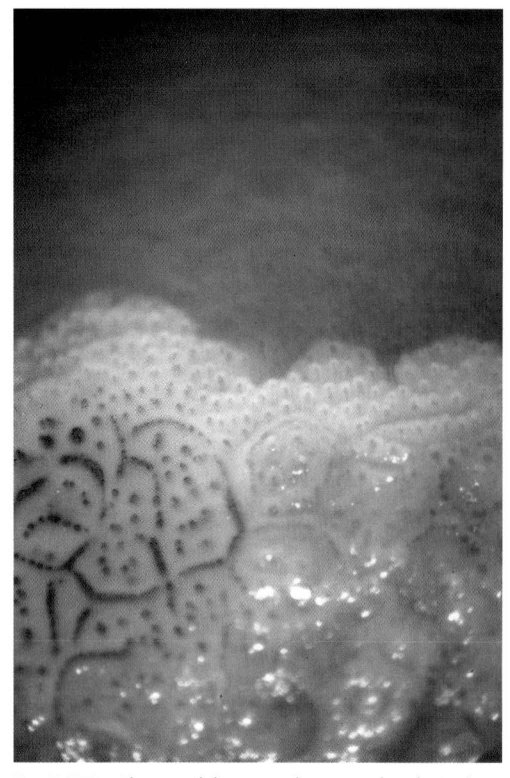

Fig. 7.**152** Flat condyloma and severe dysplasia (Pap IVa) in a 28-year-old patient.

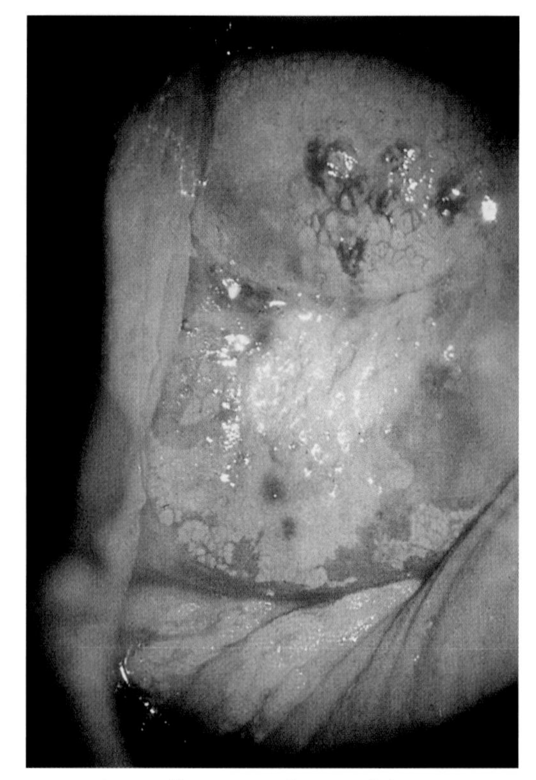

Fig. 7.**153** Papillomavirus infection of the portio vaginalis in a 28-year-old patient. Application of acetic acid revealed a mosaic on the anterior lip of the cervix and a flat condyloma (dissolving into isolated, spotlike areas) on the posterior lip and vagina.

stratified squamous epithelium of the portio vaginalis.

In individual patients though, one may find nodules also inside the cervix that become white after application of acetic acid (Fig. 7.**154**). Histologically, they correspond to lesions caused by papillomavirus infection. Here, in the transformation zone between the columnar epithelium of the endocervix and the stratified squamous epithelium of the ectocervix, infections with different pathogens may occur repeatedly, and chronic infections (*Chlamydia*) often occur as well. It is therefore not surprising that cellular oncogenes are switched on in this particular region.

From that point of view, papillomavirus infections on the portio vaginalis are of special importance. The risk of degeneration (dysplasia) is much higher here than in the vagina or in the vulvar region. It is therefore recommended that women be carefully monitored once HPV-16 and HPV-18 have been detected. Early elimination of cytologically or histologically altered cells by means of laser, cryoablation, or conization lowers the risk of carcinoma.

Special risks:

- risk of dysplasia and carcinoma (p. 97)
- possibly transmission to the newborn during delivery, resulting in the occurrence of laryngeal papillomas (HPV-11)
- risk of infecting the sexual partner.

Diagnosis:

- Colposcopy after swabbing with 3% acetic acid.
- *Detection of viral DNA.* By means of hybridization using a cellular smear or a tissue sample.
- *PCR*
- *Histology.* Possibly koilocytosis (Fig. 7.**65**, p. 97).
- *Cytology.* Pap IIw or IIID.

Therapy:

- mechanical removal by means of laser or electrical ablation, cryoablation
- denaturation (cryoablation, trichloroacetic acid, albothyl)
- immunomodulators
- interferon
- vaginal vitamin C delayed-release tablets, daily over several weeks.

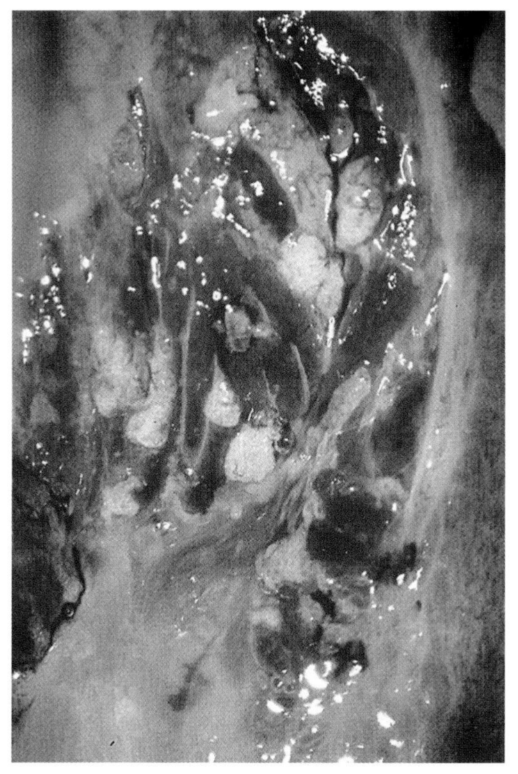

Fig. 7.**154** Intracervical papillomavirus infection in a 24-year-old patient during the 18th week of pregnancy. Several acid-white nodules are visible in the slightly opened cervix. Histologic findings support the clinical diagnosis.

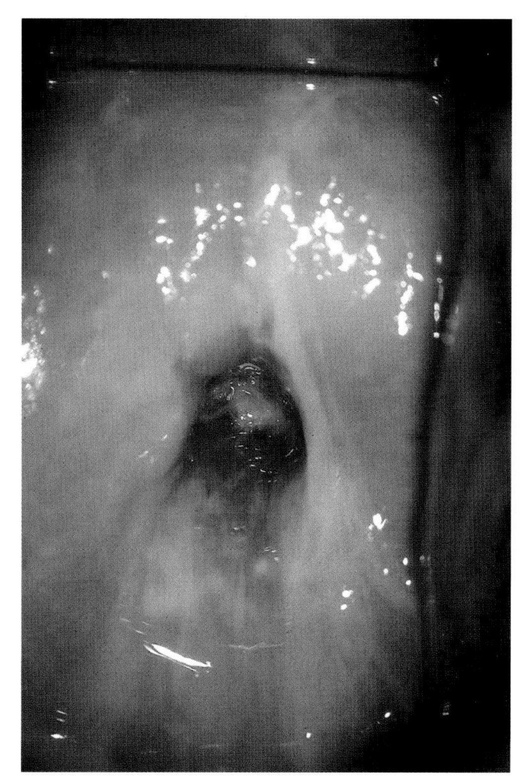

Fig. 7.**155** Apparently chronic cervicitis (lasting for six months) in a 46-year-old patient. It turned out to be a cervical carcinoma (of stage IIb).

Differential Diagnosis of Cervicitis

Cervical Carcinoma

In cases of chronic cervicitis that does not heal under antibiotic therapy, or in cases of questionable cervicitis, one should always take a swab for cytological examination. The swab is best collected from the cervical canal using a brush. If cytological examinations are inconclusive, they need to be repeated with another method or fixation—as often as it is necessary to exclude a carcinoma. Fig. 7.**155** shows the portio vaginalis of a 46-year-old patient who has been repeatedly examined over almost six months and has been treated unsuccessfully—until she changed her doctor and a cervical carcinoma of stage IIb was diagnosed. Early recognition of adenocarcinoma of the cervix or portio vaginalis is particularly difficult. In contrast to the usual infectious forms of vaginitis—which always affect large areas, if not the entire vagina or portio vaginalis—early stages of a carcinoma are initially very localized and then spread continuously. One should never hesitate too long with the histological clarification of questionable processes in the cervical region and take sufficient biopsy material.

For conspicuous features of the cervix during pregnancy, see p. 209.

Ascending Infections of the Internal Genitals

Normally, the cervix represents an excellent barrier against the penetration of pathogens into the uterus, tubes, and small pelvis.

Etiology. Only special circumstances lead to an ascending infection:

- Infections with virulent pathogens through sexual contact (e. g., *Neisseria gonorrhoeae* and *Chlamydia trachomatis*) or infections with highly virulent pathogens (e. g., streptococci of group A).
- During and after delivery, i. e., when the uterine cavity is open.
- After surgical interventions in the uterine region (e. g., abrasion, insertion of IUD, manipulations for artificial abortion).

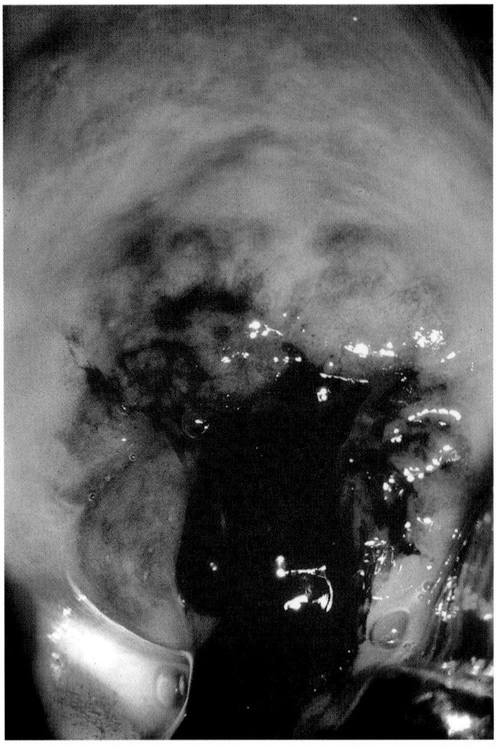

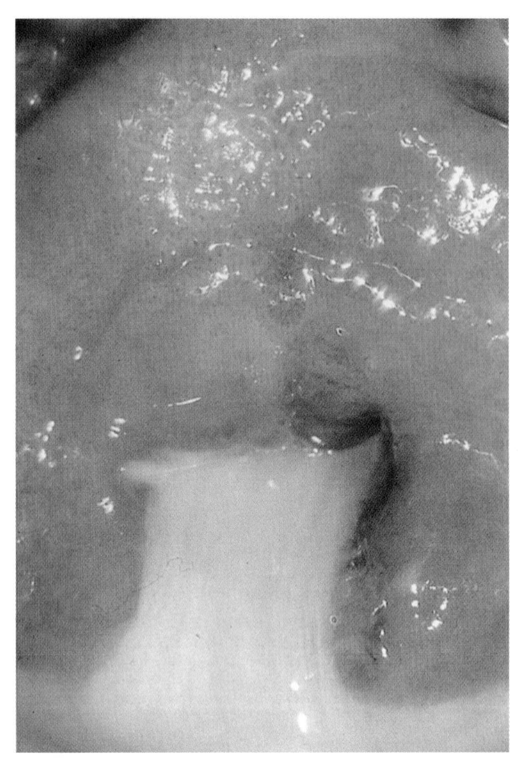

Fig. 7.**156** Endometritis caused by *Chlamydia,* (**a**) with hemorrhage in a 23-year-old patient and (**b**) with leukorrhea in a 27-year-old patient.

- Necrotic tumors (cervical carcinoma, endometrial carcinoma).
- Estrogen deficiency (only rarely).

The following factors are also known to promote ascending infections: diabetes mellitus, immunosuppression (underlying disease, carcinoma, medication, HIV infection), the period or other bleedings (polyp, submucous uterine myoma), and IUD.

The type of pathogen and the amount of pathogens that are already present in the vagina, or are introduced during manipulation, play a decisive role as well.

Course. Depending on the pathogen, the infection may run a slow and chronic course with abscess formation, as is the case with infections due to anaerobes; or it may run an extremely fulminant course (less often seen today) with death occurring within hours or a few days, as is the case with infections due to group A streptococci.

Prognosis. Infections heal better when recognized early so that treatment can be initiated in a timely fashion. This requires that the physician always considers also the possibility of an infection and orders the adequate diagnostic procedures.

Signs of infection, such as fever, leukocytosis, and above all pain, are important indicators. If they fail to develop, the body will be overwhelmed by the pathogens, mediators become activated, and the prognosis is rather poor because a diagnosis has not been established in time. In part, these cases are lethal even today, or they are survived only with considerable sequelae.

Endometritis

Inflammation of the endometrium is called endometritis. We distinguish between endometritis caused by ascending pathogens, such as gonococci and chlamydiae, and postoperative endometritis, which is caused by other pathogens and additional risk factors.

In the case of sexually transmitted pathogens, the inflammation is usually restricted to the endometrium. The main symptom of this common form of endometritis is bleeding (Fig. 7.**156 a**). Massive leukorrhea (Fig. 7.**156 b**) is the exception.

In the case of postoperative and puerperal endometritis, the pathogens and the extent and severity of the infection and inflammation actually indicate a case of endomyometritis, since areas of the myometrium are affected. This form of inflammation will therefore be discussed under postoperative and postpartal infections.

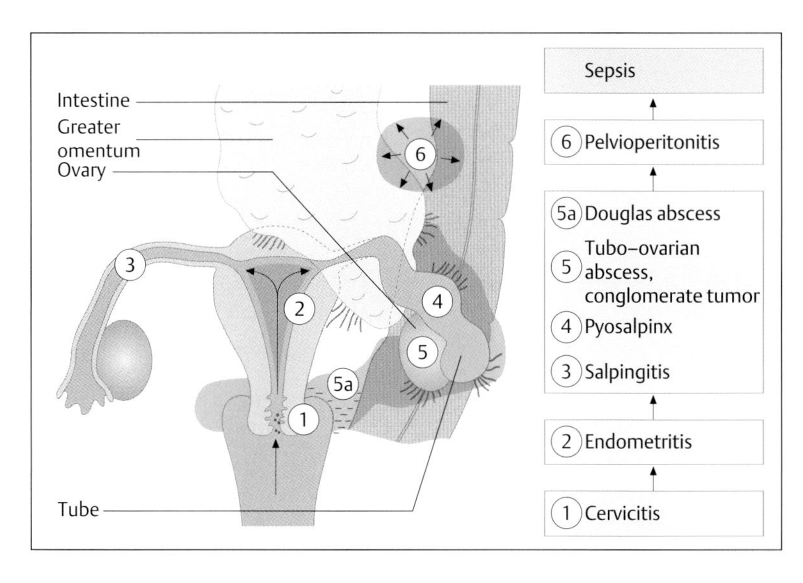

Fig. 7.**157** Ascending infections of the female genitals. Possible stages of spreading and their sequelae.

Endometritis in Outpatients

Occasionally, endometritis may occur after insertion of an IUD, or when subclinical infections of the vagina or cervix have not been recognized and considered, or—more frequently—spontaneously due to ascending pathogens, especially chlamydiae and less often gonococci. In case of the latter pathogens, endometritis is probably only a transitional stage, for these infections manifest themselves essentially in the region of the adnexa (Fig. 7.**157**). Nevertheless, this does not mean that an inflammatory response cannot occur in the endometrium. Severe symptoms, however, are rather unlikely in case of solitary endometritis.

Clinical picture. The main symptom is dysfunctional bleeding (hypermenorrhea, mid-cycle bleeding), and cervicitis is often present at the same time (see Fig. 7.**139**, p. 139) together with redness, putrid discharge, and leukocytes in the discharge (microscopic finding). Dysmenorrhea, lower abdominal pain, and subfebrile temperature may be signs of endometritis. Tenderness of the uterus during bimanual examination is only diagnostic in case of severe inflammation and pain, since pressure on the uterus is perceived as uncomfortable by the majority of women.

Diagnosis:
- assessment of the cervix
- cervical smear—if possible, from the uterine cavity—for general bacteriology (gonococci, group A streptococci), and a special smear for the detection of chlamydiae
- inflammatory parameters (blood count, ESR, CRP) for assessing the extent of inflammation
- ultrasound.

Pathogens. Chlamydiae, gonococci, group A streptococci, *Staphylococcus aureus*, intestinal flora with anaerobes.

Therapy:
- antibiotics, such as amoxicillin with β-lactamase inhibitors, doxycycline, fluoroquinolones, to attack the most important pathogens, possibly also metronidazole
- estrogens to strengthen the endometrium
- removal of the IUD in severe cases (this is not necessary in mild cases, such as chlamydial infection treated adequately with antibiotics).

Prognosis and course. Prognosis is usually good. The course of the infection can be easily assessed using inflammatory parameters (CRP).

Special Forms of Endometritis

Pyometra

Pyometra is a rare special form of endometritis, in which the accumulation of pus within the uterus leads to occlusion of the cervical canal. Preconditions include pathogens in the uterine cavity and favorable conditions for pathogen multiplication, or an existing immunodeficiency. Such conditions may exist after surgical intervention (such as conization, or abrasion in cases of endometrial carcinoma) or in the presence of a necrotic malignant tumor that occludes the cervical canal. Occasionally, pyometra is a random finding, namely, when pus is suddenly draining from the cervical canal. Ultrasound, laboratory data, cytology, and bacteriology are helpful when assessing the risk. If draining occurs, one may initially monitor its course under antibiotic therapy, if the patient's

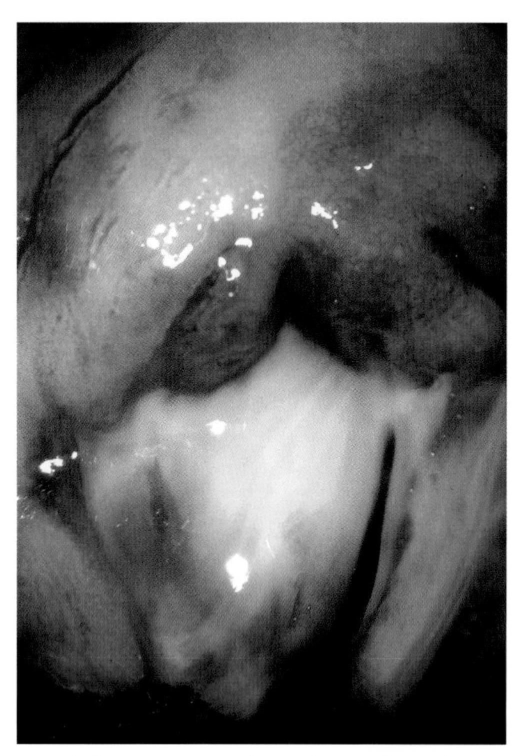

Fig. 7.**158** Pyometra, with pus draining from the cervix, in a 60-year-old patient.

condition allows for this. Mainly *Staphylococcus aureus* and anaerobes (e. g., *Bacteroides* species) are found as pathogens. Sepsis and septic shock may occur depending on the underlying disease and the additional risk, although this is very rare.

Clinical picture. There are hardly any complaints. At the most, there is yellow discharge when drainage occurs. Fever is rare.

Diagnosis:

- *Clinical picture.* Drainage of pus from the cervix (Fig. 7.**158**).
- *Microscopy.* Massive leukorrhea.
- *Ultrasound.* Fluid/pus in the uterine cavity, endometrial polyp.
- *Bacteriology*
- Inflammatory parameters for assessing the extent of inflammation.
- Exclusion of a malignant tumor (cytology, histology).
- Exclusion of peritonitis.

Therapy:

- attempt to dilate the cervical canal if there is no spontaneous drainage (caution: perforation)
- drainage of the uterine cavity under ultrasonic guidance
- systemic administration of antibiotics that will definitely attack the two pathogens mentioned above (*Staphylococcus aureus*, anaerobes)
- subsequently, further checks are necessary to exclude a malignant tumor
- if in doubt, surgical sanitation should be carried out.

Risks:

- malignant tumor
- perforation into the abdomen, followed by peritonitis or sepsis.

Endometritis Caused by Tubercle Bacilli

Endometritis due to tubercle bacilli is very rare today. It is observed almost exclusively in older women, and the diagnosis is usually established by the pathologist based on a random finding. In younger women, it may be found occasionally when diagnosing sterility. It is more often observed in women from developing countries, although it is then usually accompanied by infection of the tubes as well.

Salpingitis

Inflammation of the tubes is called salpingitis. The tubes are the main sites of manifestation of all ascending pathogens (Fig. 7.**157**).

Extent of infection and pathogens. Ascending infections are progressive inflammations that may not only affect various organs and regions but also manifest themselves as different clinical pictures depending on the pathogen and the circumstances. Starting from the inside of the tubes, these infections can affect all layers of the tubal wall and can further spread to the surrounding areas. Accordingly, the clinical picture is very complex.

The nomenclature of such an infection is confusing. It would be better to speak of a general inflammation of the upper genital tract. The term "adnexitis" used in German-speaking countries corresponds roughly to the term "pelvic inflammatory disease (PID)" used in English. Nevertheless, thanks to ultrasound and inflammatory parameters, we are now able to define the extent of such infections more precisely:

- endometritis
- salpingitis
- pyosalpinx
- hydrosalpinx
- tubo-ovarian abscess.

Salpingitis is an inflammation of the tubes caused by ascending pathogens, and a multitude of

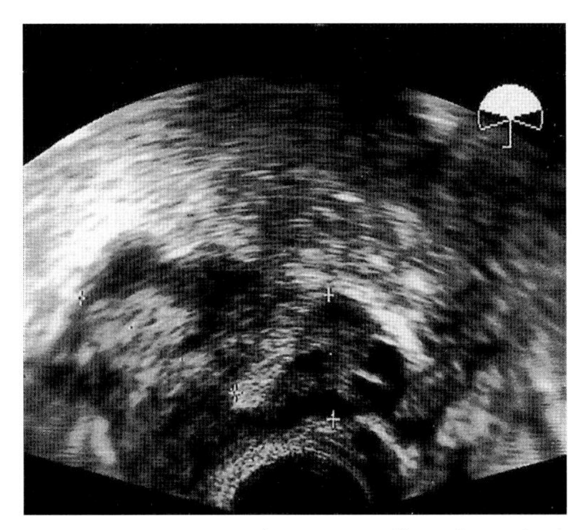

Fig. 7.**159** Sonogram showing an inflamed conglomerate tumor of the right adnexa, in a 32-year-old patient suffering from chronic PID for 10 weeks. The ovary is visible between the two white crosses.

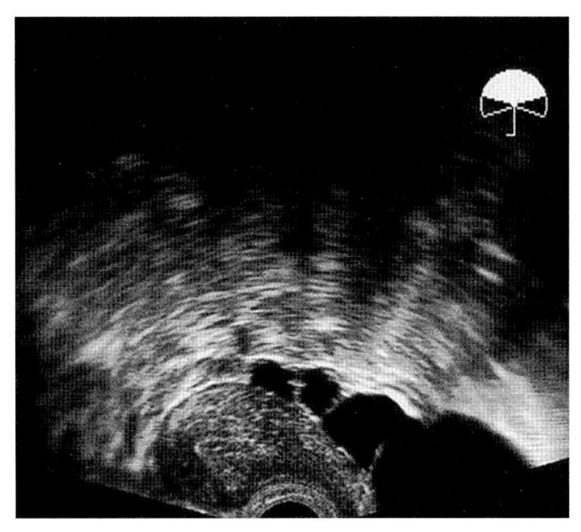

Fig. 7.**160** Sonogram showing hydrosalpinx in a 35-year-old patient suffering from primary sterility and chronic recurrent PID.

different bacteria may be involved here. This is why there are different views on the role and frequency of various pathogens as a cause of acute salpingitis.

Two pathogens have been demonstrated as a cause of salpingitis:

- *Neisseria gonorrhoeae*
- *Chlamydia trachomatis.*

The clinical pictures, including the course and the amount of damage done, differ significantly according to the biological properties of these two pathogens.

Other pathogens may be:

- herpes simplex viruses
- group A streptococci.

In addition, various other bacteria can often be isolated from tubes affected by salpingitis, for example, anaerobes (*Bacteroides* species, peptococci, peptostreptococci), and in addition *Gardnerella vaginalis*, *Escherichia coli*, group B streptococci, and others, i. e., microbes that are commonly found in the vagina as well.

Depending on the extent of the infection in the adnexal region, more or less extensive adhesions to the greater omentum, the intestine, the pelvic wall, or the abdominal wall will occur if therapy is not initiated in a timely fashion.

Acute Salpingitis

Characteristic signs for this acute form of salpingitis are sudden severe pain in the lower abdomen (usually on both sides), high temperature, and malaise. The disease affects almost exclusively young, sexually active women. Among the laboratory data, high numbers of leukocytes in the blood (up to 20 000/µL) with a hardly increased ESR are typical for the acute process. After a few doses of antibiotics, the symptoms disappear as fast as they occurred.

Pathogen. *Neisseria gonorrhoeae* is involved in 50–70% of cases. The rate of detection depends on various factors. It is the higher, the earlier bacteriological diagnostic procedures are used. Gonococci can adhere to the epithelial cells and can also penetrate them; as a result, detection of this pathogen is less successful in the pus and much more successful in tissue swabs. This is particularly true for the fallopian tubes.

Gonococci are very sensitive to antibiotics and, as a rule, are no longer detected in cultures after the first administration of an antibiotic.

Pathogenesis. Gonococci usually ascend during, or immediately after, the period when the cervix is open and the protective estrogen secretion is still absent. The adherence of gonococci to epithelial cells seems to be an important factor in inducing an inflammation of the tubal epithelium. Both, the pili and the protein 2 of gonococci play a major role here. Their ability to vary widely helps the gonococci to overcome the body's defense system.

The rapid multiplication of gonococci and the intracavitary spread lead to an almost sudden infection of the entire internal genitals. The inflammatory response induced by gonococci in the internal genitals causes severe pain and usually also high temperature.

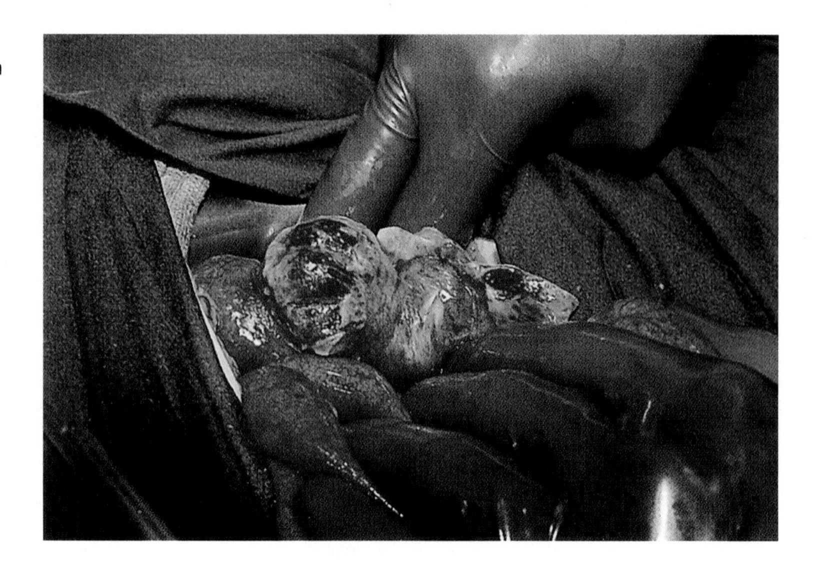

Fig. 7.**161** Conglomerate tumor associated with salpingitis in a 32-year-old patient, with *Chlamydia* detected in her cervix.

Clinical picture:
- sudden onset
- severe pain in the lower abdomen
- fever (> 38 °C)
- pain upon movement of the uterus
- pasty, dolente resistance in the region of the adnexa
- lower abdomen also tender to pressure
- guarding of abdominal muscles, depending on the extent of infection.

Special risks or sequelae:
- bacteremic spread of gonococci leading to exanthema or arthritis
- conglomerate tumor (Fig. 7.**159**)
- pyosalpinx
- hydrosalpinx (Fig. 7.**160**)
- tubo-ovarian abscess
- sterility
- increased incidence of tubal pregnancy.

Early treatment can limit the sequelae.

The gonorrheal infection usually remains restricted to the adnexa. In individual patients, however, there may be systemic dissemination involving the joints as well. Some cases of gonorrhea have only been recognized because of arthritis. A fine-spotted skin lesion may develop with systemic infection, but this is rare.

In some cases, other pathogens of the vaginal region—such as various anaerobes, various streptococci, *Staphylococcus aureus*, *Escherichia coli*, and others—ascend together with the gonococci; as a result, chronic abscess-forming processes sometimes occur in the adnexal region after the acute symptoms have subsided.

To prevent this, an antibiotic therapy is required that attacks these pathogens as well. The treatment should last for at least 10 days.

Repeated surveillance of the laboratory parameters and examination of the small pelvis by ultrasound should make it possible to recognize such development at an early stage when it can still be treated with antibiotics. In case of severe abscess-forming infection, however, only surgical sanitation of the site of infection will effect a cure.

Diagnosis:
- *Clinical picture*
- *Pregnancy test.* It should be negative
- *Microscopy.* Plenty of leukocytes (granulocytes) in the discharge; the vaginal flora is often disturbed (bacterial vaginosis).
- *Detection of bacteria in the culture* (transport medium, special growth media) if antibiotics have not yet been administered: in the cervix, or in the fimbriae if laparoscopy has been performed.
- Detection of chlamydia.
- *Laboratory parameters.* Blood count (leukocytosis); CRP (always elevated levels), ESR (initially normal, then markedly increased after a few days).
- *Ultrasound.* Thickened tubes, conglomerate tumor (Figs. 7.**159**, 7.**161**), fluid in the recto-uterine pouch (Douglas space).
- *Laparoscopy.* Reddened and thickened tubes, adhesions.
- *Clinical course.* Rapid response to antibiotics.
- *Serology* to support the diagnosis in special cases, especially in case of disseminated gonorrhea.

In every case of suspected salpingitis, one should exclude the possibility of an ectopic pregnancy or appendicitis. Arguments against acute salpingitis include the lack of sexual contact during the previous weeks, unilateral appearance of symptoms, a microscopically normal vaginal flora without leukocytes in the discharge

Recognition of acute salpingitis is difficult when the symptoms have already existed for several days and when antibiotics have already been administered. The acute leukocytosis may already be over, and only the ESR is still increased. In such cases, laparoscopy is recommended in order to secure or complete the diagnosis. This is not required in clear cases of acute salpingitis.

Therapy. Treatment depends on the extent of the infection and on the pathogens involved.

Short-term penicillin therapy is sufficient for uncomplicated gonococcal infections if applied timely.

Because gonococci are so sensitive, almost any antibiotic may be administered (exceptions: clindamycin, lincomycin). The quick response to penicillin is good evidence for a gonococcal infection caused by a sensitive strain.

One problem that needs to be considered is the fact that other pathogens usually contribute to salpingitis as well, especially when the infection has already persisted for some time. In addition, it cannot be excluded that chlamydiae may be involved at the same time. This is particularly difficult when no typical pathogens can be detected in the cervix and no laparoscopy with collection of swabs and sample excision has been performed.

In such patients, one has to take the clinical picture as a guide and design a broad therapy.

Therapy in case of gonococcus detection. Penicillin or ampicillin (i.v.) or amoxicillin (orally) and also tetracyclines should be adequate in most cases. An antibiogram is important for recognizing β-lactamase-producing strains.

Successful treatment is possible with cephalosporins of the third generation.

In addition, an antiphlogistic agent should be administered, such as diclofenac, piroxicam.

Duration of therapy: five to seven days.

After normalization of the ESR, no further measures are necessary.

Persistence of an increased ESR indicates an insufficient response, or that there may be an additional problem. Here, one might first attempt treatment with a more effective antibiotic and higher doses. Apart from that, one should search for other causes of the increased ESR, such as abnormal erythrocytes, immune disease, or other chronic diseases including a malignant tumor.

Therapy without pathogen detection:

- doxycycline (200 mg) + metronidazole (2 × 500 mg) per day
- ampicillin or amoxillin + β-lactamase inhibitors
- clindamycin (4 × 600 mg) + gentamicin or tobramycin (80 mg) per day (not for gonococci)
- cephalosporin (2–6 g) + metronidazole (2 × 500 mg) + doxycycline (200 mg) per day
- ampicillin (3 × 2 g) + doxycycline (200 mg) per day
- fluoroquinolones with or without metronidazole, depending on the drug (no metronidazole in the case of moxifloxacin)

Once the fever has subsided, treatment may be continued orally for a total of 10–14 days.

Subacute Salpingitis

Subacute salpingitis is usually associated with moderate symptoms; these vary and are sometimes so uncharacteristic that tubal infection is not considered initially. Fever is rare, and the temperature is only slightly increased, if at all. The symptoms reach from variable pain in the lower abdomen, discharge, dyspareunia, and back pain to respiratory pain and pain in the right upper abdomen and right shoulder. The laboratory data show only moderate leukocytosis (up to 12 000/μL) and a moderate increase in CRP (up to 60 mg/L; the normal value is 5 mg/L). *Chlamydia trachomatis* is the most common pathogen here. The clinical parameters in case of chlamydiae are never as pronounced as with acute gonorrheal salpingitis.

Pathogens. *Chlamydia trachomatis* is detected in about 90 % of patients with subacute salpingitis.

Less often involved are:

- gonococci
- anaerobes
- *Escherichia coli* and other *Enterobacteriaceae*
- streptococci of groups A, G, and F
- *Staphylococcus aureus*
- *Mycoplasma genitalium.*

Frequency. Subacute salpingitis is nowadays 10 times more common than acute salpingitis.

Pathogenesis. In anatomical terms, the disease causes a local inflammatory response, the severity of which is in sharp contrast to the minor clinical symptoms. The tubal endothelium is affected in particular, but inflammatory reactions may also extend over the entire tubal wall. As a result, multiple adhesions may develop in the small pelvis between tube, ovary, greater omentum, and intestine. Inflammation of the peritoneum in the

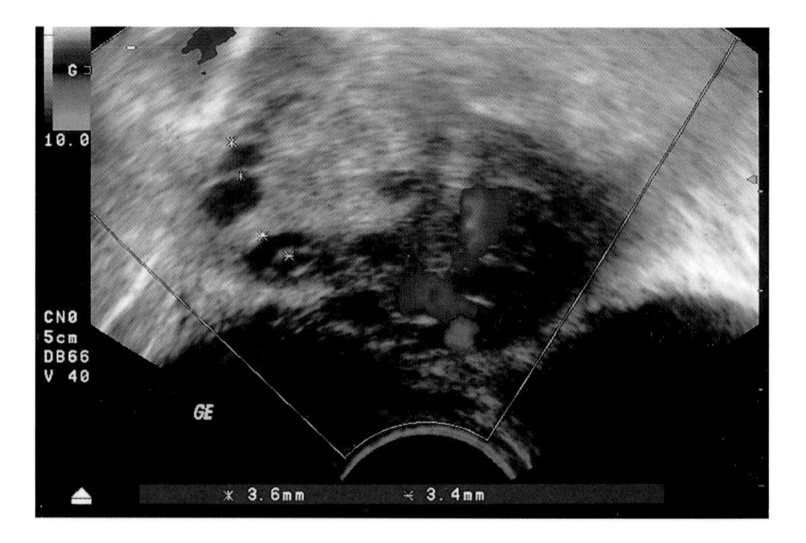

Fig. 7.**162** Sonogram of an inflamed conglomerate tumor of the right adnexa due to *Chlamydia.*

region of the liver (perihepatitis) is actually a classic complication in the abdominal cavity if subacute salpingitis is caused by chlamydiae and occurs in up to 10% of these patients. Clinically, it manifests itself as pain in the right shoulder due to irritation of the phrenic nerve.

Symptoms:

- mild, variable pain in the lower abdomen for days or weeks
- contact bleeding, dysfunctional bleeding (cervicitis/endometritis) for some time
- slightly yellowish discharge (cervicitis)
- pain during intercourse
- fatigue and weakness
- pain in the right upper abdomen and/or in the right shoulder (perihepatitis)
- sporadic back pain,
- joint pain.

Due to the uncharacteristic, variable symptoms, some patients have already accumulated a medical history of weeks or months with many consultations and preliminary examinations.

Clinical picture:

- moderate impairment of the general condition
- cervicitis with redness and yellow cervical secretion
- pain upon movement of the uterus, painful adnexal region
- palpable painful resistance of the adnexa (conglomerate tumor), but not always
- laparotomy, or better laparoscopy: inflammatory conglomerate tumor (Fig. 7.**161**).

Diagnosis:

- Medical history, clinical picture, and findings of the clinical examination.
- *Microscopy.* Leukocytes in the wet mount.
- Swab from the cervical canal for the detection of *Chlamydia* (preferred method: PCR).
- First-stream urine for the detection of *Chlamydia* (increased chance of detection).
- Cervical swab for general bacteriology (exclusion of gonococci, etc.).
- *Laboratory parameters.* Blood count, CRP, ESR.
- *Ultrasound.* Fluid in the Douglas pouch, conglomerate tumor (Fig. 7.**162**), pyosalpinx/hydrosalpinx.
- *Chlamydial serology.*
- Laparoscopy only in unclear cases without detection of a pathogen.

Laparoscopy. Laparoscopy is only justified if the diagnosis is not clear and pathogens could not be detected. Due to the improved detection of *Chlamydia* from the cervix and first-stream urine by means of amplification tests, laparoscopic clarification of acute and subacute salpingitis is rarely necessary today. Redness of the tubes may be so discrete that an inflammation restricted to the inside of the tubes is not recognized even by laparoscopy. Detection of the pathogen (*C. trachomatis*) is most often achieved from the cervix, also in cases of salpingitis. An attempt to detect chlamydiae from the fimbriae is less often successful than detection from the cervix; it is therefore not a routine approach and should be rather reserved for special cases or scientific studies.

Failure to detect the pathogen. Detection of the pathogen from the cervix in cases of chlamydial salpingitis is not always successful, especially not when the chlamydial infection of the cervix happened a long time ago or when the patient already received antibiotics, such as amoxicillin,

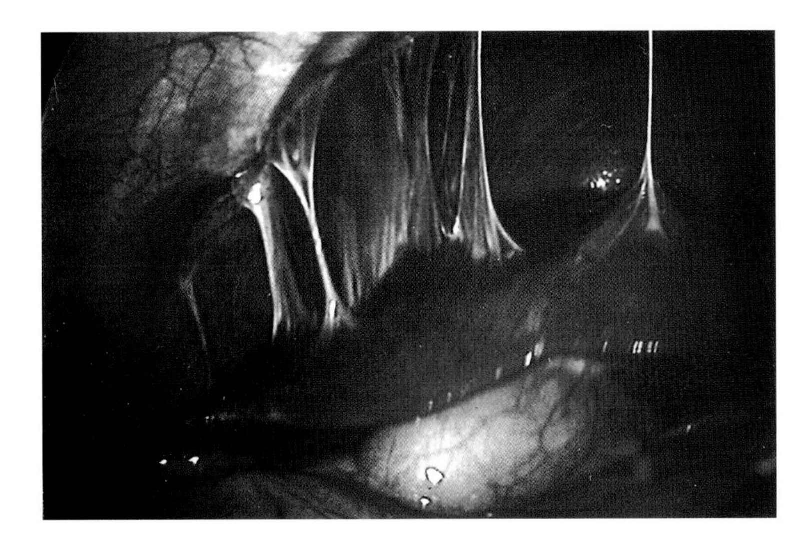

Fig. 7.**163** Condition after perihepatitis (Fitz–Hugh–Curtis syndrome) due to *Chlamydia* in a 37-year-old patient.

doxycycline, Co-Trimoxazole, which are also active against chlamydiae.

Serology may help in such patients. In 10% of women with detectable *Chlamydia*, no antibodies to *C. trachomatis* are found. Here, we are probably dealing with a superficial cervical infection. Antibodies are usually detected in cases of chlamydial infection of the upper genitals. Hence, the absence of antibodies against *C. trachomatis* in subacute salpingitis speaks, in all probability, against a chlamydial infection.

Sequelae:

- sterility, the frequency of which increases with the number of chlamydial infections (according to Weström, 1987, the incidence of sterility is 12% after the first infection, 24% after the second infection, and 54% or more after the third infection)
- tubal pregnancy
- perihepatitis (Fitz–Hugh–Curtis syndrome) with adhesions between the liver and the thoracic wall (Fig. 7.**163**)
- arthritis (large joints)
- hydrosalpinx (see also Fig. 7.**160**, p. 149),
- chronic persistent lower abdominal pain.

Therapy:

Standard therapy: doxycycline (200 mg per day for 10 days or, better, 20 days).

For other drugs, see Table 7.**10**, p. 137.

Follow-up and further care. After complete subsiding of all signs of inflammation, elimination of the pathogen, and normalization of the vaginal flora, the following examinations may be carried out: hysterosalpingography, perturbation with ultrasonic guidance, or laparoscopy with methylene blue perturbation. If the treatment has been timely and adequate, one will find completely normal tubes. Should mild intratubal constriction or occlusion have already occurred, it may still be time to render the tubes patent.

If the antibody titer is high, the course of healing can be monitored. The first check-up may take place after three month at the earliest, but it is better to do it only every six months.

Inflammatory Conglomerate Tumor, Tubo–ovarian Abscess

If the antibiotic therapy for certain pathogens comes too late or is insufficient, an abscess-forming inflammation may develop from salpingitis and from an initially inflammatory conglomerate tumor. The reason for this may be that patients present very late for an examination because there are relatively few symptoms of pain. Apart from an inflammation primarily originating from the genitals, inflammation may also originate from the intestine (e. g., diverticula or appendix), or it may even result from hematogenous dissemination of *Staphylococcus aureus* from an infected infusion site (vein).

Pathogenesis. The reason for late examination and diagnosis in outpatients lies probably in the fact that the severe inflammatory response is associated with low levels of pain. This is characteristic for *Chlamydia* infections. The body tries to limit the inflammatory process by covering it with the greater omentum and other movable organs, such as the intestine or the ovaries.

If certain additional bacteria are present, further changes may occur that are associated with increased leukocyte infiltration and abscess formation.

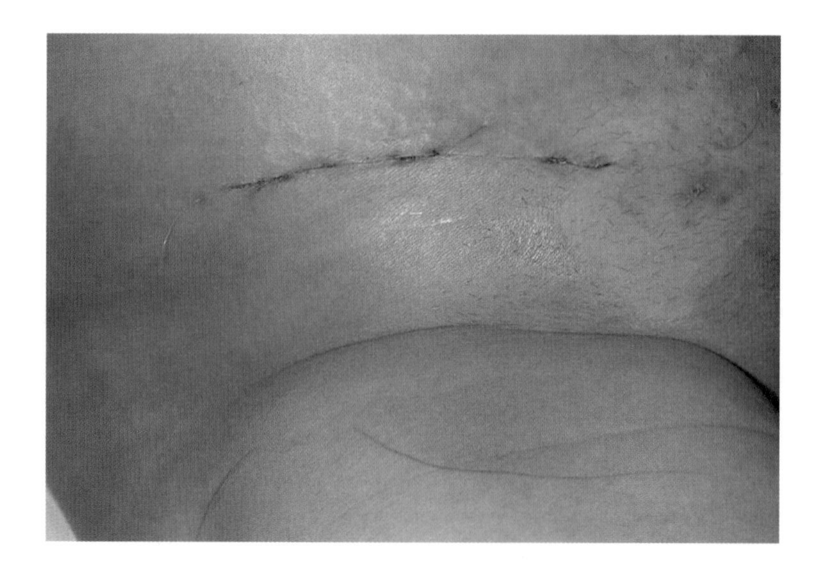

Fig. 7.**164** Wound infection caused by *Staphylococcus aureus* after removal of the inguinal lymph nodes because of a vulvar carcinoma.

Pathogens:

- sexually transmitted pathogens, such as gonococci and *Chlamydia trachomatis*
- *Staphylococcus aureus* (after surgery)
- group A streptococci (very rarely spontaneously, more often after surgery or delivery)
- *Enterobacteriaceae* and other intestinal bacteria (after surgery or delivery, and also originating from intestinal processes)
- anaerobes (see intestinal bacteria)
- actinomycetes (rarely)
- tubercle bacilli (rarely).

Diagnosis:

- *Clinical picture.* Lower abdominal pain, often only with a mild increase in temperature or none at all.
- *Laboratory parameters.* In most patients, the number of leukocytes in the blood is clearly increased, with the CRP only slightly increased and the ESR markedly increased if there are abscesses.
- *Detection of pathogen* is often unsatisfactory. One may attempt isolation from a cervical swab and, in case of laparoscopy or laparotomy, from the conglomerate tumor. Any pus should be collected with a syringe to send as much pus as possible for bacteriological tests; this will yield better gram-stained preparations, and chances are higher that the pathogen can be cultured.
- *Histology* if actinomycosis is suspected.
- *Ultrasound.*

Therapy. Treatment depends on the clinical condition of the patient and on the pathogens detected or potentially present. *Chlamydia* should always be considered in outpatients. After surgery or during childbed, one should pay more attention to *Staphylococcus aureus*, group A streptococci, and intestinal bacteria.

Conglomerate tumor:

- Antibiotics: ampicillin or amoxillin + β-lactamase inhibitors, doxycycline + metronidazole, moxifloxacin, or levofloxacin. If the patient's condition is critical, high doses of a second or third generation cephalosporin + metronidazole, or one of the carbapenems.
- Laparoscopy: only after a cure has been attempted with antibiotics. Adequate and timely treatment with antibiotics may lead to complete regression of the conglomerate tumor.

Tubo-ovarian abscess:

- Antibiotics: preferably a second generation cephalosporin + metronidazole, or one of the fluoroquinolones + metronidazole.
- Surgical sanitation (laparoscopy or laparotomy). This is the only approach that has a chance of cure in advanced chronic cases.

Wound Infection After Surgery

Frequency and prophylaxis. The frequency of wound infections depends on various risk factors and on the type of surgery. The number of infections can be markedly lowered by draining the area of the wound (important for vaginal interventions because anaerobes are common there) and by preoperative antibiotic prophylaxis.

Risk factors of an infection:

- pathogens, such as group A streptococci, *Staphylococcus aureus* (Fig. 7.**164**)
- high counts of facultative pathogens (e.g., bacterial vaginosis), intestinal bacteria

- tissue trauma, necrosis
- hematoma
- hypoxia
- long duration of surgery
- diabetes mellitus
- immunosuppression
- anemia.

Postoperative infections are less common if antibiotic prophylaxis is used. Risk factors include the type of intervention, colonization of the area of surgery, the type of bacteria, the patient's general condition, and many others (see also Antibiotic Prophylaxis, p. 239).

Infection of the Vaginal Stump Following Vaginal Hysterectomy

Infections of the vaginal stump are more common after vaginal hysterectomy than after abdominal hysterectomy because of the relatively large wound created by the simultaneously performed vaginoplasty and also because of frequent colonization of the vagina with facultative pathogens, particularly anaerobe bacteria. In the majority of cases, the infection remains localized and is therefore less severe than after laparotomy. Here, too, the pathogen is the decisive factor for the prognosis.

The risk of infection can be kept to a minimum by preoperative reduction of pathogens in the vagina by means of antibiotic prophylaxis (single dose).

A foul-smelling discharge, mild subfebrile temperature, and a slightly protracted recovery of the patient may be the only symptoms. The number of leukocytes in the blood is usually not significantly increased.

Treatment is usually sufficient if it involves good drainage and vaginal irrigation. Depending on the pathogen and the patient's condition, systemic antibiotic therapy may shorten the duration of the infection. Apart from the patient's condition, the inflammatory parameters (leukocytes in the blood, CRP) can help with assessing the severity of the infection.

Infections After Hysterectomy

Pathogenesis and frequency. Infections in the small pelvis are common after vaginal (and also abdominal) hysterectomy. Here, too, the reason is contact during surgery with areas colonized by bacteria, namely, the vagina. Complete occlusion of the vaginal stump in case of abdominal hysterectomy increases the risk of an infection with high fever. Though wound infections after vaginal hysterectomy are slightly more common than after abdominal hysterectomy, they are rather localized and thus associated with fewer symptoms. For a long time, therefore, antibiotic prophylaxis has only been recommended for vaginal hysterectomy.

Clinical picture. Fever usually occurs only two days (or later) after surgery. Patients complain of increasing pain in the lower abdomen.

Diagnosis and therapy:

- Expansion of the vaginal stump.
- Swabs for bacterial diagnosis.
- Blood cultures
- *Laboratory parameters.* Leukocytes and CRP almost always increased or rising again, thrombocytes.
- Early administration of antibiotics.

If the fever does not subside soon, abscess formation or thrombophlebitis may have already occurred in the small pelvis.

Peritonitis

The clinical picture of peritonitis may reach from a localized response in case of moderately pathogenic microbes, such as *Chlamydia*, and a small perforation of diverticula to severe peritonitis of the entire abdominal cavity accompanied by sepsis or intestinal injury. The symptoms and the pathogens detected differ accordingly.

The most severe forms of peritonitis are triggered by group A streptococci. Detection of *Escherichia coli* and other intestinal bacteria speaks rather for intestinal perforation or injury, since it happens most likely here that so many bacteria are introduced that the body can no longer cope with them.

Postoperative peritonitis due to vaginal pathogens has become rare, since we now pay attention to anaerobes in the vagina (bacterial vaginosis) and administer effective antibiotics.

Common pathogens. In case of localized inflammations in the small pelvis, the most likely pathogens are the ascending bacteria that also cause salpingitis:

- chlamydiae and, less often, gonococci
- actinomycetes (very rarely).

After surgery and post partum, the pathogens include:

- *Staphylococcus aureus*
- streptococci of groups A, D, F, G
- *Escherichia coli*
- anaerobes
- fungi, such as *Candida albicans* (rarely).

Several microbes are usually detected, and it is not easy to decide which one is the responsible pathogen and which one may be only a colonizing microbe or synergist.

Pathogenesis. The most severe forms of peritonitis are commonly caused by intestinal microbes after perforation or after surgery, such as perforation of the appendix, diverticulitis, perforation of an ulcer, gangrenous cholecystitis, gynecological laparotomy, or cesarean section.

Peritonitis is rarely caused by hematogenous spread. However, dissemination from the genital region is possible in the case of ascending infections.

In the majority of gynecological cases, peritonitis remains localized as pelvioperitonitis. In these patients, adhesions with the greater omentum and the intestine cover the focus of infection in superior direction.

Bacterial toxins cause paralysis of the intestine (subileus, ileus).

Clinical picture. Abdominal pain, nausea, vomiting, obstipation, meteorism, fever, hypotension, tachycardia, oliguria. Gravely ill appearance, guarding of abdominal muscles, absence of peristaltic, and diarrhea.

The symptoms are less severe with localized pelvioperitonitis.

Diagnosis:

- Clinical examination by means of auscultation and palpation.
- *Laboratory parameters.* Repeating the tests is essential as values change during the course of the infection.
- Leukocytosis (> 20000/μL) is rather a good sign.
- Leukopenia (< 4000/μL) is a bad sign.
- CRP is always markedly increased (> 20 times).
- Electrolyte determination: the potassium value is often reduced.
- Swabs for bacteriology taken from the site of operation are essential. Examination of feces for pathogens or toxins is only required as an additional test in case of diarrhea.
- *Radiographic examination.* Abdominal overview while standing, air–fluid level in the small intestine and/or colon.

Therapy. Surgical approach with irrigation and subsequent drainage. In cases of pelvioperitonitis (a localized process with abscess formation in the Douglas pouch), is may be sufficient to drain the Douglas pouch (large caliber).

Antibiotics: cephalosporins (e. g., cefotiam, cefuroxime, cefotaxime, ceftriaxone) + 5-nitroimidazoles (metronidazole); fluoroquinolones, or—when the patient is in critical condition—carbapenems (imipenem, meropenem).

Close monitoring by means of clinical and laboratory surveillance is essential.

Thrombophlebitis in the Small Pelvis

This condition occurs after surgery and also after uncomplicated spontaneous delivery. It is probably not rare at all, although it is mostly discovered only during laparotomy or when a leg is swollen. Treatment is usually conservative by means of antibiotics (see Ovarian Vein Thrombophlebitis p. 221).

Sepsis

Sepsis and, even more so, septic shock are the most severe infections; even today, they are highly lethal and, if the patient survives, may lead to lifelong sequelae. The avoidance of such a situation—or at least, early recognition of the danger—should therefore have high priority in the care of patients. Sepsis and septic shock are most common after surgery and after delivery. Further causes include severe oncological illness, chemotherapy with leukopenia, infected infusion access devices and also port systems for catheters, or highly pathogenic bacteria, such as group A streptococci. The main symptom is the patient's poor state of health. Fever may be absent. CRP is the most reliable inflammatory parameter for recognizing this dangerous situation.

Definition and Course of Sepsis

Sepsis is an overreaction to infection or trauma in the form of systemic inflammation, microvascular coagulation, and altered fibrinolysis. It is the most severe course a bacterial infection may take. It represents an invasion of the body, and the sooner it is stopped, the higher the chance that the patient will survive. Every day, about 1400 people worldwide die of sepsis; 30 % die within two months and 50 % within six months. Sepsis is the cause in 80 % of deaths following severe injuries.

Many bacteria are able to cause sepsis. In healthy immunocompetent individuals—including most of the gynecological patients and pregnant women—only highly pathogenic bacteria, such as group A streptococci, actually become dangerous. For example, when using proper microbiological diagnostic procedures, group A streptococci are found as a pathogen of puerperal sepsis in almost 90% of cases. What makes group A streptococci so dangerous are superantigens, and there are very different virulent strains. However, even less virulent strains may, under certain circumstances, increase their virulence and form superantigens. Hence, any detection of group A streptococci in the genitals should always be taken seriously and treated accordingly.

Symptoms like fever and increased pulse rate are not very characteristic, as they are also present with many other infections. More typical are respiratory problems, pain, hypothermia, leukopenia, and the apparent lack of a cause for the patient's poor general condition.

The starting points for sepsis occurring in an intensive care unit include the lungs, the abdomen, the kidneys, a wound, or a catheter.

Phase 1. Infection and inflammation in connection with a wound (surgery, placental adhesion site). Immunomodulators are released, and among them are also proinflammatory and thrombogenic factors as well as numerous cytokines. These cytokines provoke inflammatory reactions along the blood vessels, resulting in an increase in plasminogen activator inhibitor of type 1 (PAI–1), which reduces fibrinolysis.

Phase 2. Formation of blood clots, one of the most complex steps in the cascade of events in the patient's body. The inflammation causes the release of tissue thromboplastin (so-called tissue factor) that, in turn, generates thrombin. Thrombin promotes coagulation by forming fibrin, and this process is abnormal during sepsis because PAI-1 has been activated.

Phase 3. Suppression of fibrinolysis. Blood clots are formed in vital organs, thus leading to necrosis:

- rapid consumption of protein C
- deficit in activated protein C
- abnormal coagulation
- formation of microvascular blood clots
- necrosis
- organ dysfunction, septic shock
- death of the patient.

For treatment during phase 3, a recombinant human activated protein C (rhAPC, Xigris, Lilly) is used. Attempts to prevent the immune response to bacterial endotoxins or to strengthen the body's immune system have so far been unsuccessful. Until now, anti-inflammatory agents and TNF antagonists proved to be ineffective as well.

Pathogenesis. Common portals of entry for bacteria into the blood stream include:

- wound infection
- thrombophlebitis (site of infusion)
- urinary tract infection
- the lungs
- indwelling catheter
- port system for catheter.

Already during the early phase of sepsis, microcirculation becomes disturbed by leukocyte aggregation and endothelial damage leading to capillary occlusion. The resulting insufficient circulation promotes multiplication of the invading bacteria and thus advances the sepsis. The terminal stage of sepsis is characterized by uncontrollable multiple organ failures. Endotoxins play a decisive role in various reactions. They stimulate the complement system through activation of macrophages and the release of various mediators. These mediators include interleukin-1 and tumor necrosis factor, which play an important role in the septic process.

Pathogens:

- group A streptococci
- *Staphylococcus aureus*
- *Escherichia coli*
- *Klebsiella pneumoniae*
- pneumococci
- *Enterococcus* (may only be present as a contaminating microbe)
- *Pseudomonas* (mainly in multimorbid immunocompromised patients)
- *Candida albicans* (mainly in immunocompromised patients or after taking antibiotics, such as carbapenems)
- *Staphylococcus epidermidis* (rarely causing sepsis, usually only present as a contaminating microbe, therefore only to be considered if detected in several blood cultures).

Clinical picture. One of the main symptoms is remittent fever. Occasionally, fever may be absent, in which case the diffuse pain and the patient's grave condition are pathognomic. The spread of bacteria may affect many organs. The spleen, in particular, increases in size and becomes soft (histopathology reveals a septic spleen, or splenic tumor), and abscesses may infiltrate also the liver and kidneys and even the brain.

Hemorrhagic or pustulous foci in the skin may be caused by gonococci, *Staphylococcus aureus*, group A streptococci, and also by meningococci, but not by *Enterobacteriaceae*, such as *Escherichia coli.* The latter (namely, the gram-negative rods) frequently lead to septic shock.

Diagnosis:

- *Blood cultures.* Repeated cultures for aerobic and anaerobic bacteria are essential. Detection of bacteria in the blood (bacteremia) per se is not yet evidence for sepsis as microbes are often flushed into the blood stream, for example, just by cleaning one's teeth.
- *Clinical picture.* Poor general condition, fever with shaking chills (may also be absent), restlessness, dyspnea, confusion, and impaired consciousness, and episodic hypotension are characteristic symptoms.
- *Laboratory parameters.* Leukocytosis with shift to the left, and—depending on the point in time—also leukocytopenia or even normal leukocyte numbers. The CRP value is increased 20–100 times. Also lower thrombocyte numbers and a reduction in inorganic phosphate and raised renal and liver parameters may be found.

Therapy. The decisive factor in the treatment of sepsis is early and effective treatment with antibiotics—the same principle that applies to peritonitis, where the spectrum of pathogens is often similar.

Further measures include:

- oxygen supply
- volume replacement
- surgical sanitation of foci
- early ventilation
- digitalization in the case of cardiac insufficiency
- vasoactive substances (dopamine, dobutamine)
- wet packs around the calves.

So far, administration of steroids did not yield better results. Using heparin is another controversial measure. In addition, the effectiveness of polyvalent immunoglobulins has not yet been demonstrated unambiguously, although high doses did ease the course of the disease in individual patients. There is still insufficient experience with the use of special (and very expensive) IgM antibody preparations against certain strains of *Escherichia coli.*

Initial treatment may consist of β-lactam antibiotics (penicillins, possibly together with a β-lactamase inhibitor, or cephalosporin + aminoglycoside, possibly together with a 5-nitroimidazole). Imipenems and carbapenems are indicated during the advanced stage of sepsis.

Cephalosporins of the third generation are especially suited because they are highly effective against gram-negative bacteria and highly resistant against β-lactamase. Cephalosporins of the second generation are more effective in the case of staphylococci.

The advantage of penicillins is that they attack also enterococci; their disadvantage is that they are not resistant to β-lactamase. In severe cases, they should therefore be combined with a β-lactamase inhibitor.

As 5-nitroimidazoles are very effective against anaerobes, it is recommended that one of these compounds is always added when treating gynecologic infections.

Particularly effective drugs are the following carbapenems: imipenem–cilastatin and meropenem; they are highly effective against both aerobes and anaerobes and have the broadest spectrum.

Sequelae. In the case of bacteremia, either as a result of sepsis or due to thrombophlebitis originating from an infected access, bacteria spread throughout the body. Especially *Staphylococcus aureus* tends to colonize in organs or at sites of low resistance, where it causes abscess formation. Particularly feared is abscess formation in the brain. In every case of bacteremia due to *Staphylococcus aureus*, it is therefore recommended that antibiotic treatment lasts for at least 10 days. Other sites, such as joints, bone marrow, retroperitoneal space, or symphysis, may also be affected. One of the most characteristic symptoms is pain, and it is the more severe the more pressure is generated by the abscess if it cannot expand or drain.

Caution. Pain that cannot be controlled by analgesics should always trigger suspicion of an inflammatory process.

Septic Shock

This is the most severe form of an infection; it occurs when antibiotic treatment has been too late or when ineffective drugs have been administered. It is associated with high lethality (30%) even today.

Pathogens. Group A streptococci, *Staphylococcus aureus*, *Enterobacteriaceae* (*Escherichia coli*, *Klebsiella* and others), less often also anaerobes, such as *Bacteroides fragilis.*

Pathogenesis. Septic shock is an intoxication through bacterial toxins following the excessive multiplication of bacteria due to an infection—mostly due to sepsis that was either treated too late or took an extremely fulminant course. Septic shock is caused by certain bacteria that produce superantigens, such as group A streptococci and specific strains of *Staphylococcus aureus*, and less often by other bacteria, such as *Escherichia coli*. The massive release of cytokines induced by the bacterial toxins leads to a drop in vascular tonus and endothelial damage and, thereby, to the most severe injury of organs.

Clinical picture. The following parameters indicate septic shock:

- decrease in blood pressure, with the systolic pressure dropping to < 80
- tachycardia (> 120/min)
- heavy or spasmodic respiration
- increase in CRP by a factor of 30–100
- decrease of thrombocytes in the blood to < 100 000/μL
- decrease of leukocytes in the blood to < 4000/μL or even to < 500/μL
- increased renal parameters
- anuria.

Therapy and prognosis. Volume replacement, antibiotic therapy, replacement of coagulation factors, and intensive monitoring of the patient (central venous pressure, indwelling catheter in the bladder) are decisive in the prognosis of septic shock. The patient's general condition and the type of pathogens involved also play a role.

The chance of survival is poor if the septic shock is caused by group A streptococci or also by *Enterobacteriaceae* (*Escherichia coli* and others), whereas it is fairly good if the shock is due to anaerobes or *Staphylococcus aureus* in a patient who is otherwise in a good condition.

Toxic Shock Syndrome (TSS)

This is an acute febrile disease caused by toxin-producing bacteria, usually specific strains of *Staphylococcus aureus*. Here, the intoxication is the central symptom. Apart from high temperature, the characteristic signs are exanthema, hypotension, and exfoliation of the skin after one to two weeks. In principle, the disease can originate from any site of infection and even from bacteria colonizing the vagina. The disease has been particularly spectacular in menstruating women using highly absorptive tampons (which have subsequently been removed from the market).

Frequency. This is a rare disease that is frequently not diagnosed as such. The pathogen itself is not so rare and is often found in healthy people. Up to 90 % of adults carry antibodies to the toxic shock syndrome toxin 1 (TSST-1) antigen.

Pathogen. *Staphylococcus aureus*, namely, very specific strains (usually those belonging to phage group 1) that produce enterotoxin F (TSST-1).

Pathogenesis. The site of origin may be any local infection due to specific strains of *Staphylococcus aureus*, for example, in the region of cervix and vagina and in Pfannenstiel (suprapubic) incision, even after very small incisions like those for laparoscopy. In bad cases, multiplication of the pathogens is intensified and toxins are released at the same time. The pyrogenic toxins produced by these strains are crucial (TSST 1, enterotoxins A, B, C, D, and G). They function as superantigens and induce a massive release of cytokines, thus leading to fever, hypotension, and endothelial damage. They also stimulate many different types of lymphocytes. In addition, a series of other toxins are produced, such as hemolysins and epidermolytic toxins (exfoliative toxins).

Although less often, toxic shock syndrome occurs also in men or children, where the *Staphylococcus aureus* infection may occur locally, for example, in the pharynx. So far, no cases of toxic shock syndrome have been reported during pregnancy.

Whether or not a patient falls ill depends also on the presence of antibodies to TSST-1 in the blood. Up to 90 % of adults carry these antibodies without ever having fallen ill, with the antibodies even offering some protection.

Clinical picture. Toxic shock syndrome is a highly febrile acute disease with exanthema and multiple systemic dysfunctions:

- fever: 39 °C or more
- hypotension with symptoms of shock (superantigen toxins)
- erythema or diffuse maculopapulous exanthema which may later lead to skin exfoliation (exfoliative toxins)
- hyperemia of the oropharynx, vagina, or conjunctiva.

The following disturbances may also occur:

- vomiting and diarrhea
- confusion or sleepiness
- restricted kidney function (renal insufficiency)
- respiratory distress syndrome
- liver dysfunction
- myalgia associated with increase in creatine kinase
- thrombocytopenia
- hypocalcemia
- hypophosphatemia.

Diagnosis:

- clinical picture, if other infectious diseases have been ruled out
- detection of a *Staphylococcus aureus* strain that produces the enterotoxin TSST-1 (only

successful if a swab has been taken prior to antibiotic therapy)
- increase in antibodies against TSST-1 (late detection as antibody production takes two weeks).

Differential diagnosis:
- sepsis
- acute rheumatic fever
- leptospirosis
- scarlet fever
- Rocky Mountain spotted fever
- gastroenteritis
- hemolytic syndrome
- uremic syndrome
- systemic lupus erythematosus
- Kawasaki disease during childhood.

Therapy:
- β-lactamase-resistant antibiotics that are effective against staphylococci, such as cephalosporins of the second generation (e.g., cefotiam, cefuroxime)
- antishock therapy
- antitoxin therapy with high doses of immunoglobulin administered intravenously
- possibly cortisone.

Course of disease and complications. If treated in time, the prognosis is quite good. Prognosis depends on the underlying disease and the point in time when antibiotics are administered. Lethality has been reported to lie between 2–4%. Complications include pulmonary edema, cardiomyopathy, renal insufficiency, and encephalopathy, among others. Relapses are possible. In any case, generally, *Staphylococcus aureus* should not be in the vagina and should be removed, if possible.

Gas Gangrene Infection

This is a rare disease that occurs after surgery or injury. Whereas food poisoning due to clostridia (botulism) is not so rare, soft tissue infections occur only when sufficient amounts of these pathogens are introduced into wounds (unclean working conditions, accidents), favorable conditions for the multiplication of anaerobes exist, and no antibiotics are administered.

Pathogens. *Clostridium perfringens, Clostridium novyi, Clostridium septicum* are sporeforming anaerobes. They are widely distributed, especially in the intestine of animals.

Transmission. Usually these pathogens originate from the patient's own intestine or the perianal/vaginal region. In rare cases, they have been introduced from external sources through smear infection (accidents, injuries).

In a vaginal swab taken from the vulva (e.g., after delivery), detection of *Clostridium perfringens* is not a rare event (0.1–1%). In such patients, the pathogen has to be clinically evaluated.

Incubation time. One to four days.

Pathogenesis and clinical picture. Sudden severe pain in the surgical area. Development of a pronounced local edema with a watery, brown, sweet-smelling wound exudate. The phenomenon of crepitation occurs only later in the course of the disease.

The disease is caused by toxins—proteinases, collagenases, and lecithinases—which lead to necrotic liquefaction and gas formation. These toxins also result in general intoxication with a very grave clinical picture. The body temperature is only moderately increased (about 38°C). However, the heart rate is clearly increased (> 120/min).

Diagnosis:
- *Microscopy.* Large gram-positive rods in the wound smear (Fig. 1.2, p. 7); they can easily be mistaken for lactobacilli.
- *Culture.* Detection of clostridia.
- *Radiographic examination.* Penniform, striated pattern of muscles.
- *Clinical picture.* Crepitation during palpation of the affected tissue area (however, this is also found without gangrene after surgery).
- *Laboratory parameters.* Usually leukocytosis, often thrombocytopenia.

Therapy:

The most important measure is surgical revision and opening of the infected area to facilitate extensive drainage. Further multiplication of the anaerobic clostridia can be inhibited by ventilating the tissue. In very serious cases, hyperbaric oxygenation therapy may be carried out, which is only possible in surgical centers (especially in military hospitals):
- antibiotic therapy with penicillin G (20 million IU per day)
- other options are cephalosporins, metronidazole, tinidazole
- effective antitoxin treatment is not available.

Urinary Tract Infections (UTI)

Urinary tract infections are among the most common infections in gynecologic patients. The majority of infections are uncomplicated mild cystitis and, sometimes, asymptomatic bacteriuria. These infections occur most frequently after surgery, especially when a catheter has been used, or when an indwelling catheter has been applied for many days.

In general, urinary tract infections are the most common nosocomial infections.

The extent of a urinary tract infection depends on the mechanisms of bacterial virulence and the patient's immune responses. Mechanisms of virulence include special features for adherence and penetration (e. g., P antigen-recognizing fimbriae), the production of toxins (e. g., hemolysin), antihumoral activity (e. g., the ability of *Proteus mirabilis* to inactivate IgA antibodies), and the ability to accumulate nutrients (e. g., iron) against a concentration gradient.

Immunodeficiencies, which may be genetically based, increase the risk of infection in the affected individual. For example, dysfunction of neutrophilic granulocytes may lead to an increased occurrence of renal scars after pyelonephritis. Such dysfunction may be due to reduced expression of interleukin-8 receptors, thus interfering with the migration of neutrophilic granulocytes to the site of infection.

Complicated urinary tract infections may lead to urosepsis if the complicating factors and the infection are not treated adequately.

Frequency and etiology. In addition to genetic factors, personal habits of cleaning and care combined with the special activities in this region play a decisive role. During pregnancy, urinary tract infections are more frequently seen because of the slightly depressed immune system and due to hormonal and mechanical changes. The number of urinary tract infections increases with age and with the number of births, involving up to 10 % of all pregnant women.

In addition, women with urinary incontinence and anatomical changes in the urethral region tend to have more urinary tract infections.

Coitus promotes cystitis as well, especially when the vagina is short (e. g., after hysterectomy) and when hormonal deficiency causes additional atonicity of the tissue.

Contraception by means of diaphragm and spermicide (nonoxynol-9) increases the risk of urinary tract infection. Nonoxynol-9 promotes the growth of *Escherichia coli* in the vagina, is toxic for epithelial cells, and promotes the adhesion of *Escherichia coli*, enterococci, and group B streptococci to these cells. Nonoxynol-9 kills some lactobacillus strains, particularly those producing hydrogen peroxide, whereas gram-negative bacteria are not affected.

Bacteriuria

Every spontaneously voided urine contains low numbers of bacteria from the external regions of the urethra and vulva. Under the microscope, large lactobacilli can therefore be occasionally recognized in the urine of women. To evaluate increased counts of bacteria in the urine independently of the way it has been obtained, the following threshold values have been introduced:

Significant bacteriuria:

- midstream urine: 10^5 bacteria/mL
- catheter urine: 10^4 bacteria/mL.

Dip-slide culture tests for the determination of bacterial counts in the urine have been developed (e. g., Uricult, Urotube); they provide culture media for the most common bacteria. The colonies develop within 24 hours and may be read directly or shipped to a bacteriological laboratory for assessment and further processing.

One disadvantage of premanufactured culture media is that not all pathogens grow on them. If one suspects urinary tract infection and cannot detect any microbes, it is essential that freshly voided urine be sent as soon as possible to a bacteriological laboratory.

If the urine is shipped and this takes a prolonged period, the microbes rapidly multiply since urine is a good culture medium.

Uncomplicated Infection of the Lower Urinary Tract (Cystitis)

Clinical picture. In the majority of patients, cystitis is combined with urethritis. Solitary urethritis is more likely caused by specific pathogens, such as chlamydiae. Patients with cystitis complain of dysuria, frequent urination, and pain above the symphysis.

In cases of uncomplicated urinary tract infection, complications or sequelae are rarely observed. In a healthy person, a number of physiological defense mechanisms prevent infections in the urinary tract. In women, these include the maintenance of a low pH in the vagina, the flow of urine through ureter and urethra, the production of antibodies and proteins (e. g., Tamm–Horsfall mucoprotein), as well as cellular immune responses (e. g., targeted leukocyte migration).

Diagnosis:

- *Chemical tests.* The use of urine reagent test strips offers a quick and reliable orientation

Table 7.**11** Spectrum of pathogens and resistances associated with urinary tract infections (bacteriuria) (Women's Hospital at the University of Freiburg, Germany)

Type of pathogen	Number of isolates	Frequency	Resistance against different antibiotics				
			Ampicillin	Co-Trimoxazole	Tetracycline	Gentamicin	Norfloxacin
Escherichia coli	270	57.0%	18%	10%	23%	2%	0%
Enterococcus	53	11.1%	2%	2%	45%	100%	33%
Staphylococcus							
– coagulase-negative strains	41	8.6%	68%	25%	52%	10%	3%
– *S. aureus*	16	3.4%	75%	16%	6%	0%	6%
Proteus mirabilis	33	7.0%	9%	16%	97%	0%	0%
– *P. morgani*	3	0.6%	67%	33%	67%	0%	0%
– *P. vulgaris*	2	0.4%	100%	0%	0%	0%	0%
– other *Proteus* species	2	0.4%	50%	50%	100%	0%	0%
Klebsiella pneumoniae	23	4.8%	100%	6%	13%	0%	0%
Pseudomonas aeruginosa	14	3.0%	100%	100%	100%	0%	0%
– other *Pseudomonas* species	5	1.1%	100%	100%	20%		
Enterobacter cloace	3	0.6%	100%	0%	0%	0%	0%
Citrobacter diversus	3	0.6%	100%	0%	0%	0%	0%
– *C. freundli*	2	0.4%	100%	0%	0%		
Acinetobacter anitratus	2	0.4%	50%	0%	0%	0%	0%
Group B streptococci	2	0.4%	0%	0%	0%	0%	0%
Corynebacterium species	1	0.2%	0%	0%	0%	0%	0%
Total	475		32%	13%	33%	12%	4%

whether or not the urine is pathologic. In the presence of *Escherichia coli*, which is detected in > 60% of all urinary tract infections (Table 7.**11**), the test is mostly positive for nitrite. In case of leukorrhea, the test strip indicates an increased protein content. More modern strips indicate fairly well also an increase in leukocyte numbers. Positive detection of blood outside of period and childbed suggests cystitis.

- *Microscopy.* If the examination of freshly voided urine (no sediment) shows bacteria, erythrocytes, and above all more than three leukocytes per visual field at 400× magnification, this is a sure sign of cystitis.
- *Bacteriology.* Dip-test cultures are good for determining the bacterial count, isolating the bacteria, and establishing an antibiogram. Detection of yeast in the urine is usually due to contamination from the vulvar region. Detection of several types of microbes suggests contamination.
- Further diagnostic steps in case of chronic infections include ultrasound, cystoscopy, and intravenous pyelography.
- *Laboratory parameters.* They are normal in cases of uncomplicated urinary tract infection.

Pathogens. *Escherichia coli* is isolated in 70–95% of all patients with acute uncomplicated cystitis, and *Staphylococcus saprophyticus* in 5–15% of cases. In some instances other intestinal bacteria (e.g., *Proteus mirabilis*, *Klebsiella* species, or enterococci) have been isolated. A very similar distribution is observed also for acute uncomplicated pyelonephritis.

Therapy. Treatment does not normally pose a problem, since the infection is superficial and almost all antibiotics are eliminated through the kidney and are therefore present in the urine in high concentration:

- amoxicillin (3 × 750 mg), during pregnancy
- Co-Trimoxazole (2 × 1 g)

- fluoroquinolones in case of problem pathogens (do not use during pregnancy or for children)
- oral cephalosporins.

Duration of therapy: one to three days.

In case of uncomplicated cystitis, single-dose therapy is sufficient when a potent antibiotic with a long half-life, such as a modern fluoroquinolone, is administered (healing rate: >90%). If an antibiotic with a short half-life (one hour) is used, the healing rate is lower, and treatment should therefore be extended to three days.

A follow-up after eight days is recommended. If the cystitis is not cured after short-term treatment of sensitive pathogens, one is dealing with a complicated urinary tract infection, which is diagnosed in 5–10% of these patients.

In case of recurrent cystitis in mature women, additional estrogen replacement therapy and pelvic exercises are recommended, once metabolic and other underlying diseases have been excluded. In young women, more attention should be paid to normalization of the vaginal flora, changes in sexual practices, and proper skin care in the anal and vulvar regions (e. g., use of petroleum jelly).

In case of recurrent cystitis after coitus, which may occasionally occur if the vagina is shortened due to hysterectomy, the dreaded relapse can be avoided by taking a single dose (one-half to one tablet) of Co-Trimoxazole or amoxicillin, or one of the quinolones during the first hours after coitus. Here, too, the decisive factor is the vaginal flora and can be influenced by proper skin care.

Vaccination for strengthening the local defenses is also available (Uro-Vaxom). It leads to long-term freedom from relapses in some patients.

Differential diagnosis:

- chlamydial urethritis (use the first 10–30 mL of the morning urine for detection of *Chlamydia* by means of PCR)
- recurrent genital herpes in the urethral region (see Fig. 7.**49**, p. 90)
- vaginitis
- vulvitis
- skenitis
- malignant tumor
- interstitial cystitis.

Uncomplicated Infection of the Upper Urinary Tract (Acute Uncomplicated Pyelonephritis)

Acute pyelonephritis occurs more frequently in women than in men. Ascending pathogens may reach the kidneys especially during pregnancy, but also after surgery.

In case of acute uncomplicated pyelonephritis, patients complain of fever, shaking chills, and malaise. Diagnosis is established based on flank pain, pyuria, and bacteriuria. In almost all patients, pyelonephritis is unilateral. Symptoms of an infection of the lower urinary tract like those with acute cystitis may be present at the same time, since acute pyelonephritis is usually an ascending infection. Acute uncomplicated pyelonephritis occurs mainly in women; particularly at risk are pregnant women with asymptomatic bacteriuria and patients with vesicoureteral reflux.

Diagnosis. The same as with cystitis. Microscopic signs of severe inflammatory reactions include an increase in leukocytes and urinary casts in the urine. (Here, the examination of sediment makes sense.)

Pathogens. See uncomplicated infection of the lower urinary tract.

Therapy. In case of acute uncomplicated pyelonephritis, 14 days of antibiotic therapy is recommended for serious cases. In moderately severe and mild cases, seven days of therapy are sufficient. In mild cases, patients can be treated with oral antibiotics in an outpatient clinic. In case of moderately severe and severe pyelonephritis with serious systemic symptoms, such as nausea and vomiting, initial treatment is carried out with parenteral antibiotics in a hospital until the patient is free of fever. The antibiotic should be selected according to the antibiogram, the kinetics, and the tolerance. Once the symptoms have improved, parenteral therapy should be switched as soon as possible to oral therapy. At this point, also chemically unrelated antibiotics may be used.

Caution. The clinical symptoms are often minimal in case of chronic pyelonephritis.

In case of recurrent urinary tract infection with resistant pathogens, one should always consider also an involvement of the kidneys, i. e., an infection of the upper urinary tract.

Complicated Urinary Tract Infections

Here, too, we distinguish between infections of the *lower* urinary tract (cystitis) and the *upper* urinary tract (pyelonephritis). In response to targeted questioning, the medical history raises the suspicion that the patient may have a complicated urinary tract infection. The clinical findings of complicated urinary tract infection are often modest. In addition, the pathogens of complicated urinary tract infections are sometimes less virulent. In disabled or geriatric patients in nursing homes, typical symptoms may be absent even in case of severe urinary tract infection. Accompanying symptoms, such as a paralytic ileus or respiratory insufficiency may serve as a guide.

Complicated urinary tract infections are those where anatomical changes promote the onset and maintenance of a urinary tract infection. These include:

- urinary incontinence
- obstructions
- urolithiasis
- renal and cardiac insufficiency
- diabetes mellitus
- pregnancy.

Repeated antibiotic therapy in case of recurrent urinary tract infection causes a shift in pathogen composition and a selection of pathogens, thus leading to colonization of the urinary tract with problematic pathogens.

Diagnosis. Specific urological diagnostic procedures should then be used in order to detect the complicating factors in the urinary tract or to exclude them. The following are essential:

- urinalysis
- bacteriology, including the determination of antibiotic sensitivity.

During **pregnancy**, urinary tract infections of the mother represent a risk factor, since they may be associated with amnionitis, preeclampsia, maternal anemia, and an increased incidence of premature births (< 37 weeks of gestation) and stillbirths.

Only about 7% of women with bacteriuria show typical symptoms of urinary tract infection before or after delivery.

Pathogens. Clearly, the spectrum of pathogens is very broad. Pseudomonads, enterococci, and coagulase-negative staphylococci play a role in addition to *Escherichia coli* and other *Enterobacteriaceae* (e.g., *Proteus*, *Klebsiella*, *Enterobacter*, *Citrobacter* species).

One therapeutic problem is created by certain pathogens (e.g., *Pseudomonas aeruginosa*, staphylococci, etc.) that in combination with foreign material (e.g., indwelling catheters, stones) can form a biofilm. This leads to an altered metabolic situation and protects the microbes from the body's defense system.

Therapy. Antibiotic therapy can only provide a cure if also the complicating factors can be effectively treated. In case of severe urinary tract infection, the first step is an empirical antibiotic treatment that is as effective as possible. At the same time, one should aim for interdisciplinary diagnosis and therapy of the complicating factors. This includes the restoration of urinary flow in case of urinary retention, complete sanitation of biofilm surfaces, if possible (e.g., urinary calculus, necrotic tissue, catheter, splints), and the treatment of concomitant medical conditions and risk factors (e.g., diabetes mellitus). If this cannot take place, successful treatment will usually be temporary, and relapses will most likely occur.

Antibiotic treatment of complicated urinary tract infection should last much longer, namely, about 10–14 days, since these infections reach into deeper tissue layers. Isolation of the pathogen and determination of antibiotic sensitivity are always required. In some patients, long-term prophylaxis over weeks and months with low doses of antibiotics (e.g., 250 mg Co-Trimoxazole) is recommended.

Antibody-coated Bacteria

Antibody-coated bacteria are mainly found in case of bacteriuria and can therefore contribute to the localization of infections in the lower or upper urinary tract.

Here, we are dealing with bacteria surrounded by antibodies. They are only associated with infections inside tissues (e.g., kidney, prostate), which can be demonstrated by immunofluorescence microscopy. In such patients, a more intensive antibiotic therapy is required.

Chronic Interstitial Cystitis

This pain syndrome is associated with frequency and urgency of urination. It affects mainly women. The cause is unknown. Etiologic studies suspect infections, changes in the urinary mucosa, exogenous noxa, as well as neurological, hormonal, vascular, allergic, and autoimmune disorders. Diagnosis is based on the clinical picture; it is a diagnosis by exclusion. Cystoscopic

Table 7.**12** Mycobacteria and the diseases caused by them

Pathogen	Disease
Obligatory pathogens: "typical" mycobacteria	
M. tuberculosis	Tuberculosis
M. bovis	Tuberculosis
Facultative pathogens: "atypical" mycobacteria (> 20 species)	
M. kansasii	Primarily pulmonary infection
M. avium complex	Pulmonary infection, lymphadenitis, sepsis (in AIDS patients)
M. intracellulare	Serious systemic disease in AIDS patients
M. marinum	Skin infection and other diseases
M. simiae	Pulmonary infection
M. szulgai	Pulmonary infection
M. xenopi	Pulmonary infection
M. scrofulaceum	Lymphadenitis in children, rarely pulmonary infections
M. fortuitum	Abscesses, osteomyelitis, and other diseases
M. ulcerans	Skin infection
M. leprae	Leprosy

examination reveals mucosal bleedings, while histologic examination shows mast cell infiltration. Therapy varies according to the symptoms.

Tuberculosis

General Comments

In the 19th century, tuberculosis was still widely distributed in Europe and claimed up to 30% of the population. It has now almost disappeared from this region thanks to improved living conditions, more effective chemotherapeutics, and vaccination. Recently, with the advent of acquired immunodeficiency syndrome (AIDS) and the increased mobility of people, tuberculosis not only has returned with increased prevalence, but the spectrum of pathogens has also been changing. In addition to the typical mycobacteria (*Mycobacterium tuberculosis* and the now rare *Mycobacterium bovis*), which have been the predominant types until recently, atypical mycobacteria (*Mycobacterium avium/intracellulare* complex) are increasingly being isolated from AIDS patients. In contrast to the typical pathogens of tuberculosis, these are only facultative pathogens (Table 7.**12**).

Today, tuberculosis is a disease of poor people and of immunocompromised patients. It is increasingly reintroduced to the industrialized world from third-world countries.

Apart from its occurrence in AIDS patients, tuberculosis is often found in people from developing countries. Here, genital tuberculosis still plays a major role as a cause of sterility. Otherwise, it is occasionally discovered by chance during surgical intervention or suggested as a tentative diagnosis by the pathologist.

Genital Tuberculosis

Pathogen. *Mycobacterium tuberculosis* (> 90%) and *M. bovis.* These are facultative intracellular bacteria.

Frequency. Genital tuberculosis is a rare disease; there are no data available on its frequency. In 2001, 6740 cases of tuberculosis have been reported in Germany. This number includes many cases of introduction from countries with higher incidences.

Transmission and pathogenesis. In Germany, the lung is the primary portal of entrance in up to 95% of cases. The pathogen then spreads through the blood stream into the tubes. From the tubes it spreads to the neighboring organs, i. e., the ovaries (33%) and the uterus (80%), and to the cervix (10%). The initial foci in the tubes spread only very slowly, thus causing no complaints despite considerable tissue destruction. The result is tubal sterility.

Clinical picture. If there are any symptoms at all, they are uncharacteristic. Pain or dysfunctional bleedings may occur. The clinical picture of acute salpingitis is rather rare. Nodules or conglomerate tumors are typical, but they are detected more by chance (Fig. 7.**165**).

Diagnosis. Due to the extremely slow reproduction of the pathogen—the doubling time is 24 hours (instead of 20–30 minutes as with normal bacteria)—these bacteria also grow very slowly in culture, thus making results available only after weeks. The use of PCR allows one to shorten the culture process, since this method requires only very small amounts of cultured mycobacteria. Direct detection in the tissue is still very limited

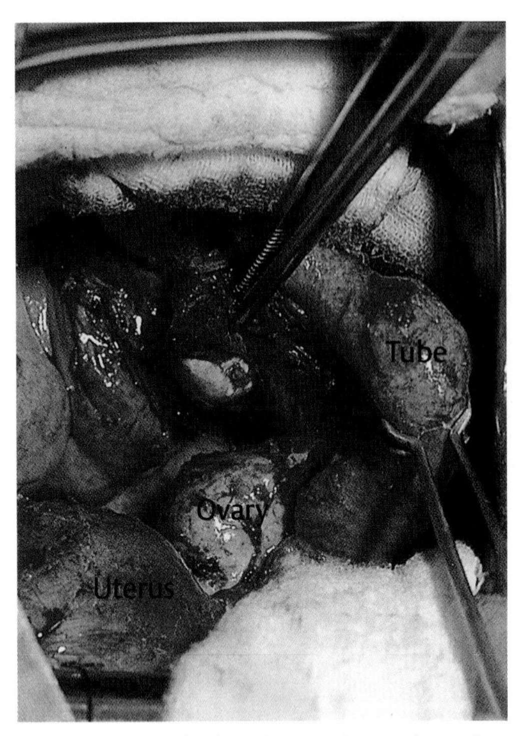

Fig. 7.**165** Genital tuberculosis with granular, yellow material in the swollen tubes in a 29-year-old patient suffering from primary sterility.

due to the low numbers of bacteria and the difficulties in obtaining material.

The first step is the skin test; it clarifies if there is an infection at all.

Since only cellular immune responses develop, only intracutaneous tuberculin tests are meaningful.

Tuberculin test (e. g., TB tine test). The test is positive if swelling and redness of the skin occur after 24–48 hours. It may be false negative in old people or immunocompromised patients.

The second step is the search for sites of infection. It includes identification of the pathogen, which is essential for deciding on the therapy.

Chest radiograph and, if possible, *identification of the pathogen* in the sputum and, if genital tuberculosis is suspected, also in endometrial biopsies, abrasion material, and menstrual blood. Several samples should be examined because of the low pathogen numbers:

- fluorescence test (sputum)
- Ziehl–Neelsen staining (sputum)
- PCR
- culture on special media (positive results are not obtained before 2–3 weeks, and negative results only after 6–8 weeks)
- typing and antibiogram require six more weeks
- possibly, animal experiments.

Histology. Occasionally, a tentative diagnosis of tuberculosis is suggested by the pathologist on the basis of the occurrence of Langerhans giant cells, etc.

Therapy. Combination therapies are used to prevent the development of resistances: isoniazid + rifampicin + ethambutol during the first three months, followed by isoniazid + rifampicin, or by antibiotics according to the results of the antibiogram. As a rule, treatment is carried out in an outpatient clinic and lasts for about half a year.

Prophylaxis. A BCG vaccine with live, attenuated tubercle bacilli is used for prophylaxis of meningitis and miliary tuberculosis, but only in tuberculin-negative patients after testing or in newborns. Protective immunity is about 80 % (see also p. 242).

Notifiable disease. Disease and death must be reported.

Tuberculosis and Pregnancy

Tuberculosis (usually pulmonary tuberculosis) has hardly any effect on the course of a pregnancy. The prognosis for mother and child is good if treatment is initiated early enough. Tuberculosis acquired at birth is extremely rare today. An infection of the child in utero is most likely when a pregnant woman falls ill with primary tuberculosis or, in the worst-case scenario, with miliary tuberculosis. Diaplacental transmission is possible but rarely occurs. Children may be infected through aspiration of the amniotic fluid during delivery, or later at home. The symptoms of connatal tuberculosis are uncharacteristic (e. g., abdominal complaints, anemia, lethargy). Direct detection of the pathogen in the newborn is more likely to be successful than the intracutaneous tuberculin test, which becomes positive only after six weeks.

Conception under tuberculostatic treatment is neither a reason for discontinuing the therapy prematurely nor for terminating the pregnancy. In addition, the requirement for treatment is no cause for concern or even termination of the pregnancy.

Therapy during pregnancy. Florid infections should and can be treated with isoniazid, rifamycin, and ethambutol without any risk during the entire pregnancy. If an active infection is questionable (only seroconversion of the tuberculin test), one will be more reserved and restrict the treatment to monotherapy with isoniazid.

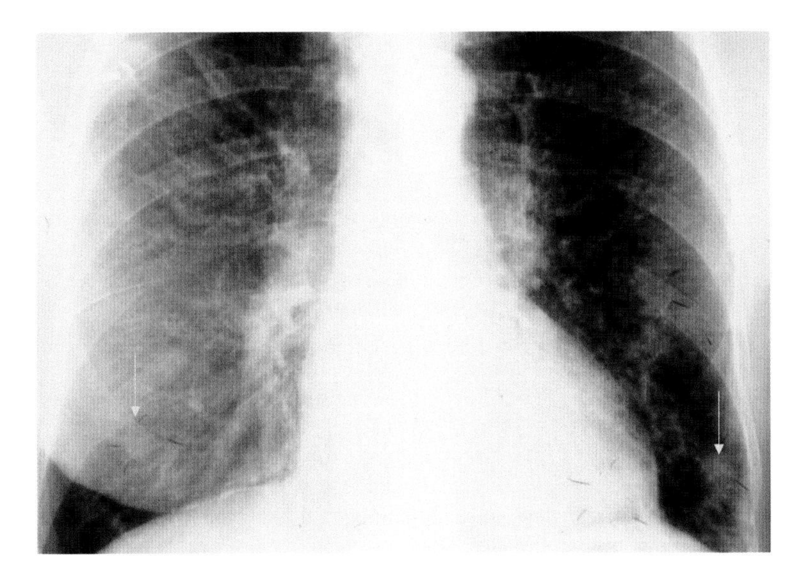

Fig. 7.**166** Round foci of aspergillosis in the lungs of a patient with advanced ovarian carcinoma and fever.

Isoniazid during pregnancy, however, may be hepatotoxic. Laboratory tests and close monitoring are therefore recommended.

Members of the household must be monitored as well and treated, if necessary. If there is any risk, the newborn should be vaccinated with BCG prior to being sent home.

Infections in Immunocompromised and Neutropenic Patients

New infections like AIDS (HIV) and the increased use of more radical chemotherapy in cancer patients with extreme leukopenia—but also other medical developments, such as radical surgery and organ transplantation with iatrogenic immunosuppression—increasingly pose problems with respect to infections.

Harmless microorganisms suddenly become dangerous pathogens when the immune system is suppressed or inactivated.

This applies to fungi—reaching from *Candida albicans* and *Candida glabrata* to *Aspergillus niger*—as well as bacteria and protozoa.

Two aspects are problematic here:

- these microorganisms are widely distributed and are therefore often detected
- many of these microorganisms are more resistant against the usual anti-infectives than common pathogens.

Aspergillosis

Aspergillosis occurs in immunocompromised cancer patients after chemotherapy and leukopenia with fever.

Pathogen occurrence. Ubiquitous in the air.

Invasive Aspergillosis

Multiple round lesions in the lungs (Fig. 7.**166**).

Clinical picture. Fever, increase in CRP, reduced function of the lungs.

Detection:

- chest radiograph
- bronchoalveolar lavage for cultures.

Therapy. Itraconazole (2 × 200 mg per day, for three weeks), amphotericin B, or the new and better-tolerated voriconazole.

Aspergilloma

Encapsulated tumor in the lung.

Detection. Chest radiograph, CT. Cultures are of no use; antimycotics are ineffective because there is no dissemination.

Therapy. Surgical removal.

8 Infections During Pregnancy

General Introduction

Infections during pregnancy are especially feared because they may not only endanger the mother but also her child. Some infections take a more severe course during pregnancy, or even occur only during this time or during and after delivery. In addition, pregnancy is an extremely sensitive phase in the life of a woman, and any infections and their sequelae should be taken seriously.

Pathogens may infect the child:

- by means of the blood (hematogenous infection, only in case of primary infection)
- by ascending from the vagina through the fetal membranes (mostly bacteria)
- by passing through the placenta (transplacental infection) at the end of the pregnancy, especially during labor (e. g., HIV)
- during passage of the child through the birth canal (hepatitis B virus, cytomegalovirus, HSV, HPV, gonococci, chlamydiae, group B streptococci, *E. coli*, etc.).

During pregnancy the mother has a higher risk of infections (malaria, puerperal sepsis, catheter infections) and other diseases.

The following **complications of infections** may occur in particular:

- direct damage to the child by infection in utero (embryopathy, fetopathy)
- indirect damage to the child by premature delivery
- infection of the child during birth
- exacerbation of an infection of the mother
- reactivation of latent infections of the mother
- ascending infections of the mother (endometritis, sepsis)
- death of the child
- death of the mother.

Viral infections during pregnancy, especially during the first trimester, pose the most serious **danger to the child.** Bacterial infections are particularly threatening during birth, but so are some viral infections, such as varicella (chicken-

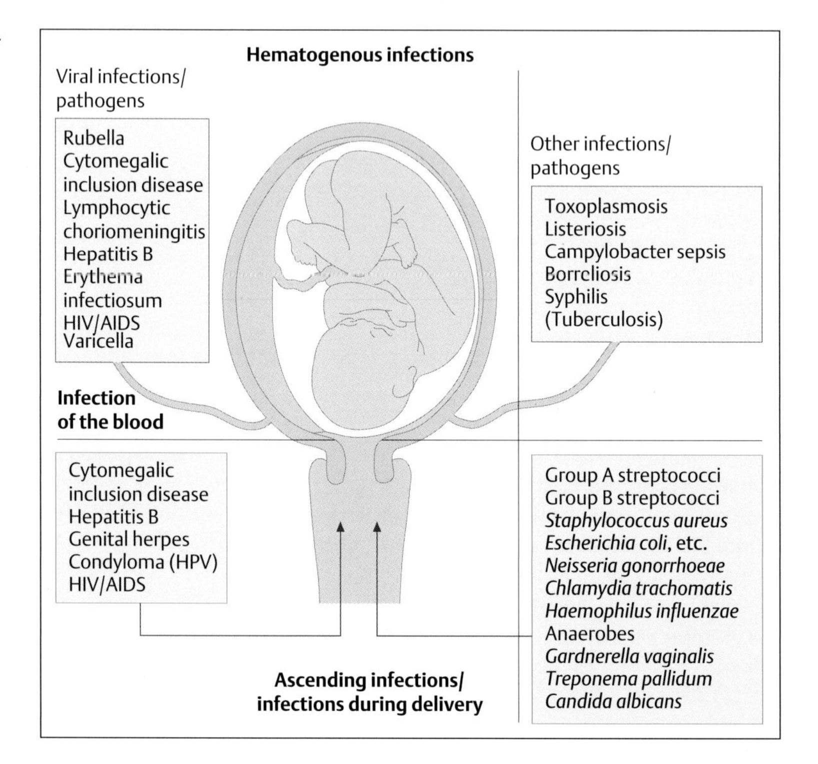

Fig. 8.1 Diagram illustrating the most common hematogenous and ascending infections during pregnancy and during delivery.

pox), cytomegalic inclusion disease, hepatitis B, and herpes simplex (Fig. 8.**1**).

Viruses normally destroy the cells in which they have multiplied. They are therefore especially feared during the embryonic phase as they may cause irreparable embryopathies. Among the known viral infections, a high percentage of damage is done by the rubella virus; but also the virus causing erythema infectiosum and the LCM virus threaten the life of the child (see Fig. 8.**2**).

Bacterial infections endanger the child by inducing severe inflammatory responses during the fetal period.

Treatment options. Any care for a pregnant woman aims at saving her and her child from damage due to infections. However, this is only achieved when the infection can be recognized and when therapeutic agents are available.

This does not apply to all infections. There are a number of infections that may run their course without producing symptoms, and there are pathogens (viruses) for which we do not have any effective drugs.

Another problem during pregnancy is the *reactivation* of latent infections; this holds true especially for herpes viruses (HSV, CMV, EBV, VZV), papillomaviruses, and also other pathogens. Here, there is hardly any risk of hematogenous infection as the pathogen is inactivated by antibodies in the blood. A dangerous situation exists only when there is direct contact with pathogens excreted into the birth canal or when pathogens pass through the placental barrier.

The distinction between primary infection and reactivation occasionally creates problems. Diagnostic serology relies only rarely on a significant rise in titer ($>$ 2 titer steps) in case of primary infection; it is often based only on the detection of IgM antibodies. This is problematic in case of chronic persistent infections, such as toxoplasmosis, cytomegalic inclusion disease, and other herpes virus infections, since IgM antibodies may be produced over many years.

By determining the strength of antigen–antibody binding (avidity), the start of an infection can be narrowed down more closely. Alternatively, this is done by means of a western blot, since the number of visible bands increases with the duration of the infection, reflecting the fact that antibodies are produced against an increasing number of pathogen structures.

Viral Infections

General Remarks

Forms of infection, frequency, and risks for the child. Viral infections are common, also during pregnancy. Although all viral infections pose a risk theoretically, only a few pathogens surpass the 1 % threshold of posing a risk for the child.

The overview in Fig. 8.**2** lists different viral infections during pregnancy, their frequencies, their risks of damage, as well as the periods of highest risk.

Estimated values had to be used for some of the infections listed, either because data simply do not exist or because documented data on frequencies and risks are not available despite various studies performed.

Due to the limited therapeutic options for viral infections, only the following **consequences** are available at present:

- *Termination* of the pregnancy. This should only be performed—with proper indication and at the parents' requests—if the risk of damage to the child is significantly increased. If the mother is endangered, termination is possible at any time under German law.
- Administration of *immunoglobulins* to avoid hematogenous spread of the virus. This measure is only worthwhile if immunoglobulins are administered early (one to four days after the initial contact with the virus).
- Administration of *virostatics.* Aciclovir is still administered with some reservation, although virustatics are now standard procedure if the mother is infected with HIV.
- *Serological exclusion* of certain infections that pose an increased risk often provides sufficient reassurance to the patient.
- *Informing the patient* about the actual, and usually minor, risk of the current viral infection.

Rubella (German Measles)

Infection with the rubella virus is the most feared complication during early pregnancy, since this virus—unlike any other virus—causes irreversible damage to the child in a high percentage of cases. For historical aspects, see Table 8.**1**.

Pathogen. The rubella virus belongs to the togaviruses; only one serotype is known. Its nucleic acid is single-stranded RNA, and its sensitive envelope contains hemagglutinin. Stability of the virus outside the cell is low. Replication of the

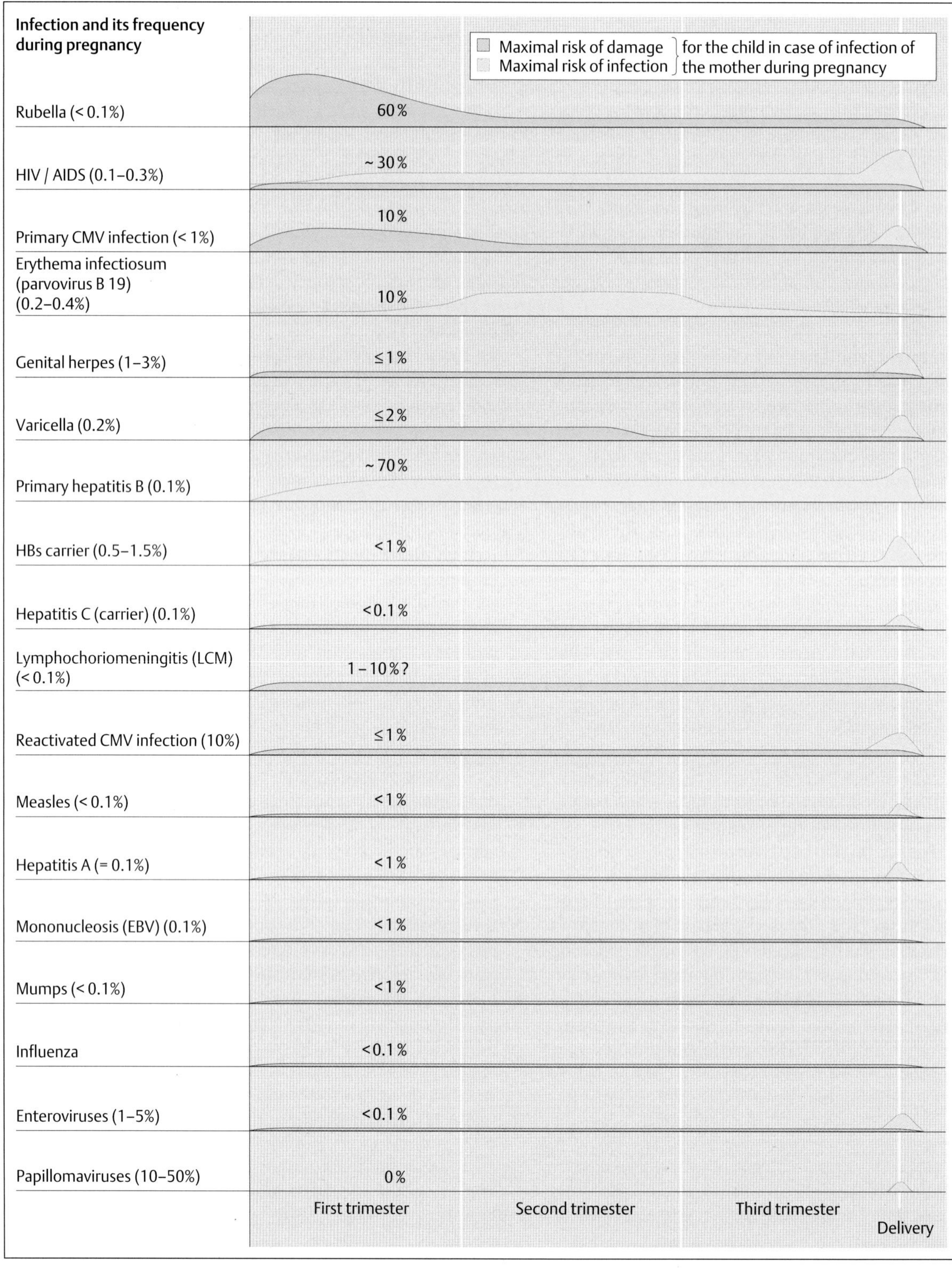

Fig. 8.**2** Viral infections during pregnancy. In addition to the estimated frequencies of various infections during pregnancy, the diagram illustrates the risks of damage and infection for the child. Although the frequency of infection cannot always be separated from the frequency of damage, an attempt was made to illustrate by color-coding the different risk types of specific infections over the course of the pregnancy.

Table 8.1 Rubella

Year	Important historical facts
1941	*Gregg* (Australian ophthalmologist): discovery of cataracts after a rubella epidemic *Gregg:* triad of cataract, deafness, and heart defect
1962	Isolation of the rubella virus
1964	Rubella epidemic in the United States 250 000 pregnancies affected 13 410 cases of fetal death or death of the newborn 20 000 children damaged
1966	Development of rubella vaccine
1975	Vaccination on a wide scale

virus in cell cultures does not induce a distinct cytopathic effect.

Frequency. Rubella infections have become rare because of vaccination. Over 90% of adults possess antibodies against the rubella virus. During recent years, about five rubella-induced embryopathies per year have been reported in Germany.

Transmission. Droplet infection, or transplacental infection in case of viremia during pregnancy.

Incubation time. Two (or three) weeks.

Clinical picture. This is a mild childhood disease, with 50% of infections taking an uneventful course without exanthema and with mild respiratory symptoms, at the most.

Typical symptoms include temporary, small-spotted exanthema, swelling of the lymph nodes behind the ears and on the neck, and arthralgia (more common in adults) (Fig. 8.**3**).

Risks for the child. Rubella infection during the first weeks of pregnancy causes a high percentage of embryopathies. Depending on the time of infection, it affects the eyes (cataract), the heart (malformations), the inner ear (deafness), and possibly the central nervous system (mental retardation, which is often recognized only much later) (Fig. 8.**4**).

If there is clear evidence of rubella infection during the first 14 weeks, it is now common practice in Germany to terminate the pregnancy because the risk of damage is higher than 10%, and even higher than 50% during the first few weeks.

If there is the urgent desire to have a child, the risk may be assessed by means of prenatal diagnostics (see p. 37) as the child is not always infected.

Diagnosis (Table 8.2):

Serology:

- *Hemagglutination inhibition (HAI) assay.* This is the standard test for determining permanent immunity. Two samples of blood are required for detecting a fresh infection: the first one as early as possible, and the second one eight to 10 days after the appearance of the exanthema. Evidence for a fresh rubella infection is either the very first occurrence of antibodies in the second blood sample, or a titer rise between the first and the second blood sample by at least a factor of four.
- ELISA. It yields high titers and is more suitable for the detection of IgM antibodies (it may yield false positive results).
- Hemolysis-in-gel test. This test is carried out for confirmation when the titer in the HAI assay is lower than 1:32 because the HAI assay is not absolutely reliable in the lower range.
- Complement fixation test (CFT). It plays only a role in diagnosing a fresh rubella infection. High titers (1:80 and higher) raise suspicion, but they are no proof.
- *Detection of rubella-specific IgM antibodies.* This test is always required when samples for

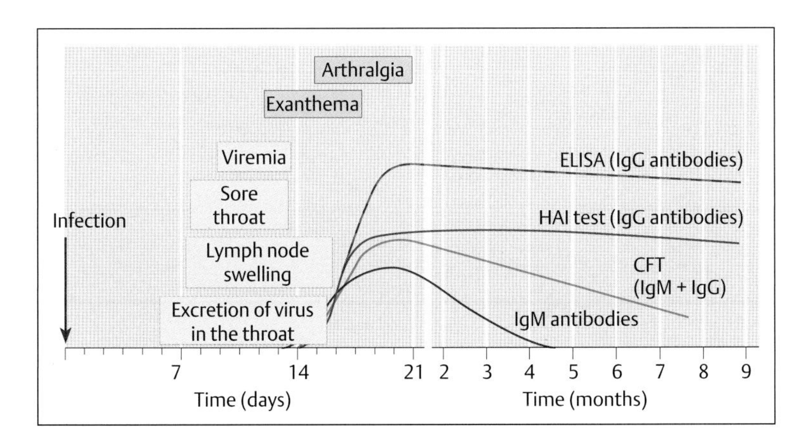

Fig. 8.**3** Rubella infection. The diagram illustrates the period of infectiousness (viral excretion in the throat of contact persons, viremia during pregnancy), various clinical symptoms, and the time course of various antibody classes as detected by various methods (laboratory tests).

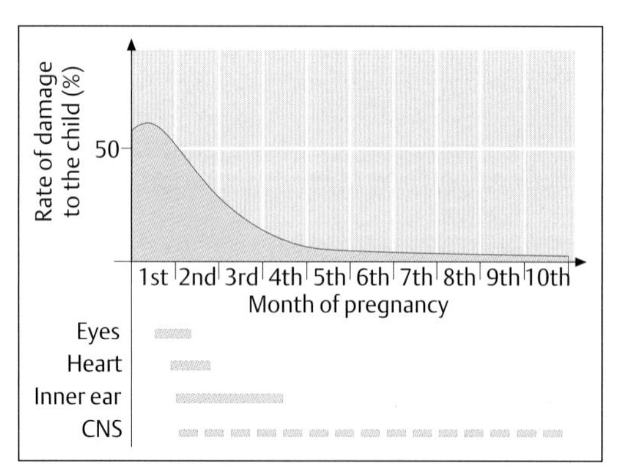

Fig. 8.**4** Rubella infection during pregnancy. Level of damage and types of damage during the course of the pregnancy.

serology are collected only after exanthema has developed and the antibody titer is already high. In this case, only the detection of specific IgM antibodies can prove that the exanthema was caused by a rubella infection.

Pathogen detection:

- *Detection of the virus in cultures.* This is expensive and does not play a role in diagnostics.
- *Polymerase chain reaction (PCR).* This method is used for the detection or exclusion of the virus, particularly in the amniotic fluid.

Prenatal diagnosis. If there is the desire to have a child and the child's risk of infection is low, infection of the child may be excluded with increasing success in special laboratories. This can be either by amniocentesis for the detection of rubella virus in the amniotic fluid by PCR, or—from the 22 nd week of pregnancy on—by puncture of the umbilical cord for the detection of IgM antibodies.

Diagnosis of congenital rubella infection:

- persistence of rubella-specific antibody titer in the newborn: no titer fall six to eight weeks after birth (Fig. 8.**5**)
- detection of rubella-specific IgM antibodies in the cord blood, or later in the newborn
- detection of rubella virus from a throat swab. Rubella virus may be excreted over many months, sometimes over one to two years.

Prophylaxis prior to a pregnancy. The immune status (rubella titer) is determined by means of the HAI assay (> 90 % of women of childbearing age possess antibodies). A titer of more than 1 : 16 is reliable and indicates sufficient protection. A titer of 1 : 8 is unreliable (due to the nature of the method). Detection of rubella-specific antibodies in the hemolysis-in-gel test or by ELISA indicates protection. To be on the safe side, rubella vaccination is recommended. If the titer check does not yield a titer rise after eight to 12 weeks, no further measures are necessary as one can assume that there is sufficient immunity.

If the rubella titer is negative (lower than 1 : 8) and the hemolysis-in-gel test is negative as well, vaccination is necessary. A titer check is required after eight to 12 weeks. If there is no measurable titer, vaccination should be repeated.

Table 8.**2** Problems with rubella diagnosis during pregnancy

Diagnosis/Problems	Findings/Approach
Antibody titer prior to pregnancy	No risk or minimal risk
First titer determination during pregnancy	Possible risk
– HAI titer 1 : 32 to 1 : 256	Immunity is assumed
– HAI titer < 1 : 16	Checks are required
– HAI titer > 1 : 256	IgM determination to exclude a fresh inapparent infection
Titer monitoring or further tests	– If the HAI titer is < 1 : 16, monitoring is required during weeks 16–20 of pregnancy to exclude an asymptomatic infection during the first trimester – If the IgM antibody test is positive, further tests are required to confirm that rubella IgM antibodies are actually present, since false positive results are common with IgM antibody tests. Consultation with the laboratory is essential prior to discussing the risk with the patient
Establishing the patient's history	– Questioning about symptoms, vaccination, contact with exanthematous persons
Problems	– Possibly reinfection: very low risk, if at all (no cases of damage are known) – False positive ELISA–IgM test, e. g., wrong test or cross-reaction in case of EBV infection – IgM antibody persistence (very rare)
Recommendations: prenatal diagnostics in unclear cases and involvement of a special laboratory	

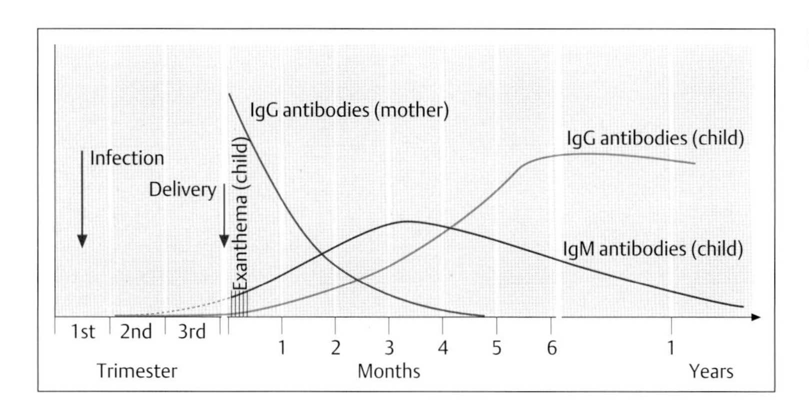

Fig. 8.**5** Congenital rubella infection. Time course of antibody production by the child.

If the titer remains negative, no further measures are required, as one may assume that very low amounts of antibodies do exist, thus preventing the live vaccine from working. Nevertheless, a check-up during pregnancy is recommended (16th week of pregnancy).

Vaccination against rubella is exclusively done for building up immunity to prevent rubella infection during the planned pregnancy. It is carried out by subcutaneous injection of a live vaccine into the upper arm.

In very rare cases, there are mild side effects resembling a rubella infection (mild flulike symptoms, exanthema, arthralgia).

Antibody production after vaccination is slightly slower than after natural rubella infection. The outcome of the vaccination should therefore not be checked before eight weeks, preferably after 12 weeks. For documentation of the rubella titer, it is essential to check the titer after each vaccination.

Only in rare cases does vaccination fail to induce a measurable titer of rubella-specific antibodies. The reason for this may be that immunity already exists, although at such a low level that it cannot be verified by means of the HAI assay. On the other hand, the vaccine—a heat-sensitive live vaccine—may have been inactivated to such an extent that the remaining amount of viable viruses is no longer sufficient to trigger an immune response.

There are also individuals who have an increased infection threshold. In particularly stubborn cases, vaccination may be repeated with a double dose to be on the safe side.

Vaccination should never be performed during pregnancy, and a new pregnancy should not start earlier than eight weeks after vaccination.

However, if vaccination has been carried out by mistake during an existing pregnancy, or if a pregnancy did start within the waiting period of eight weeks, this is of *no* consequence. There is no reason at all to terminate the pregnancy, for the risk from the attenuated virus in the vaccine is extremely low.

In over 800 well-documented cases in which vaccination occurred during early pregnancy, there has not been a single verified case of damage due to the vaccine virus. The warning against becoming pregnant should therefore be viewed as a precautionary measure only.

Prophylaxis during pregnancy:

- ▶ Determination of immune status, if this has not been done earlier.
- ▶ Seronegative women without rubella exposure should have a titer check between the 14th and 16th weeks of pregnancy to make sure that there has been no rubella infection in the meantime.
- ▶ Seronegative women with recent rubella exposure (one to three days ago) should receive rubella-specific hyperimmune globulin (15 mL) as soon as possible. A titer check should follow after three weeks, and then again after six weeks, in order to confirm that a rubella infection did not take place (Table 8.**3**). The antibodies administered may yield a temporary titer of 1 : 8 to 1 : 16, at the most.

If a persistent antibody titer develops, an infection did take place. It is then essential to discuss with the patient the issue of prenatal diagnostics—and, possibly, termination of the pregnancy. However, timely administration of antibodies can reduce the risk by a factor of three.

Erythema Infectiosum (Fifth Disease)

Erythema infectiosum is the fifth exanthematous childhood disease after rubella, measles, varicella, and scarlet fever. The pathogen, parvovirus B19, has been identified only in 1983 as the cause of erythema infectiosum. This disease has been regarded for a long time as a harmless infection that needed to be differentiated from rubella by serological means. Today, this infection is feared during pregnancy, since the child may die

Table 8.3 Effects of timely administration of 15 mL rubella hyperimmune serum

- ▶ Absence of clinical rubella symptoms
- ▶ Reduction in the rate of infection
- ▶ Diminished virus replication in the throat
- ▶ Reduction/suppression of viremia
- ▶ Low antibody response (titer level)
- ▶ Reduced risk of damage to the child
- ▶ Seronegative women with rubella contact several days ago (> 5 days): no administration of immune globulin because it is already too late; antibody monitoring, but no sooner than at least three weeks after the presumed contact.
- ▶ Women with unknown immune status and rubella contact a short time ago (one to three days): Collection of blood samples for antibody determination, administration of immune globulin. If it turns out that antibodies are present, no further measures are required. If no antibodies are present, titer checks after three and six weeks.
- ▶ Women with unknown immune status and rubella contact six to 14 days ago: no administration of immune globulin, because it is already too late. If negative, titer check after three weeks; if positive, no further measures because immunity already exists.
- ▶ Women with unknown immune status and rubella contact more than 14 days ago: if antibody titer is high, determination of rubella-specific IgM antibodies, titer check after eight days (titer rise is very rapid within a few days).

because of anemia following the state of fetal hydrops.

Pathogen. Parvovirus B19 is a member of the family Parvoviridae. It is a relatively stable virus without an envelope. Its genome consists of linear single-stranded DNA.

Frequency. Endemic infection is higher than originally assumed. Antibodies against parvovirus B19 are present in 50–70% of adults. The frequency during pregnancy is estimated to be one in 400.

Transmission. Droplet infection; infection caused by banked blood and plasma products is also possible, though rare.

Pathogenesis. The B19 virus is transferred by the blood via the placenta to the fetus. The infection affects the bone marrow, thus leading to inhibition of erythropoiesis. In addition to this inhibition, the infection leads to hemolysis in the fetus; as in adults, this may cause hemolytic anemia and aplastic crisis. Finally, generalized fetal hydrops develops. The virus probably also infects other organs. Its involvement in chronic polyarthritis and Schönlein–Henoch purpura has been suggested.

Clinical picture. The course is asymptomatic in almost one third of the infections. Flulike symptoms with fever, headache, malaise, and nausea occur during the prodromal stage, followed by a maculopapulous erythema with a tendency to confluence. The erythema affects arms, legs, and trunk symmetrically but usually spares the palms and soles. Mild pain in the joints, especially in the small joints, myalgia, and lymphadenopathy may also be present. These may persist for weeks and months (in about 20% of cases). The seasonal peak of infection is during winter and spring.

Risk groups for serious infection are pregnant women, patients with congenital or acquired anemia, and immunocompromised persons.

Complications. The frequency of developing severe anemia with fetal hydrops in the event of erythema infectiosum infection during pregnancy is reported as lying between 4–17.5%. The highest risk is between the 14th and 24th weeks of pregnancy, since this is the time of the highest density of P antigen on fetal erythrocytes to which the B19 virus binds. Erythrocyte transfusion is only rarely required after the 26th week of pregnancy.

Diagnosis:

- ▶ *Indication.* Serodiagnostics should be performed if a pregnant woman develops exanthema, if erythema infectiosum is present in the woman's surroundings, and in the event of fetal hydrops.
- ▶ *Serology.* Enzyme or fluorescence tests for the determination of IgG and IgM antibodies by means of recombinant antigens. Further tests include immunoblot tests for the determination of IgG and IgM antibodies.
- ▶ *Pathogen detection.* Growth in culture is not possible. Detection of viral DNA by means of

PCR (especially in the amniotic fluid, blood, serum, and other body fluids).
- *Distinctive features of laboratory parameters.* Reticulocytopenia, low hemoglobin levels, often neutropenia with lymphocytopenia and thrombocytopenia, occasionally eosinophilia.

Therapy. Treatment is only symptomatic and includes erythrocyte transfusion in the event of severe anemia. Inhibition of viral replication is not possible.

Approach in case of exposure to erythema infectiosum. Infections usually occur as an epidemic disease in nurseries or schools:
- Determination of the immune status of the pregnant woman. If there are no antibodies, she should stay away from the source of infection, and serology should be repeated after three and six weeks because asymptomatic infections do occur.
- In the case of infection during pregnancy (disease, or only detection of IgM antibodies), the fetus should be closely monitored (once a week) by ultrasound for eight to 10 weeks.
- When the first signs of hydrops appear, cordocentesis (percutaneous umbilical blood sampling) and amniocentesis should be performed for diagnosing the infection of the fetus, followed by intrauterine erythrocyte transfusion. Despite an increased survival rate of the children treated this way, this approach is partly controversial because of theoretical immunological risks. Termination of the pregnancy is not justified, since no damages have been observed so far in the surviving children. The child either dies in utero or is born healthy.
- If a child is born with fetal hydrops, antibodies against parvovirus B19 are determined in the mother; if present, the amniotic fluid (which may be stored frozen) is examined in a special laboratory for the presence of B19 DNA.

Prophylaxis. An active vaccine is in the making. Passive vaccination with standard immune globulin is possible. However, there are hardly any indications for this.

HIV Infection (AIDS)

Hardly any other infection has triggered such a quick and intensive research as this disease, which was first diagnosed more than 20 years ago. Due to the rapid development of new antiviral compounds, the prognosis and life expectancy for individuals infected by HIV have much improved, although neither a vaccine nor a cure have been found. In gynecology, HIV now plays only a role in the care of infected pregnant women. The care of HIV-positive patients has now been so well established that severe genital infections or malignant diseases because of HIV infection hardly ever occur today.

History and frequency. This infection posed a new problem for medicine. It occurred at the beginning of the 1980 s and has affected to a considerable degree the work of gynecologists and obstetricians.

The infection has probably been transmitted from animals to humans some 50 years ago. Only through massive dissemination of the infection by special risk groups (homosexuals, drug addicts) has it become so widespread that it became visible as an epidemic disease. In Africa and other third world countries, transmission of the infection is predominantly heterosexual, and the women in these countries become as frequently infected as men. The main reason for the alarmingly high prevalence in these countries (up to 20% of the population) is poverty, the lack of information and understanding, and the occurrence of other genital infections that promote transmission.

Pathogen. The human immunodeficiency virus (HIV) belongs to the group of lentiviruses, which have been known for some time and cause chronic diseases of the central nervous system in animals (sheep). It is a retrovirus (Retroviridae), i. e., it possesses RNA as genetic material, which must first be transcribed in the cell into DNA. For this purpose, the virus carries its own enzyme, the reverse transcriptase.

The virus has a complex structure (Fig. 1.**1**, p. 3) with a lipid-containing envelope, and it is therefore very sensitive to alcohol and environmental factors.

The virus is extremely variable and changes its envelope continuously. None of the isolates are identical, not even those from the same patient. So far, we distinguish two types: HIV-1 and HIV-2; the latter is still rare and largely confined to West Africa. The pathogenicity of HIV-2 seems to be lower than that of HIV-1.

So far, the variability of the virus has frustrated any attempts to develop an effective vaccine. The ability of the virus to develop drug resistance is also very high, and new compounds need to be designed continuously. For the same reason, combinations of compounds are more effective than monotherapy.

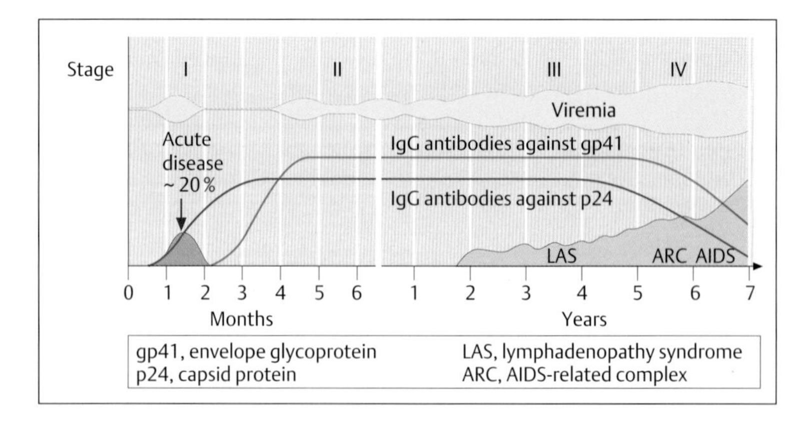

Fig. 8.**6** HIV infection. Diagram illustrating the infectiousness (viremia) and the production of antibodies during the clinical course of HIV infection without therapy.

Transmission. The risk of transmission depends on the viral load of blood and tissues, and it is enhanced by local inflammations because of the increased presence of leukocytes. The risk of transmission rises also with the advance of symptoms.

- Anal intercourse. The likelihood of injuring the single-layered intestinal epithelium, the presence of HIV target cells in the mucosa, and the higher viral load in the semen than in the cervix increase the risk.
- Sexual contact. Inflammation in the genital region increases, the risk because an increase in leukocytes leads to increased excretion of the virus.
- Through the placenta (depending on the viral load, membrane permeability, and uterine contractions).
- During delivery (70–80 % of child infections).
- Contact with blood (injuries, contaminated needles, open wounds) (the risk is 1 : 100 to 1 : 1000).
- Banked blood (the risk is about 1 : 10^6).
- Breast-feeding. Though there is little experience, the virus can be detected in the mother's milk (the risk of transmission is about 10 %).
- So far, no transmission has been observed through social contacts. The risk is extremely low, although a causal connection is difficult to recognize because the infectiousness of the virus is low and the latency period is long (years).
- No transmission through immunoglobulin preparations.

The risk of infection during sexual intercourse is increased by having contact with intravenous drug users, bisexuals, partners from areas where the disease is endemic, partners with infections that are usually sexually transmitted, partners with multiple applications of blood products, and promiscuity with unknown partners.

Incubation time:

- acute disease: two to four weeks
- antibody production (Fig. 8.**6**): three to 12 weeks, in extreme cases up to two years (measurable amounts of antibodies)
- complete clinical picture of AIDS after eight months to 20 years.

Pathogenesis. This is a very complex process involving many cell types including those of the immune system, and it ends with the breakdown of cellular immunity. This disease develops slowly over many years. The virus infects cells carrying the main receptor (CD4) on their surface, especially T4 cells, and cells of the central nervous system. The viral particle is taken up by the cell and undergoes uncoating. A DNA copy is then produced by the viral transcriptase and covalently integrated into the cell's genome.

Using the viral DNA as template, RNA copies are transcribed and appear in the cytoplasm where they are assembled into viral particles. These are finally budding from the cell membrane that provides them with an envelope into which virus-specific proteins are integrated.

Due to the virus-specific antigens on their surface, T4 lymphocytes are recognized and eliminated by the body's defense system, thus causing a gradual decline in T4 cells. Infected cells in the brain are destroyed as well. In addition to the increased susceptibility to opportunistic pathogens, cerebral defects associated with changes in personality may occur relatively early in about 40 % of the affected individuals. Finally, extreme wasting and death occur.

The virus itself is extremely variable due to errors made by the reverse transcriptase. As a result, none of the isolates are identical. This explains why the HIV virus repeatedly dodges the body's defenses, thus leading to progression of the disease.

Clinical picture. Here we must clearly distinguish between an asymptomatic virus infection and the full-blown disease. Thanks to increasingly more effective drugs, severe disease is becoming rare in industrialized countries.

The clinical course of the infection has been subdivided into four stages, although it is not yet known whether only 40–60% of the infected individuals reach stage IV or whether all of them fall ill after an extended period of time (> 10–20 years). New drugs have considerably improved the prognosis, with many of the infected persons remaining at stage II for a long time.

Stage I. Acute disease, with about 20% of the infected individuals showing flulike symptoms similar to those of mononucleosis, usually two to three weeks after transmission.

Stage II. Latent infection without symptoms.

Stage III. Lymphadenopathy.

Stage IV. Complete clinical picture of AIDS, with either opportunistic infections (*Pneumocystis carinii*, *Toxoplasma gondii*, cryptococci, mycobacteria), virus infections (CMV, HPV, herpesviruses [Fig. 8.**7**]), changes in the central nervous system with encephalitis and atrophy, or malignant diseases. The gastrointestinal tract, the lungs, and the central nervous system are especially affected.

All four stages are infectious, although infectiousness increases during the progression of the disease.

The disease varies considerably: it may run a very quick course, or it may be very mild and without any subjective impairment of the patient. Much has changed to the better with the therapeutic possibilities available today.

Risks for gynecological patients

Thanks to the increasingly more effective drugs and the reduction in viral load, the risks posed by AIDS patients to others have become much lower. Even the severe genital infections and increased rates of malignant disease initially observed have almost completely disappeared in industrialized countries.

Apart from that, other infections may accelerate the course of the disease, and genital infections pose an increased risk of infecting the sexual partner. Today, HIV-positive women can only receive normal gynecological care if they undergo regular examination by physicians specializing in HIV infection.

Consistent use of condoms with both HIV-negative and HIV-positive partners is recommended. Uptake of other HIV mutants from a positive partner may accelerate the course of the disease.

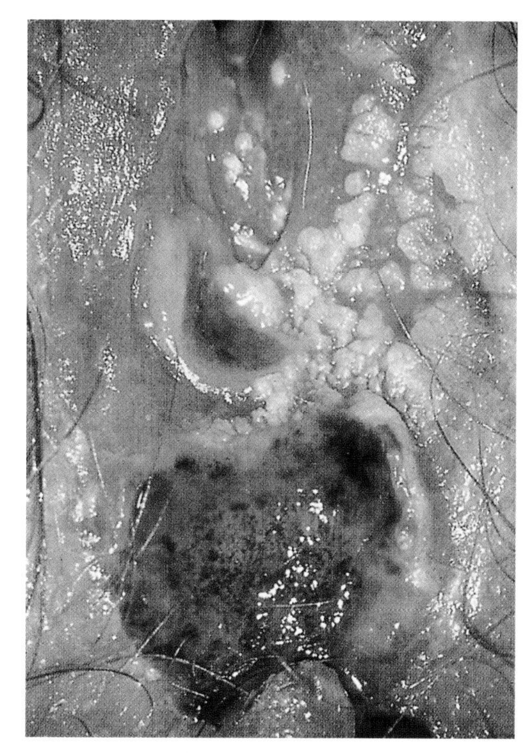

Fig. 8.**7** Terminal stage of AIDS in a 21-year-old patient with severe recurrent genital herpes and condylomas.

Diagnosis:

Serology:

- *Enzyme immunoassay.* Indirect or competitive ELISA is used as a screening procedure (specific for HIV-1 and HIV-2).
- *Fluorescence test* (some cross-reaction between HIV-1 and HIV-2).
- *Western blot* (p. 34). Based on the appearance of different antibodies against individual viral components, it can provide information on the duration of an existing infection.

Detection of pathogen:

- Cultures from blood (heparinized), semen, or cervical secretion. So far, this very expensive procedure is only used for research purposes, since only few virus particles per mL of blood are present. In contrast to infections with hepatitis B virus, where there may be up to 10^{12} virus particles per mL, there are perhaps only 10^4/mL in case of HIV infection.
- DNA hybridization by Southern blot technique.
- PCR (determination of viral load).

Diagnosis of HIV infection is established by serological tests. A very sensitive, but not absolutely specific, ELISA test is used as a screening procedure; it yields more positive results than HIV

Table 8.**4** Prophylaxis and treatment of HIV infection during pregnancy

Prophylaxis	Treatment
Mother without symptoms	Mother with symptoms
CD4 > 250/μL and RNA copies < 10 000/μL	CD4 < 250/μL and RNA copies > 50 000/μL
From the 32nd week of pregnancy onward	From the 13th week of pregnancy onward
Preferably: zidovudine (AZT) + lamivudine (3TC)	Nelfinavir (250 mg/day)
or zidovudine + didanosine (DDI)	Nevirapine (200–400 mg/day)

infections are actually present. For this reason, every positive ELISA has to be confirmed by a western blot.

In view of the far-reaching implications of the diagnosis and in order to eliminate any human error, the diagnostic tests should be repeated with a second serum sample. If this sample is also positive in all tests, the diagnosis is established.

Determination of viral load. This is carried out by means of PCR on a blood sample. The viral load is now regarded as a measure for infectiousness and prognosis.

Determination of sensitivity. The rapid development of drug resistance by the HIV virus requires combination treatment. Nevertheless, in special cases—above all if the antiretroviral therapy is unsuccessful—determination of sensitivity to the drugs used for the particular patient may become necessary. For economic reasons, this will be restricted to special cases.

HIV and Pregnancy

Now that severe genital infections have become rare thanks to improved HIV therapy, pregnancy has become the most common reason why gynecologists see HIV-positive women.

The pregnancy itself does not have a negative influence on the course of the HIV infection. There is also no increase in the rate of premature delivery. Infection of the child is considered the main risk during pregnancy. While initially relatively high at 50%, it is now below 5% with prophylaxis. The initially high rates of transmission were due to more advanced stages of infection with high viral loads and to insufficient prophylactic measures.

Today, the care for HIV-positive pregnant women can definitely be provided in a gynecological practice. Assessment of the stage (diagnostic procedures) and recommendations for treatment and prophylaxis should be carried out by specialists or in medical centers, or at least in consultation with them.

Results of studies indicate that about 35% of child infections occur during the last weeks of pregnancy (after the 32nd week), and about 65% occur during delivery. The increasing permeability between mother and child and the contractions during labor promote transmission of the virus.

The risk for the child depends on the stage of the disease in the mother. Declining titers of p24-specific antibodies correlate with an increase of virus particles in the blood and cervical secretion and, hence, with an increase in the viral load. The viral load is determined today by means of PCR on blood samples. Inflammation, uterine contractions, and premature delivery further increase the risk of transmission.

With the increase in experience and as the result of further studies, generally accepted recommendations for the care of HIV-positive pregnant women have been established. The aim is to keep both risks as low as possible: the risk of transmitting the virus to the child and also the risk of damaging the child by means of drugs.

Treatment during pregnancy. When deciding on a therapy, one has to choose between health issues of the mother and those of the unborn child. With the establishment of increasingly highly active antiviral compounds (see p. 47), a new problem has been created because the undesired effects of these compounds on the fetus are largely unknown.

Antiretroviral therapy is recommended for all pregnant women, since it has been observed that, even with a load of 1000 HIV-RNA copies per μL of blood, the rate of transmission can be lowered from 9.8% to 1%. Today, antiretroviral combinations (Table 8.**4**) are recommended, as they should lower the development of resistances.

Resistance screening during pregnancy is controversial. In general, such a test is recommended in case of acute infection, increase in viral load during therapy, or viral persistence in the blood.

The second approach to reducing HIV transmission is cesarean section in the event of uterine inertia.

These days, prophylaxis with zidovudine (AZT) (5 × 100 mg) or better Combivir from the 32nd week on and continuing peripartal is recommended (see Table 8.**4**)—together with a generous decision toward early primary cesarean section (in the 38th week). Precautionary measures are required prior to delivery. Breast-feeding is discouraged as transmissions have been reported.

Approach if a pregnant women is already undergoing antiviral treatment:

- If the pregnancy is discovered after the first trimester, treatment should be continued.
- If the pregnancy is discovered during the first trimester, the treatment may be discontinued and then continued after the end of the first trimester. At the very least, compounds that carry an increased risk for the child should be discontinued (e. g., efavirenz or delavirdine).

If the antiretroviral therapy is only started after delivery, the newborn is also treated for six weeks. There have been no studies on the treatment of newborns from mothers who did not receive prophylactic treatment. Starting AZT administration 48 hours after birth is thought to be moderately effective.

Other potential problems with HIV during pregnancy. The effect of methadone is reduced by protease inhibitors (e. g., nevirapine), though not by indinavir.

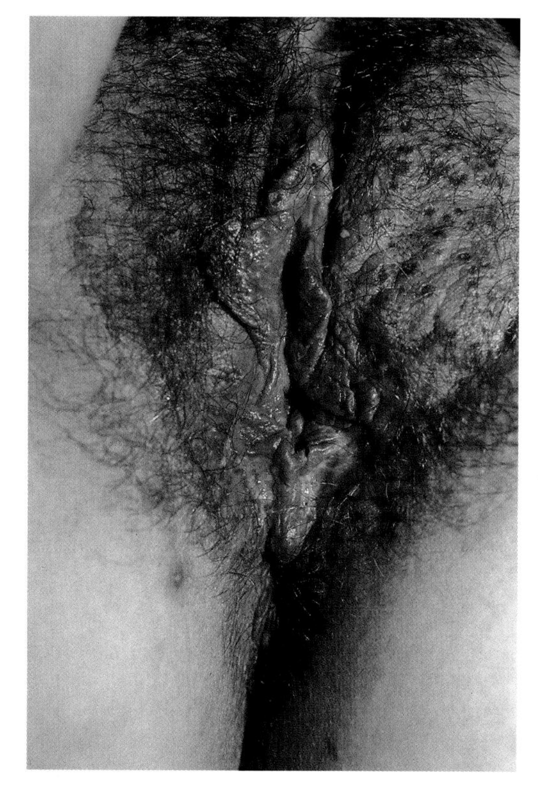

Fig. 8.**8** Primary genital herpes in a 33-year-old patient during the 21st week of pregnancy.

Genital Herpes

Genital herpes during pregnancy is a dreaded situation, particularly at the time of delivery, because it may cause serious disease in the newborn. In Central Europe though, the fear is greater than the actual risk. With about one in 25 000 births, neonatal herpes is much less common here than in the United States. There also seem to be differences regarding the viral types, since both types of HSV now occur with similar frequencies in Central Europe, whereas type 2 is still predominant in the United States with 70 %.

In principle, one needs to distinguish during pregnancy between the rather rare form of primary genital herpes, which poses a high risk for the child (about 30–50 %) at the time of delivery, and the more common form of recurrent genital herpes, which has a much lower risk for the newborn—especially when sufficient amounts of antibodies are present.

Hence, only the children of seronegative mothers are in danger. These children may be infected due to a possible primary infection of the mother just before delivery or, because they do not have any protection provided by the mother, after birth by hospital personnel or visitors (herpes labialis).

Primary Genital Herpes

Primary genital herpes is always accompanied by clinical symptoms (Fig. 8.**8**). However, the lesions are not always interpreted correctly, and this may become dangerous in the peripartal period.

The intensity of symptoms depends in part on the serostatus of the patient. Except during the time of birth, even primary genital herpes seems to pose a very low risk for the child.

Early during pregnancy, the route of infection is probably hematogenous, although this is a rather rare event. Only very few isolated cases have been described. It is more likely that such cases result in the death of the fetus rather than in any damage to the child, since a slightly increased rate of abortion has been reported.

A congenital herpes simplex syndrome is not known.

The **main risk** for the child consists of infection during birth through the infected birth canal. Here, the risk for the newborn of contracting the disease is up to 50 %. After rupture of the fetal membranes, an ascending infection in utero is also possible, and even cesarean section (e. g., four hours later) may not prevent the infection of the child.

Severe neonatal herpes infection is altogether a rare event. According to US figures, it is now observed at a frequency of only one in 7500 births. In Europe, it seems to be even much less frequent with one in 25000 births. Since effective treatment of herpes with aciclovir is possible today, the rare event of primary genital herpes is no longer that dangerous. However, as with all infections, it is important to initiate treatment or prophylaxis in time.

If the mother has primary genital herpes, the risk of infection for the child is:

- < 2% during the first trimester
- about 10% during the third trimester
- about 50% at the time of birth.

Recurrent Genital Herpes

Much more frequent than primary genital herpes infection is recurrent genital herpes. As it is often asymptomatic, it may not be noticed by the patient. The excretion of herpesviruses can only be detected by examining cultures from vaginal and cervical swabs, or by PCR.

Virus excretion during pregnancy has been detected in over 10% of pregnant women known to have recurrent genital herpes.

The endemic genital infection with herpes simplex virus (HSV-2 and HSV-1) is up to 20–30% in Germany. One may therefore assume that about 2% of all pregnant women excrete herpes simplex virus at some point during the pregnancy.

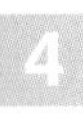

According to these figures and to studies carried out by Yeager (1984), 0.3% of pregnant women excrete virus into the birth canal at the time of delivery.

Whether or not an infection of the child actually takes place depends on the amount of virus particles excreted and on the antibody titer of the mother.

Yeager was able to demonstrate that infection of the child occurred only in those patients in which the mother showed a very low antibody titer in the serum. According to Brown, the child becomes infected in 5%, 1,2% after cesarean section and 7,7% after vaginal delivery, the child becomes infected only in 5–10% of women with florid recurrent genital herpes at the time of delivery.

If the mother has recurrent genital herpes, the risk of infection for the child is:

- < 0.1% during the first trimester
- < 1% during the third trimester
- < 5% at the time of birth.

Treatment during pregnancy. Teratogenicity of aciclovir at normal dosages has not been demonstrated in animal experiments. Experience with aciclovir treatment of herpes infections in pregnant women has been documented in the international registry of aciclovir use during pregnancy. Worldwide, 1060 pregnant women with herpes infection have so far been treated with aciclovir and evaluated, according to data provided by the original manufacturer (June 30, 1997). According to these data, there is no increased risk of malformation after taking aciclovir during pregnancy.

Nevertheless, there is a relative contraindication for treating herpes infection during pregnancy with aciclovir, i. e., the risks and benefits must be carefully considered and accurate diagnosis is imperative. Treatment should only be initiated in the following cases:

- primary genital herpes during pregnancy
- avoidance of cesarean section by prophylactic administration of aciclovir during delivery
- severe herpes zoster during pregnancy.

To be on the safe side, aciclovir should not be prescribed during early pregnancy (1st to 14th weeks) if possible, since not enough patients have been observed so far to exclude completely any risk.

Approach if genital herpes is suspected during pregnancy up to two weeks before delivery:

- Confirmation of the diagnosis: isolation of the virus through culture (duration: two to three days), detection of antigen in the fluorescence test (one to two hours), ELISA (five to six hours) or better PCR.
- Blood samples for determination of antibodies against genital herpes: to distinguish between primary and recurrent genital herpes and, at the same time, to determine the antibody titer.
- If the serological test is negative, it should be repeated after four weeks (prior to birth, at the latest) to know whether the child will have protection.
- In case of primary genital herpes: oral treatment with aciclovir (5 × 200 mg) for five days, close monitoring of the child after birth.
- In case of recurrent genital herpes: no aciclovir treatment, reassurance of the patient, close monitoring of the child after birth.

Approach in case of genital herpes at the time of delivery:

- If clinically clear, extensive herpes lesions are present (above all, during primary infection) and the immune status is unknown: cesarean

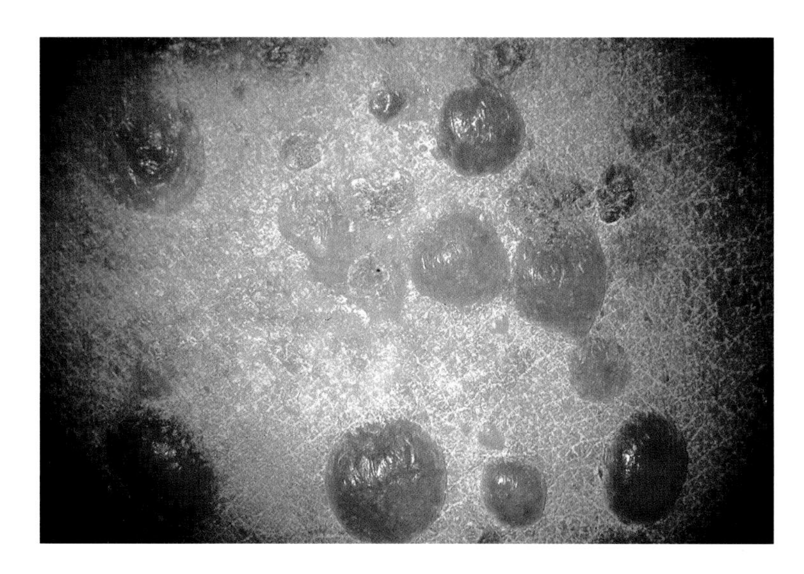

Fig. 8.**9** Herpes gestationis in a 30-year-old patient during the 34th week of pregnancy.

section makes only sense if the rupture of the fetal membranes happened less than four hours ago. Aciclovir treatment of the mother, prophylactic aciclovir treatment of the newborn.
- If lesions are known to be due to recurrent genital herpes and the antibody titer is high: vaginal delivery is possible under aciclovir treatment of the mother. Close follow-up of the child is essential, with administration of aciclovir to the newborn as soon as the slightest symptoms occur.

Prophylaxis for children after birth if the mother has a florid infection:
- swab of the nasopharynx
- immune globulins if the titer of the mother is low
- possibly aciclovir treatment.

Herpes Gestationis

This disease should be correctly called pemphigoid gestationis. The clinical picture of blistering skin (Fig. 8.**9**), occurring in various regions of the body, is so different from lesions caused by herpes simplex virus that it cannot be mistaken. It is probably an autoimmune disease, and the vesicobullous skin lesions may also be absent. The diagnosis used so far, which is based on the detection of C3 deposition along the basement membrane in a skin biopsy, is increasingly being replaced by the detection of antibodies against BP180 autoantigen in the serum. Treatment consists of 0.3–0.5 mg of prednisolone/kg body weight.

Bullous Pemphigoid

(Differential diagnosis: genital herpes, candidiasis, and folliculitis)

This is a rare mild immune disease with blisters, and it is not easily recognized. It may also start on the vulva (Fig. 8.**10**). Diagnosis is established by means of biopsy and detection of immune complexes in the biopsy or serum. Treatment consists of administration of prednisone or azathioprine.

Cytomegalic Inclusion Disease (CID)

The cytomegalovirus (CMV) belongs to the pathogens most commonly transmitted to newborns. This is because, in 10 % of pregnant women with florid CMV infection, the virus is excreted in the urine and in the cervical secretion. Fortunately, the course of peripartal infections is usually asymptomatic or benign, with damages to the child being rare. Infection of the fetus, however, may be a serious disease with grave consequences. In such cases, the only possible option is termination of the pregnancy. So far, there is no effective, well-tolerated therapy available for this virus.

Cytomegalic inclusion disease is a sexually transmitted infection.

Frequency. Infection with the cytomegalovirus is one of the most common florid infections during pregnancy. Antibodies against CMV are present in 50–60 % of adults, with the virus still remaining in the body. Suppression of the immune system

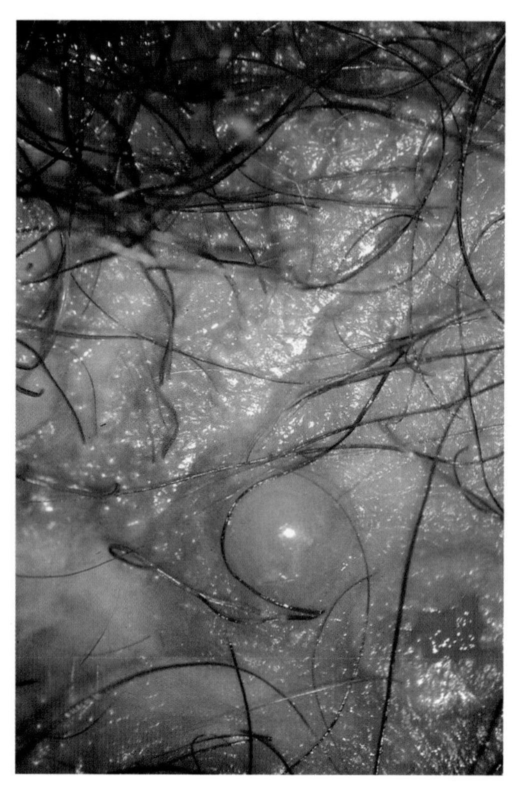

Fig. 8.**10** Pemphigoid of the vulva in a 45-year-old patient.

during pregnancy causes reactivation of the virus in 20% of women carrying CMV.

One should therefore expect to find a florid CMV infection in about 10% of all pregnancies. About 10% of the children of these mothers become infected during birth, corresponding to about 1% of all newborns. In Germany, slightly more that 20 congenital infections are reported every year.

Pathogen. The cytomegalovirus belongs to the group of herpesviruses. It is a relatively large DNA virus with a lipid envelope, which makes it extremely unstable. Various subtypes have been described.

Clinical picture. The symptoms of cytomegalic inclusion disease are uncharacteristic; they include fatigue, weakness, swelling of the lymph nodes, and occasionally also mild fever. In immunocompetent persons, the disease usually takes a mild course. In immunocompromised persons—and this includes the fetus—the virus may cause serious damage (hepatitis, myocarditis, encephalitis, blindness). Apart from the unborn child, this group includes patients undergoing immunosuppression (e. g., after kidney transplantation) and especially people with AIDS. Reactivation of the virus poses a threat to AIDS patients.

As with other herpesvirus infections, the CMV is usually not eliminated after the infection but persists in the lymphocytes and in the kidneys. Due to the depressed immune system during pregnancy, the virus is often reactivated. As during primary infection, specific IgM antibodies are detected here as well. In addition, CMV is excreted in the urine and often also in the cervical secretion.

Risk for the child. During primary CMV infection of the mother, transmission to the child is by the hematogenous route, and infection may occur anytime during the pregnancy. Fetal damage is likely to be more severe if the infection occurs early during the pregnancy.

In case of primary infection of the mother during the first trimester, the rate of fetal infection is estimated at 10–20%. Transmission is probably more frequent during late pregnancy, though the damages are less severe.

Up to 90% of children with congenital cytomegalic inclusion disease (CID) exhibit sequelae.

As with other pathogens, transmission of the cytomegalovirus to the child occurs less often during early pregnancy and more frequently during late pregnancy. If there is evidence of fetal infection, the risk of damage is about 20%. Early during pregnancy, this may trigger a discussion about terminating the pregnancy.

The risk posed by reactivation of a CMV infection during pregnancy is far below 1%.

Based on the serological finding, it is a major problem to discern whether the detection of IgM antibodies during the first test indicates a primary infection or reactivation of the virus. This is why tests—or, at least, the collection of serum samples—before the pregnancy are helpful.

Studies using more recent methods indicate that congenital CMV infection in cases where the mother already possessed antibodies to CMV before she became pregnant may not be the result of viral reactivation in the mother, but rather that of reinfection with another CMV type during her pregnancy.

A typical sign for congenital CMV infection is hepatosplenomegaly, which can be discovered already in utero by means of ultrasound, and also after birth.

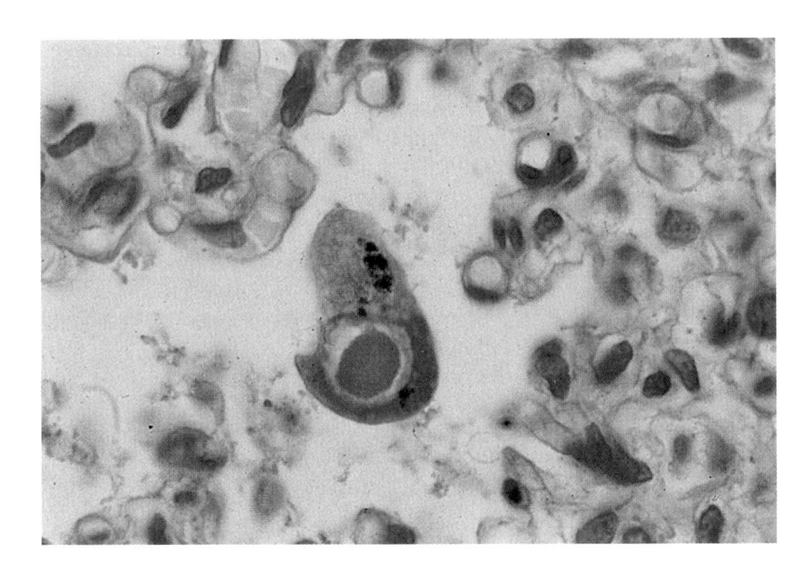

Fig. 8.**11** Cytomegalovirus infection. The child died in the 30th week of pregnancy. The typical owl-eye cells found in the lungs support the diagnosis. (Micrograph by courtesy of Prof. Dr N. Böhm, Department of Pathology, University of Freiburg, Germany.)

Primary CMV Infection During Pregnancy

Diagnosis:

- seroconversion from negative to positive (fluorescence test, ELISA)
- rise in the IgG antibody titer by a factor of four. Possible clues:
- high IgM antibody titer (may also be high in the event of viral reactivation)
- high numbers of CMV particles excreted in the urine; however, the only clear evidence for primary CMV infection is seroconversion from negative to positive, indicating the first appearance of CMV-specific antibodies.

Frequency during pregnancy. Less than 1 %, perhaps 0.1–0.3 %.

Congenital CMV Infection and Disease

This is a rare but serious disease of the newborn due to hematogenous transmission of the virus. In the acute stage, the child exhibits hepatosplenomegaly, petechial bleedings due to thrombocytopenia, increased transaminases, massive CMV excretion in the urine, pronounced inflammatory reactions with typical giant cells in the placenta (which may weigh more than 1000 g). Persistent cerebral damages (microcephaly) are common.

The infection may already take its course in utero during the second and third trimesters. Hepatosplenomegaly and ascites can be detected by ultrasound. Cases of fetal hydrops have also been described. This may lead to the death of the unborn child, in which case the histological examination reveals the typical owl-eye cells (Fig. 8.**11**) in various organs.

Premature cesarean section in such patients does not have any advantage, only disadvantages.

If the infection takes place earlier during pregnancy, it may have already healed by the time of birth—or premature birth, which is more often the case—and only the lasting damages are found (e. g., microcephaly and cerebral retardation). The prognosis of these children is altogether moderate to poor.

Frequency. About 25 congenital CMV infections per year have been reported during recent years in Germany. One may therefore expect at least 100 CMV-damaged children per year. Since there are no measures available apart from terminating an early pregnancy, this disease is considered tragic.

Prophylaxis. Pregnant women should avoid risk areas where they may be infected with the CMV virus, especially if they did not develop antibodies against it. Such areas include dialysis units, transplant units, and pediatric wards. When dealing with children (day care, kindergarten), direct contact with urine should be avoided. There is no effective vaccine available at present.

Approach if primary CMV infection is suspected or confirmed during the first trimester. Intrauterine infection of the child occurs only in about 20 % of these pregnancies. The infection can be recognized (or excluded) by the presence (or absence) of CMV in the amniotic fluid into which the virus is excreted by the kidneys. In the past,

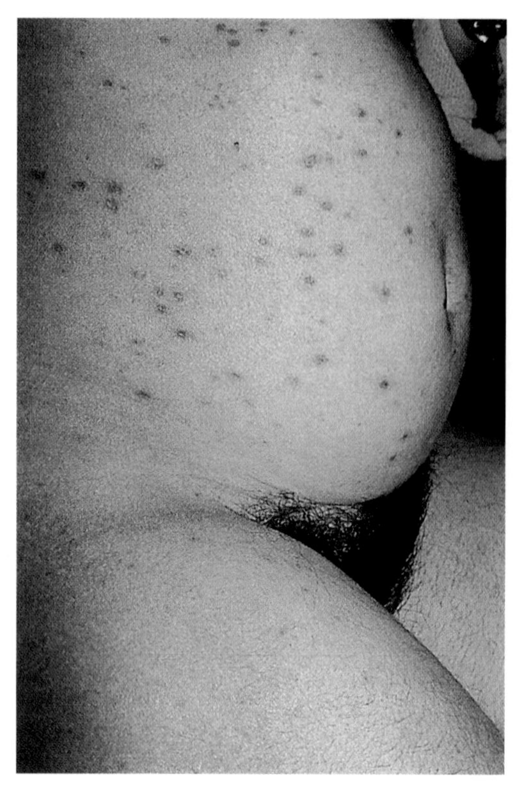

Fig. 8.**12** Varicella in a 34-year-old patient during the 32nd week of pregnancy. The child was born healthy.

detection of the virus in the amniotic fluid required culture methods; today, the virus is detected by means of PCR.

Cord puncture for the detection of IgM antibodies in the fetus is possible from the 20th to 22 nd weeks of pregnancy onward, but it is difficult and not necessary.

If the PCR test is negative, and possibly also the test for CMV-specific IgM antibodies, the mother may be encouraged to carry on with the pregnancy, since the residual risk is extremely low.

Reactivation of CMV Infection During Pregnancy

Risk for the child. In 20% of pregnant women with a previous CMV infection, reactivation of the latent CMV infection may occur during pregnancy, or the latent infection is still florid. Close to 50% of pregnant women carry the CMV, and almost 10% of them exhibit a florid CMV infection with detectable IgM antibodies and with CMV excreted in the urine.

About 10% of the children of these women become infected with the virus during birth. This means that about 1% of all children become infected with CMV during birth. Clinical signs of CMV infection develop in only 10% of the infected children, which corresponds to one in 1000 newborns. Here, the late sequelae are much less common and severe than with congenital CMV infection due to primary infection of the mother.

The signs for reactivated CMV infection during pregnancy include:

- detection of CMV-specific IgM antibodies in the serum of the mother
- no or only a slight rise in the already high titer of IgG antibodies
- no or only minor CMV excretion in the urine
- absence of clinical symptoms
- detection of CMV-specific IgM antibodies with known IgG antibody titer before the pregnancy.

Persistence of CMV-specific IgM Antibodies and the Desire to Have Children

If antibodies against CMV are present already before the start of the pregnancy, they provide a relatively high level of protection against congenital infection by hematogenous transmission. There remains a potential risk for the child, since recent data show that the mother may become reinfected with another CMV strain.

In view of the very low risk, pregnancy is not a contradiction. Further serological checks should *not* be carried out because they do not provide new information and have no implications. Exceptions are manifestation of the disease in the mother and unusual ultrasonic findings in the child.

Varicella (Chickenpox)

Varicella does not seem to be a harmless disease after all. It takes a severe course in 16% of the patients, and complications occur in 6% of these patients. As varicella is very contagious, most of the infections take place at the preschool age. Varicella during pregnancy (Fig. 8.**12**) is rather rare, since 90–95% of adults have already developed antibodies against the varicella–zoster virus. Like every virus infection, varicella is feared during pregnancy.

At the start of the pregnancy, the virus is transmitted to the fetus in about 20% of all cases, and toward the end of pregnancy in 80% of cases. However, the risk of damage to the child is low and exists only in the first half, being about 2% until the 20th week of pregnancy.

Frequency. The incidence of varicella infection during pregnancy is reported to be 0.1–0.5 %.

Pathogen. The varicella–zoster virus (VZV) belongs to the group of herpesviruses, all of which have a tendency to persist in the host.

Clinical picture. This is an exanthematous disease with symptoms that are not always characteristic enough to rely on the patient's history and the clinical appearance. The coexistence of fine vesicles, nodules, and crusts (starry sky distribution) associated with itching is typical. Depending on the stage, the vesicles may be so discreet that they can be recognized only under the colposcope (Fig. 8.**13**), and the exanthema as such may be assessed incorrectly. Here, negative serological tests with subsequent determination of the titer, or detection of IgM antibodies, bring clarification.

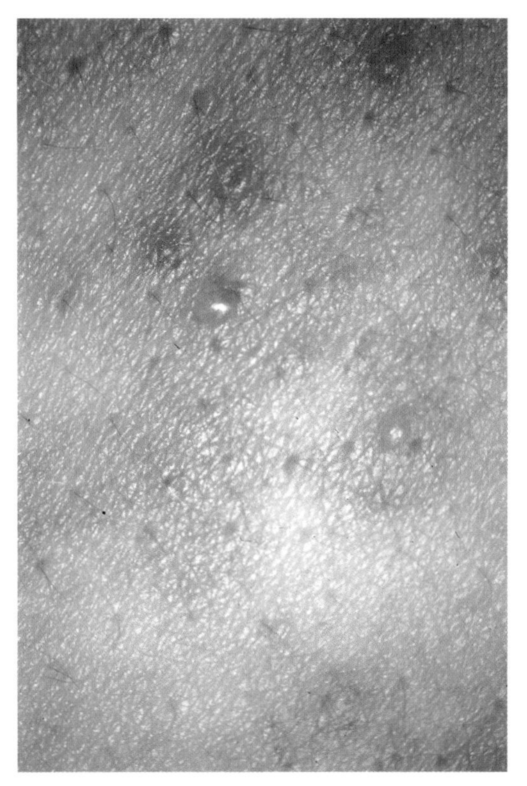

Fig. 8.**13** Varicella in a 26-year-old patient during the 24th week of pregnancy. The vesicles are visible only under the colposcope.

Congenital Varicella Syndrome

Fetal damage is rare; it is about 2 % until the 20th week of pregnancy. So far, there has been experience with 1739 patients (Enders, 1988).

Termination of the pregnancy is not generally justified, since the rate of damage caused by florid varicella infection during pregnancy is low, even in the first trimester. Only if there is evidence that the fetus has been damaged, termination of the pregnancy should be discussed with the parents (Table 8.5).

Table 8.**5** Symptoms associated with congenital varicella syndrome*

Symptoms	Frequency
Skin lesions (scars, scarring, ulcers)	100 %
Skeletal anomalies/hypoplasia of extremities	86 %
Eye defects (cataract, Horner syndrome)	64 %
Neurological defects (spasm, retardation)	42 %
Chorioretinitis	41 %
Cerebral atrophy	29 %
Lethality	47 %

* According to Enders 1988.

Perinatal Varicella of the Mother

Varicella occurring at the time of delivery is especially dreaded. There is an increased risk of severe neonatal disease with high lethality of the child early on. In theses cases, about 20 % of the newborns become infected while still in utero. With adequate measures, the risk of disease or damage to the child has now become low, even with varicella at the time of delivery. Postponing a spontaneous birth is not justified in view of today's options.

Risk for the child. If the maternal varicella-induced exanthema appears in the period between four days before and three days after delivery, very severe varicella may develop in the child. The risk is about 8 %.

Although the infection may have been transmitted to the child while still in utero, the mother has not yet produced protective antibodies to be passed on to the child before delivery.

Therapy. Since the disease manifests itself in these children only after nine to 10 days, the children should receive varicella–zoster immune globulin (VZIG; 1 mL) at the time of delivery in order to compensate for the lack of maternal antibodies. In addition, aciclovir as a therapeutic

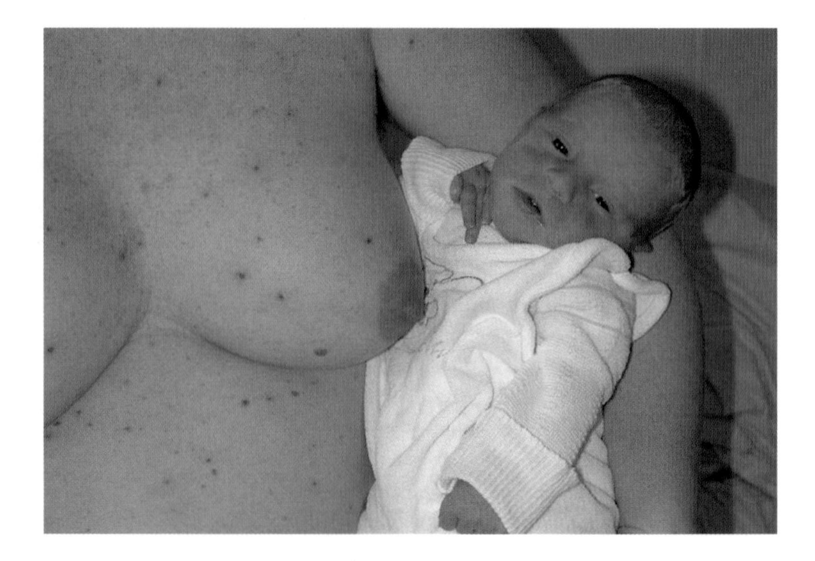

Fig. 8.**14** Puerpera with varicella and her two-day-old newborn baby. The exanthema started three days before delivery.

agent is now also available for varicella, albeit at high doses.

Approach to varicella during pregnancy and after delivery:

- Varicella during the first trimester up to six days prior to delivery: no measures, but reassurance of the pregnant women.
- Varicella four to five days prior to delivery: no speeding up and no forcible postponing of labor, possibly aciclovir orally (5 × 800 mg) until delivery (see below).
- Varicella at the time of delivery and up to three days thereafter:
  - VZIG administered to the child
  - breast-feeding is permitted
  - close monitoring of the newborn
  - aciclovir i. v. at the first signs of the disease.

Administration of hyperimmune globulin to a pregnant woman with visible exanthema does not make any sense. At this point, viremia has already occurred days before and, hence, a possible infection of the fetus as well.

As shown in Fig. 8.**14**, even florid varicella of the mother and careless contact with the newborn do not always lead to infection of the child (who did receive VZV-specific immune globulin).

Approach in case of exposure to varicella during pregnancy:

- Determination of the immune status of all pregnant women either for reassurance (when positive) or for appropriate measures (when negative).
- If the immune status is negative and exposure to varicella was less than four days ago, VZIG (0.3 mL/kg body weight) is administered up to the 20th week of pregnancy. It prevents varicella in 50% of these patients.
- If the immune status is negative and exposure to varicella was up to three days ago, at the most, active vaccination of the pregnant women is possible. A titer check is recommended after four weeks.
- If the immune status is negative and exposure to varicella was nine days ago, aciclovir treatment (5 × 800 mg) may be considered in special risk patients (although aciclovir in the amount required is not without risk during pregnancy).

Prophylaxis if the serostatus is negative. Active vaccination with live varicella vaccine (Varilrix, Varivax) before the start of a pregnancy is recommended by STICKO (Permanent Commission for Vaccination). In Germany, there is so far no recommendation for the vaccination of all children.

Herpes Zoster (Shingles)

Pathogenesis and risks for the child. Herpes zoster is normally a local reactivation of the varicella–zoster virus in the affected neurotome, and antibody titers in the blood are usually high. Hence, there is no measurable risk, since varicella (chickenpox) poses only a minor risk itself. Special measures or limitations are therefore not required, neither during pregnancy nor post partum.

In rare cases, generalized herpes zoster may occur during pregnancy (Fig. 8.**15**). Because of the intense pain, treatment with aciclovir (5 × 800 mg) is advised. It leads to quick relief from pain and to regression of the disease.

Epstein–Barr Virus Infection (Infectious Mononucleosis, Glandular Fever, Pfeiffer Disease)

Pathogenesis and clinical picture. The acute disease is characterized by high fever, sore throat, and generalized lymphadenopathy.

About 60–90% of adults have developed antibodies against the Epstein–Barr virus (EBV). As with other herpesviruses, EBV infection leads in the majority of patients to persistence of the virus in B lymphocytes. Reactivation during pregnancy is therefore possible.

At present, little is known about EBV infections during pregnancy. Only a few, poorly documented cases of damaged children have been reported in the literature. It should be noted though that there has been very little research into EBV infections during pregnancy.

Risk for the child. All we can say at present is that EBV infection during pregnancy poses a very small risk for the unborn child. As neither preventive nor therapeutic options are available and termination of the pregnancy is unjustified, this infection has no implications.

Diagnosis. Serological detection of IgG, IgM, or IgA antibodies against early and late antigens is carried out by means of fluorescence tests or other tests.

Therapy. No treatment is available.

Special measures during pregnancy are not required. Cases for observation should be referred to an infectious diseases hospital.

Infection with Human Herpes Virus Type 6 (HHV-6)

Pathogen, pathogenesis, and clinical picture. This virus has been discovered in 1986 in cells of HIV-infected persons. Like HIV, it predominantly infects CD4 and B lymphocytes, as well as glial cells. It is the pathogen that causes exanthema subitum (three-day fever, roseola infantum, sixth disease) and is assumed to cause also chronic postinfectious fatigue syndrome. The endemic infection in adults is 50–80%.

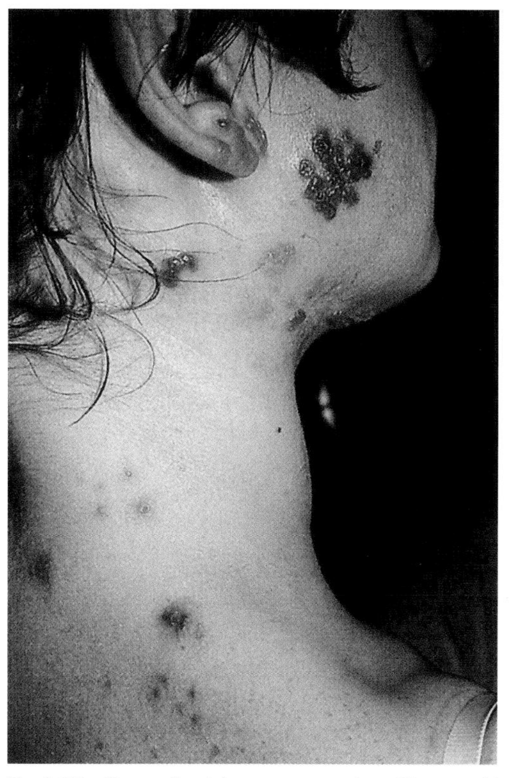

Fig. 8.**15** Generalized herpes zoster in a 22-year-old patient during the 29th week of pregnancy.

Risk for the child. So far, no risks are known.

Diagnosis. Immunofluorescence test, ELISA.

Measles (Rubeola)

Pathogen and frequency. The measles virus is a paramyxovirus of the genus *Morbillivirus*. Measles infection during pregnancy is very rare, since about 98% of adults have antibodies against the virus.

Clinical picture. This is a highly contagious acute illness with fever, cough, conjunctivitis, and maculopapulous exanthema. The prodromal stage of measles is an oral exanthema (Koplik spots). The course of a measles infection during pregnancy is not more severe than it is during childhood.

Risk for the child. A congenital measles syndrome is not known. Cases for observation seen in connection with measles have been unconfirmed special cases.

It has not been established whether miscarriage, stillbirth, or premature delivery may be linked to measles.

Only if the mother has measles at the time of delivery, severe neonatal measles may develop. In this case, the newborn should receive specific immune globulin immediately after birth.

Diagnosis:

- *Serology* (ELISA). The presence of IgG antibodies indicates immunity after measles infection or measles vaccination. Seroconversion (conversion of IgG test from negative to positive) and the presence of IgM antibodies indicate a fresh measles infection.
- *Detection of pathogen* is possible by means of PCR, but this is not a routine procedure.

In case of exposure to measles during pregnancy, the immune status of the woman should be determined. A positive status will reassure the patient that she can no longer fall ill with measles.

Mumps (Epidemic Parotitis)

Pathogen. The mumps virus is a paramyxovirus of the genus *Rubulavirus.*

Clinical picture. This is an acute disease with moderately high fever and painful swelling of the salivary glands, especially the parotid gland.

Risk for the child. The endemic infection with mumps in adults is very high, namely, about 95%. Mumps infections during pregnancy are therefore rare.

So far, neither a typical congenital mumps syndrome nor an increased rate of fetal damage during pregnancy has been observed. Hence, mumps infection during pregnancy has no implications.

If the mother has mumps at the time of delivery, the risk of severe neonatal mumps may be lowered by administration of mumps hyperimmune serum immediately after birth. If the mother has been exposed to mumps during her pregnancy, determination of her immunity to mumps will further reassure her.

Complications. After reaching sexual maturity, 20% of male patients who have mumps develop orchitis, which may lead to sterility. It is not known whether oophoritis in female patients may lead to sterility as well.

Diagnosis:
Serology. The immune status is determined by means of ELISA. Detection of IgM antibodies is also an option.

Infections Caused by Enteroviruses (Poliovirus, Coxsackievirus, Echovirus)

Frequency. Thanks to vaccination, infections with poliovirus have become extremely rare. By contrast, infections with coxsackievirus and echovirus are common, particularly during the hot summer months; occasionally they cause exanthema. The known sequelae include encephalitis, cardiac dysrhythmia, and diabetes mellitus.

Risk for the child. Intrauterine damages by echovirus or coxsackievirus have been assumed occasionally, but they have not been confirmed.

However, infection of the child together with severe meningoencephalitis or myocarditis, even with lethal outcome, may occur through transmission of the virus by the mother during delivery, or even by the nursing personnel during the first days of life. Isolated epidemics in neonatal units have been described.

Diagnosis. Isolation of the virus through culture, preferably from the feces. Serology is of no significance here.

Therapy. Specific hyperimmune serum globulin is administered if there is an epidemic in the neonatal unit, otherwise treatment is only symptomatic.

Rotavirus Infection

Rotaviruses play a certain role as pathogens of diarrhea in newborns.

Diagnosis. Detection of the virus in the feces:

- electron microscopy
- solid-phase erythrocyte aggregation test
- thin-layer immunoassay (TIA).

Therapy. Treatment is only symptomatic. Inhibition of the virus is not possible.

Hepatitis

We currently distinguish between at least six different forms of hepatitis. Hepatitis B is the one that demands special attention by obstetricians. Table 8.**6** provides an overview.

Hepatitis A

Pathogen and transmission. Hepatitis A is caused by a stable RNA virus (Fig. 1.**1**, p. 3) and is

Table 8.6 Types of hepatitis during pregnancy

Hepatitis/ pathogen	Viral-genome	Transmission	Incubation time (days)	Pregnancy	Complications	Prophylaxis
A (HAV, picornavirus)	RNA	Fecal–oral	12–90	Effects unknown	Fulminant hepatitis	Vaccination
B (HBV, hepadnavirus)	DNA	Parenteral, sexual, perinatal	40–180	Chronic disease of the child	Chronic disease, liver cirrhosis, liver carcinoma	Vaccination
C (HCV, flavivirus)	RNA	Parenteral, possibly sexual	3–140	Effects unknown	Chronic disease, liver cirrhosis, liver carcinoma	No immunoprophylaxis
D (HDV)	Incomplete RNA	Parenteral, perinatal	21–49	Effects unknown	Chronic disease	Same as for hepatitis B
E (HEV)	RNA	Drinking water, possibly fecal–oral (Asia, Africa)	20–65	Especially dangerous	Lethality in pregnant woman: 10–20 %	None

transmitted by the fecal–oral route. Other routes of transmission include contaminated foods, such as mussels and crustaceans, and drinking water contaminated with feces, especially when traveling in countries with high rates of endemic infection (Africa, Asia, Middle and South America).

Frequency. Only 10 % of small children (up to five years old) fall ill, as opposed to 70–80 % of adults. The endemic infection is low (10–20 % of adults) in the industrial countries of Western and Northern Europe and in North America, whereas it is very high (up to 90 %) in developing countries of Africa and Asia, and in South America due to poor hygienic conditions.

Clinical picture. Hepatitis A does not differ from other viral forms of hepatitis. After a nonspecific prodromal stage of several days, the following symptoms occur: jaundice, darkening of the urine, and lightening of the feces, and these are usually accompanied by general malaise, occasionally also by fever.

The symptoms disappear after four to six weeks. A severe course is rare (< 0.1 %), and chronic cases are unknown, although some cases drag on over months.

Risk for the child. Infection of the child with hepatitis A may occur in utero.

Transient enlargement of the fetal liver as well as ascites has been observed in a case of florid hepatitis A infection of the mother. The child was normal at birth.

Damage to the fetus caused by hepatitis A infection has not been described so far. Nevertheless, administration of specific immune globulin is recommended in case of exposure to hepatitis A during pregnancy.

Diagnosis:

- ▶ detection of the virus in the feces by means of immunoassay, or by PCR (which is not a routine procedure)
- ▶ detection of antibodies in the serum: fourfold increase in IgG antibodies (ELISA), detection of IgM antibodies (ELISA).

Therapy. Treatment is symptomatic. Inhibition of the virus is not possible at present.

Prophylaxis. Active vaccination with inactivated hepatitis A virus. Three injections (repeat injections after four weeks and after six to 12 months) provide protection for five to 10 years. Also available is a combination vaccine with hepatitis B. Standard immune globulin i.m. (5–10 mL) provides protection for three to 12 weeks (half-life of antibodies: three weeks).

Hepatitis B

Hepatitis B is a sexually transmitted disease. It can be prevented by vaccination and, therefore, also many of its sequelae. Because of the high risk of chronic disease in the newborn, screening for hepatitis B is part of the prenatal care in Germany.

Pathogen. It is a DNA virus with a relatively unstable envelope. The virus carries its own DNA polymerase. The most important antigens are HBsAg, HBcAg, and HBeAg.

Frequency. In Germany, about 5–10 % of the adult population have developed antibodies to HBcAg, while in Mediterranean countries the frequency is 10–30 %, and in Africa and Asia it is 70–90 %.

About 0.5–1 % of the population in Germany are infectious carriers of HBsAg, in the

Mediterranean countries 2–10%, and in Africa and Asia 10–20%. The risk of transmission is recognized by the detection of antigens (HBsAg or HBeAg) in the blood, and now it is also possible through the detection of viral DNA by means of PCR.

Incubation time. It ranges between 40 and 180 days.

Clinical picture. Hepatitis B is often clinically asymptomatic. The disease begins with unclear abdominal complaints, then fever occurs, followed by exanthema, joint pain, and finally jaundice. The disease protracts over weeks, with the infection persisting in 10–90% of patients, depending on the age of the person.

Special cases of infection have become known in which there is extreme viral replication, with viral excretion even in the sweat, without the affected persons feeling ill or knowing that they have been infected. Such individuals pose a high risk of transmission and are therefore disqualified from working in the medical field. This situation can be avoided through timely vaccination.

Diagnosis. In case of the hepatitis B virus, we have to distinguish between the antigen of the surface protein in the envelope (HBsAg), the antigen of the core protein (HBcAg), and the antigen of the HBe protein (HBeAg), the detection of which indicates high infectiousness, though its function is still unknown:

- anti-HBc antibodies are the best markers of a previous hepatitis B infection
- anti-HBs antibodies indicate that the infection has run its course. They are detected also after vaccination in cases where anti-HBc antibodies are absent
- HBs antigen indicates that viral replication is taking place and the infection is still florid
- HBe antigen indicates a severe form of florid infection.

Diagnosis of acute hepatitis B is established serologically by the detection of anti-HBc IgM antibodies.

Anti-HBs antibodies can be detected only after three to six weeks following the start of the infection. They are absent in chronic HBsAg carriers.

After vaccination, only anti-HBs antibodies are found. The vaccine contains only HBsAg because HBcAg and HBeAg do not protect against reinfection.

Anti-HBc IgG antibodies indicate a previous hepatitis B infection. If the HBs antigen is detected in these patients while anti-HBs antibodies are absent, we are dealing with an infectious chronic HBs carrier.

Risks for the child. There are two possible routes of infection:

1. Hematogenous transmission in utero, resulting from acute HBV infection of the mother. As with most viral infections, the risk of transmission to the child is 10–20% during the first trimester and 80–90% during the third trimester. The result is congenital infection, although this is a rare event. A congenital hepatitis B syndrome is not known.
2. Peripartal transmission of the virus due to virus excretion by the asymptomatic mother. This is the most common route of infection. The newborn can be largely protected against this infection by means of immediate vaccination.

Peripartal infection takes a chronic course in over 90% of infected newborns. This can be prevented, and hepatitis B screening during pregnancy is therefore of special importance. Due to the predominantly sexual transmission, which is only partly restricted to risk groups, screening of all pregnant women has been introduced.

If HBV infection of the newborn takes a chronic course, it may lead to liver cirrhosis (about 20%) and to hepatoma (about 5%) after 10–30 years. In isolated cases, fulminant hepatitis B may result in death after four to five months.

By comparison, infection of adults with the hepatitis B virus causes chronic persistent disease in only about 10% of infected individuals, at the end of which the above-mentioned late damages may develop.

Approach if HBs antigen is detected during pregnancy:

- Additional search for the HBe antigen and determination of liver parameters in order to check the severity of the infection.
- Examination of the partner and, depending on immune status and clinical picture, vaccination or treatment (interferon).
- Simultaneous vaccination of the newborn immediately after birth: passive vaccine against hepatitis B (1 mL hepatitis B hyperimmune globulin within 12 hours after birth) and the first dose of active hepatitis B vaccine. After four weeks and after one year, the second and third doses follow. In this way, the incidence of hepatitis B infection of the child can be reduced by 80–90%.
- The result of HBsAg testing is recorded in the maternity passport because, without such an entry, the child will receive active vaccination only.
- Breast-feeding is permitted after hepatitis B vaccination.

Screening during pregnancy and measures during delivery

In 1993, obligatory screening has been introduced in Germany. It is aimed at testing for the presence of HBs antigenemia after the 32 nd week of pregnancy. All children of HBsAg-positive mothers receive simultaneous vaccination immediately after birth. Unfortunately, there is no entry in the maternity passport of almost 20% of delivering mothers. Children of these mothers are vaccinated within 12 hours after birth. If follow-up tests of the mother show that she is HBsAg-positive, the child receives a passive booster vaccination within seven days. Special precautionary measures for pregnant women who are positive only for HBsAg, are not required as they pose a very low risk: only 10% of their children become infected. Pregnant women who are also HBeAg-positive, pose an increased risk for their surroundings, especially during delivery and during the early puerperal period: about 90% of their newborns become infected. Here, the rules of hygiene are imperative, and these are best achieved by providing a private bathroom.

Hepatitis C

Pathogen and transmission. The main pathogen of the disease—previously called nonA, nonB hepatitis—is the hepatitis C virus (HCV). It is a moderately stable RNA virus belonging to the flaviviruses and is surrounded by a lipid envelope. Several subtypes are known; their frequencies differ from region to region. Infections with genotypes 2 and 3 have a better prognosis.

Transmission is through blood, although blood products are considered fairly safe after general testing of samples has been introduced in Germany in 1990. Sexual and perinatal transmissions are rather rare and depend on the number of virus particles in the blood.

Viral transmission through mother's milk seems to be extremely rare (< 1%). Enders and Braun (2000) found HCV RNA only in one out of 150 samples of mother's milk from HCV-infected mothers, despite high viral loads in some patients.

Frequency. The incidence of infection in Germany is estimated at 0.6%. Mainly drug addicts (about 90% are HCV-positive) and dialysis patients (about 10% are HCV-positive) are affected.

Diagnosis:
- Serology
- PCR, especially for determining the viral load in the blood.

Clinical picture. The course of the disease is mild and often without jaundice. Nevertheless, chronic inflammation of the liver occurs in over 60% of these patients. This may turn into liver cirrhosis and even hepatoma in about 10% after 20 years, and in about 20% of patients after 40 years. The rate of mortality is 1–4%. The progression is even faster if there is coinfection with HIV and HBV or massive alcohol consumption; in these patients, liver cirrhosis and hepatocellular carcinoma appear much earlier.

Therapy. So far, treatment has consisted of administering recombinant α-interferon. In 40% of treated individuals, the liver parameters become normal. It is still unclear whether combination with virostatics, such as ribavirin, is of any advantage.

Risk for the child during birth and breast-feeding. Little is still known about the risk for the unborn child or newborn, and the same is true about what effect the pregnancy may have on the course of hepatitis C. Studies describe the risk of transmission to the child during delivery as being 3–7%, although it should be considered that many of these data were derived from HIV-positive pregnant women who were at higher risk anyway.

The risk for the child is likely to be low in general, and the currently available data do not allow for any recommendations. This applies also to breast-feeding. In women with a high viral load, one might rather tend toward cesarean section—if this is what the patient prefers. The decision of how to proceed lies with the parents, after they have been informed on the circumstances and the statistical risk.

Detection of HCV RNA in the cord blood does not mean that the newborn is permanently infected. However, detection of HCV RNA in the child after three months or detection of HCV antibodies after 12 months does indicate an infection.

Hepatitis D

Here, we are dealing with a defective virus (HDV) that occurs only in combination with hepatitis B.

Hepatitis E

The hepatitis E virus (HEV) contains a single-stranded RNA genome. It is common in tropical and subtropical countries, from where it is occasionally introduced to temperate climates. Diagnosis through detection of viral RNA by means of PCR or detection of antibodies has only become possible in recent years in special laboratories. Clinically, hepatitis E is similar to hepatitis A, and it is transferred by means of smear infection from animals or from the drinking water.

In contrast to other forms of hepatitis, hepatitis E is particularly dangerous for pregnant women and their children. Up to 20% of maternal deaths during the third trimester and, frequently, abortion during early pregnancy have been described.

A chronic course is not known, and there is no treatment.

Hepatitis G

This is caused by a recently detected virus. It belongs to the group of flaviviruses and is distantly related to the hepatitis C virus. In contrast to the latter, it does not seem to cause clinically recognizable hepatitis. About 1–2% of healthy blood donors carry this virus, and so do 10–20% of all hemophiliacs who regularly receive donor blood.

Like the HIV virus, hepatitis G virus (HGV) infects lymphocytes, but it multiplies very slowly. Hence, one explanation for the protective effect of this virus against HIV infection might be that the two viruses interfere with each other in the lymphocytes. On the other hand, HGV might inhibit certain cytokines or affect the number of cytokine receptors on the cell surface. These receptors are essential for entry of HIV into the cell.

Lymphocytic Choriomeningitis (LCM)

Pathogen. This disease is caused by the LCM virus, an arenavirus.

Frequency. Infections with this virus are relatively rare in Germany. About 1–9% of adults possess antibodies against the virus. This infection does not play a major role in terms of numbers and would be captured only by means of broad-scale screening studies.

Transmission. The infection is transmitted by golden hamsters or mice, the majority of which are infected with this virus.

Clinical picture. The clinical symptoms reach from asymptomatic infection (about 35%) to mild or severe choriomeningitis. Lethality is rare. Normally, this viral infection is not included in the testing during pregnancy. In individual studies, however, is has been shown that an infection with the LCM virus during early pregnancy may lead to abortion and, at a later time, to meningoencephalitis, chorioretinitis, hydrocephalus, or mental retardation. The neurological damages are irreversible. The distinctive features can easily be confused with symptoms caused by *Toxoplasma gondii* or by cytomegalovirus.

Diagnosis:

Detection of the pathogen:

- isolation of the pathogen in cell culture (in special laboratories)
- detection of the pathogen's RNA by means of PCR.

Detection of antibodies:

- immunofluorescence test (IFT), enzyme immunoassay (EIA), complement fixation test (CFT), neutralization test (NT).

Therapy. Treatment is symptomatic. Inhibition of the virus is not possible.

Prophylaxis. As this infection is transmitted only by golden hamsters or mice, contact with these animals should be avoided during pregnancy. In questionable cases of hydrocephalus, the search for antibodies against the LCM virus may help with identifying the cause.

Central European Encephalitis (CEE)

This is a mild form of tick-borne encephalitis, first noted in Central Europe.

Pathogen. It belongs to the group of flaviviruses and is transmitted by ticks. It is present in the tick's saliva. In endemic regions, 1% of the ticks are infected.

Clinical picture. After an incubation time of one to two weeks, 10–30% of the infected people show flulike symptoms. After a symptomfree interval, the fever reappears together with neurological symptoms (meningitis/meningoencephalitis) in 10% of patients. Irreversible neurological damages occur in up to 20% of adults.

Therapy. Treatment is only symptomatic.

Prophylaxis:

- quick removal of the tick
- active vaccination with inactivated vaccine
- passive vaccination with immune globulin after exposure has not been approved for children less than 14 years old, since an unfavorable course has been observed 96 hours after passive vaccination. For the same reason, passive vaccination during pregnancy should be avoided.

Risk during pregnancy. Direct damages to the unborn child are not known. Protecting the mother has therefore priority.

Influenza (Flu)

In contrast to the common cold, which is caused by various viruses and bacteria, the real flu (influenza) is a severe virus infection with high fever. During the great pandemics occurring after an antigenic shift, mortality can be quite high. For example, more people died during the influenza pandemic of 1918 than in World War I. Due to the special structure of influenza viruses, which contain several genomic RNA segments, recombination is possible with other orthomyxoviruses (including those of animals), thus creating viruses that are altered to such an extent that they undermine the prevailing immunity in the population.

Pathogens. The influenza virus belongs to the group of orthomyxoviruses. It is a complex RNA virus with an envelope, and it contains eight segments of genomic RNA. The hemagglutinin and neuraminidase molecules on its surface play an important role in the pathogenicity of the virus. There are three main varieties of influenza viruses: A, B, and C.

Clinical picture. The acute respiratory disease is accompanied by high fever, rhinitis, and severe malaise. It manifests itself in epidemics.

Detection. The pathogen is detected in cell cultures or by PCR, or serologically by a rise in titer (first serum from the disease phase, second serum from the recovery phase).

Therapy. A neuraminidase inhibitor, such as zanamivir, is administered by inhalation.

Risk for the child. Damage to the child, if any, is very rare and rather due to the illness of the mother.

There are some who maintain that there is a greater risk caused by therapeutic measures taken during pregnancy than by the pathogen itself.

Bacterial Infections and Zoonoses

With regard to bacterial infections during pregnancy, we have to distinguish between two types of pathogens (Fig. 8.**1**, p. 168): those transmitted by the hematogenous route (e. g., infections with *Listeria* or *Treponema*, as well as various zoonoses), and those ascending in the cervix, thus endangering the fetus. The latter infections may lead to premature birth or may cause peripartal and postpartum diseases in the mother, with the majority of pathogens originating from the body's own intestinal or cutaneous flora.

Syphilis (Lues)

See also p. 100.

Because of the serious sequelae, syphilis is part of the obligatory screening during pregnancy. Unfortunately, data on positive patients thus recorded are not available. In Germany, the number of pregnant women with positive syphilis serology has clearly increased recently due to the influx from Eastern Europe. Many women with positive TPHA test results during the obligatory screening are neither aware of having suffered from syphilis nor of having undergone specific antibiotic treatment.

Obligatory screening for syphilis with the TPHA test during pregnancy detects florid as well as healed infections. The need for treatment and its success are determined with the VDRL test and various IgM antibody tests. It is known from the preantibiotics era that up to 50% of syphilis infections heal even without antibiotics. Antibiotics are now also administered for other reasons, and many antibiotics are effective against *Treponema*. In case of doubt, one should always be generous with recommending a treatment, especially during pregnancy.

Clinical picture. In the case of primary infection, after an incubation time of about three weeks, one or several primary lesions will occur in the form of an ulcer or indurative edema, associated with painless regional lymph node swellings if the primary lesion is located in the region of external genitals. Unfortunately, this is not a reliable sign, for most of the women with positive syphilis serology do not know about their early infection.

Frequency. In Germany, the number of reported patients of congenital syphilis has been relatively constant in recent years, with about five patients per year. In 2000, 11 patients were reported. In 1997, we have seen in our clinic a case involving fetal death during the 28th week of pregnancy (the woman belonged to an ethnic risk group), where the infection of the mother probably occurred during the 20th week.

Risk for the child. Infection of the child with *Treponema pallidum* can probably occur at any time during the pregnancy. The greatest risk for the child is when the mother has the **primary infection** during pregnancy. Early during the pregnancy, this will lead to abortion or intrauterine fetal death. Clinically manifest congenital syphilis develops only during the fourth month and later.

If the mother is infected during pregnancy, the likelihood of infecting the child is between 70–100%. Only about half of the children born alive by a syphilitic mother show clinically manifest congenital syphilis.

If there is a primary lesion in the birth canal at the time of vaginal delivery, a primary lesion may appear on the head or neck of the child.

Since the primary and secondary stages of syphilis are infectious, infection during pregnancy may still occur even if the primary infection of untreated or inadequately treated syphilis occurred one to two years ago.

Such children can be detected through syphilis serology.

We distinguish between two forms of infection in the newborn:

- *early congenital syphilis* usually corresponds to the secondary stage of syphilis, its clinical manifestation is already clear
- *late congenital syphilis* where clinical manifestation occurs during later childhood or early adulthood.

Both forms occur at about the same frequency. The characteristic clinical picture of the so-called Hutchinson triad (Hutchinson teeth, diffuse interstitial keratitis, and labyrinthine deafness) is now extremely rare.

Diagnosis. It can be reliably established by means of antibody detection. The safest way of detecting a previous syphilitic infection is by means of the TPHA (or TPPA) test. However, the test can only provide information about acute and florid infections if it detects a significant titer rise—which is rarely the case.

Whether the infection is florid and thus requires treatment, can be determined by using the VDRL test and various IgM antibody tests.

Therapy. We distinguish between a fresh syphilis infection in need of immediate and adequate treatment, and syphilis that had occurred some time ago, in which case treatment is carried out more for safety reasons.

The infection is florid during the first two years and as long as IgM antibodies can be detected. Up to 50% of syphilis infections heal even without antibiotics. In case of doubt and during pregnancy, one should always provide generous treatment.

The drug of choice is *penicillin* because treponemes are extremely sensitive to penicillin.

Since the child has to be treated as well, and the child's plasma level can only reach about 20–30% of that of the mother, the dose has to be rather high.

Due to the slow division rate of *Treponema* (24 hours), treatment needs to be prolonged:

Clemizole penicillin: 1–2 million IU per day over 21 days is the best treatment, although it has been largely abandoned due to low patient compliance, especially with patients for which the treatment represented more a safety measure in case of unclear serology.

Benzylpenicillin benzathine: 2.4 million IU i.m., distributed to both buttocks, three times at one-week intervals. (This is currently the drug of choice.) Some experts doubt that this form of treatment is sufficient during pregnancy because the levels achieved in the child are only 20–30% of those of the mother. This aspect should be considered whenever the risk of fetal infection is high.

In case of *penicillin allergy*, it should be confirmed by means of intracutaneous testing that an allergy to penicillin actually exists—after all, penicillin is the most effective drug against syphilis. As macrolides are not sufficiently effective, especially not during pregnancy, only treatment with 2 g ceftriaxone per day i.m. or i. v., over 15 days, is recommended as an alternative.

In case of antibiotic treatment during pregnancy one should warn against a Jarisch–Herxheimer reaction. The rapid death of treponemes causes side effects (fever, headache, and myalgia) two to six hours after administration of penicillin, lasting for up to 24 hours. Careful follow-up of the first administration is therefore advised.

Regular monitoring of the therapeutic results is necessary for at least one year. In case of late syphilis, the serological follow-up takes over two years because the fall in titer is slower here. A titer fall after three months by four titer steps indicates that the treatment was successful. A titer rise indicates insufficient treatment.

Screening during pregnancy. Whereas serological screening is still mandatory in Germany, it is now only a general recommendation in many other countries.

Recently, the incidence of syphilis that needs to be treated has dropped to below 1:20000. Positive cases occur 10 times more often in highly populated areas or in ethnic risk groups, as compared with the total population or with that in rural areas. Hence, restriction of the screening to pregnancies at risk seems to make sense.

Follow-up of the Newborn

As far as I know, the majority of newborns from mothers with positive syphilis serology during pregnancy do not receive treatment, since positive serology is usually classified as a mere serological scar.

The newborn should always be treated if the mother has a florid, though treated, infection during pregnancy, since chances are high that the child has been infected and adequate treatment in utero cannot be guaranteed. Additional reasons for treating the child include detection of IgM antibodies in the child, a fourfold increase in the IgG antibody titer of the child as compared with that of the mother, signs of infection or disease in the child, and any further suspicion or uncertainty regarding an infection of the child. Examination of the cerebrospinal fluid is recommended if congenital infection is suspected, since the central nervous system may be affected even in cases of asymptomatic infection (but positive serology).

One may refrain from treating the child if the mother exhibits only serological scars, i. e., if only the TPHA test is positive, while the VDRL test is negative and IgM antibodies and clinical symptoms are absent. Of course, for reassurance and safety, these tests also need to be carried out for the newborn immediately after birth and, depending on the risk, should be repeated after four and 12 weeks. A titer fall in the TPHA or TPPA tests indicates maternal immunity. Together with close pediatric monitoring of the children, these tests ensure that congenital infections are not missed.

This recommendation may apply to the majority of newborns from mothers with positive syphilis serology.

Radiographic examination of the skeleton quickly confirms the diagnosis in cases of stillbirth due to syphilis.

Listeriosis

Pathogen. *Listeria* species are small, motile (flagellated), gram-positive rod-shaped bacteria. Only *Listeria monocytogenes* is an important pathogen. These bacteria are occasionally confused morphologically with small lactobacilli, *Gardnerella vaginalis*, or corynebacteria. Seven serotypes are known (O and H antigens). *Listeria* bacteria are relatively resistant and widely distributed. They normally occur in the soil.

Transmission. Infection is transmitted by animals or animal products, usually milk and dairy products (cheese). The pathogen is killed by pasteurization of the milk prior to cheese production, although the area in which the cheese is produced may be contaminated. Other foods may be contaminated as well, such as canned foods, meats, and vegetables. Contaminated foods are frequently the cause of small epidemics.

Pathogenesis. *Listeria* is transported by the bloodstream from the intestine to the fetus. Transmission of *Listeria* might already be possible during the third month, as we have now received several reports of *Listeria*-induced febrile abortions prior to the 13th week of pregnancy. About one to two infections per 1000 pregnancies are to be expected.

Prognosis for the child is good if the mother is treated in time. Transmission to the fetus does not always take place, and healing of the infection in the child is to be expected.

Clinical picture. Frequently, there are no symptoms. In particular danger are pregnant women, unborn children or newborns, immunocompromised persons, and the elderly. They fall ill with flulike symptoms, fever, bacteremia, and meningitis. In case of meningitis during pregnancy, listeriosis is always the first disease to be considered. The pathogen can be detected in the cerebrospinal fluid.

Differential diagnosis. Symptoms of meningitis during pregnancy may also indicate HSV encephalitis, although this is very rare.

Course of the disease during pregnancy. Unclear, flulike symptoms are followed by persisting low or moderately high recurrent fever, which increases again after eight to 10 days. Signs of infection of the amnion together with uterine contractions signal fetal expulsion, and this is followed by sudden recovery of the mother.

Risks for the child:
- ▶ mild subclinical infection
- ▶ fetal death in utero
- ▶ premature birth
- ▶ perinatal listeriosis (a very serious disease)
- ▶ the infection is associated with high mortality.

Diagnosis. *Detection of pathogen* is the only evidence of an infection.
Pathogen detection in the mother:
- ▶ Blood culture (fever during pregnancy).
- ▶ Amniotic fluid (abortion, rupture of fetal membranes, puncture).

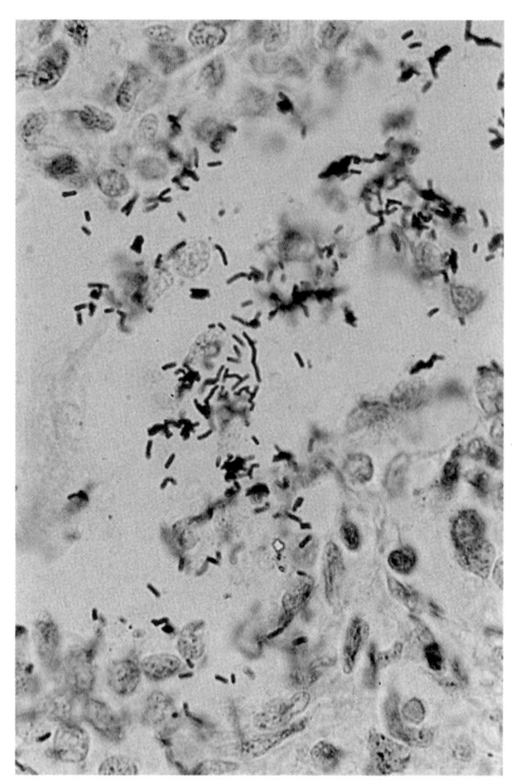

Fig. 8.**16** Listeriosis during pregnancy. The child died in the 22nd week of pregnancy. Although cultures from the mother contained listeriae, their detection in the child was possible only after silver impregnation of histological sections from all organs. The figure shows a section through the lung. (Micrograph by courtesy of Prof. Dr. N. Böhm, Department of Pathology, University of Freiburg, Germany.)

- Cerebrospinal fluid (meningitis of the mother).
- Cervical swab (while of little use as long as the amnion is intact as the dissemination is hematogenous, it makes sense after rupture of the membranes).
- Detection of the pathogen in the feces, though this is of limited value as listeriae may occur in up to 5% of adults without causing disease or providing a prognosis.
- Serology is completely unsuitable for diagnosing acute listeriosis because of the strong cross-reaction with other bacteria. Clarification of a questionable abortion later is also not possible by serology. About 50–70% of adults have developed antibodies against listeriae.

Pathogen detection in the child:

- blood
- cerebrospinal fluid
- possibly in the feces
- histological detection of *Listeria* by means of special staining methods (silver impregnation) (Fig. 8.**16**).

Every *late abortion,* especially *febrile abortion,* and every stillbirth should trigger a search for listeriosis as the cause.

Isolation of the pathogen is the safest way to arrive at a diagnosis. If inflammatory reactions are present in the placenta or in the fetus, the histological preparation usually contains bacteria, which might also include *Listeria.*

However, there are cases in which the infection of the child is so fulminant that it does not cause any histologically detectable inflammatory reactions.

In these children, the diagnosis can still be established through pathogen detection in organs of the dead child by means of silver impregnation (Fig. 8.**16**).

Therapy. Successful treatment of listeriosis during pregnancy is not an indication for termination of the pregnancy. Treatment has to start early. Treatment after expulsion of the fetus is normally not necessary.

The drug of choice is ampicillin with 3 × 2 g (up to 5 g) per day for two weeks. (Cephalosporins are ineffective.)

In case of penicillin allergy: erythromycin, Co-Trimoxazol.

Prophylaxis. Unpasteurized milk as well as cheeses made of unpasteurized milk should be avoided. One should also avoid eating the rind of soft cheese and blue cheese, as it is more likely contaminated (if the production area has been contaminated) than in inner part of the cheese. Storing the cheese in the refrigerator does not reduce multiplication of *Listeria.*

Borreliosis (Lyme Disease)

Ticks (Fig. 8.**17**) transmit any number of pathogens. The most common pathogen is probably *Borrelia.* Other pathogens transmitted by ticks include the Central European encephalitis (CEE) virus, species of *Ehrlichia*, and also protozoa.

Borreliosis is also known as Lyme disease, named after the site of first description in the United States, in 1975.

Frequency. Official data for Germany are not available. The incidence is estimated at 16–140 infections per 100 000 individuals per year. In regions at risk, the rate of clinical and subclinical infections determined by serology is 1.5%.

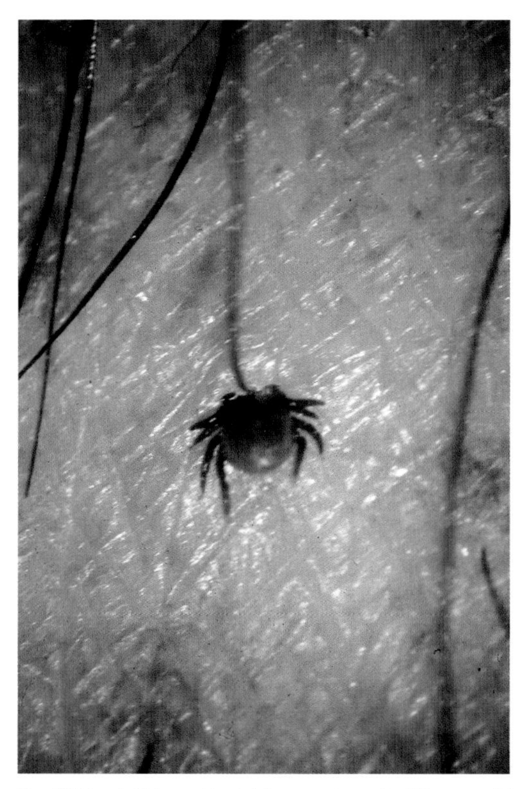

Fig. 8.**17** A tick on the labium majus of a 28-year-old patient.

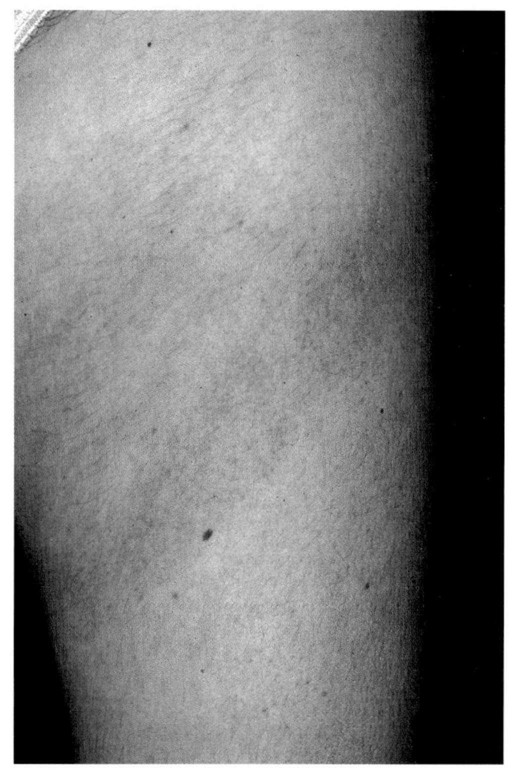

Fig. 8.**18** Erythema chronicum migrans on the left thigh of a 29-year-old patient during the 8th week of pregnancy.

Antibodies against *Borrelia* can be detected in about 15% of adults.

Pathogen. The disease is caused by *Borrelia burgdorferi* (in the wider sense), a spiral bacterium (see Fig. 1.**2**, p. 7) of the family *Spirochaetaceae.* Three genospecies occur in Germany: *Borrelia burgdorferi* (in the narrow sense), *Borrelia afzelii*, and *Borrelia garinii*, which show slightly different manifestations.

For the gynecologist, this infection is in so far important as the pathogen is related to the pathogen of syphilis and may be transferred to the child during pregnancy.

Transmission. Up to 10% of ticks are infected in Germany. The pathogen lives in the midgut of the tick. The danger of infection therefore correlates with the duration of sucking. The risk of transmission by an infected tick is about 20%.

Incubation time. Seven days to several months.

Clinical picture. The disease has several stages, but not every infected person may manifest all stages.

Stage 1 is called erythema chronicum migrans, a centrifugal migrating redness (Fig. 8.**18**) around the site of the tick bite. It starts after several days and may last for several weeks. Other nonspecific symptoms of the early stage are pseudomeningitis, fever, and myalgia. The accumulation of cases during the summer months (June and July) is characteristic.

Stage 2 begins weeks or months after the tick bite with lymphadenosis benigna cutis or with serous meningitis, which is often accompanied by peripheral facial paralysis.

The most common disease during the advanced stage (*stage 3*) is chronic recurrent arthritis (Lyme arthritis), which typically affects one of the large joints and often jumps from joint to joint. This stage first manifests itself months or years after the tick bite. Many cases of borreliosis are only recognized at this stage. Other manifestations are meningopolyneuritis, myocarditis, acrodermatitis chronica atrophicans.

Diagnosis. A tentative diagnosis is first established clinically. At the stage of erythema chronicum migrans, antibodies are detected in no more than 50% of infected persons.

Laboratory diagnostics:

- *Serology.* Immunofluorescence test (IFT), ELISA. Antibodies are only produced slowly, and the detection of IgM antibodies is not always successful. The results are confirmed by western blot. If the test is negative, it should be repeated after several weeks. High titers are also found in the puncture fluid obtained by arthrocentesis.
- possibly *culture*
- *PCR*
- Other *laboratory parameters.* These are nonspecific and include accelerated ESR, leukocytosis, and—depending on which organ is affected—increase in transaminases.

Therapy. Treatment is always indicated if clinical cues are present or when IgM antibodies can be detected serologically.

- amoxicillin (3 × 1 g per day)
- doxycycline (200 mg per day)
- erythromycin (1.5–2 g per day)
- ceftriaxone (2 g per day).

Duration of treatment. Fourteen days or longer.

Risk for the child. Because *Borrelia* is closely related to the pathogen of syphilis, its transmission to the child during pregnancy cannot be excluded.

Until now, little is known of the type and frequency of damage, since confirmed cases are rare. Isolated cases of stillbirth, incomplete development, premature birth with exanthema, or syndactyly have been reported in the literature.

As a precaution, early treatment with amoxillin is recommended if erythema migrans or other evidence of this infection is present during pregnancy; it is also important to avoid late sequelae in the mother. It is not known whether the child is endangered during the chronic stage of the infection, which manifests itself through recurrent joint effusions.

Prophylaxis. Early removal of ticks and avoidance of exposure are recommended. A vaccine has been approved in the United States—but not in Europe, since another species is involved.

Ehrlichiosis

Species of *Ehrlichia* have been known since 1945. Initially, they were found only in animals, especially ruminants, as the pathogen of febrile diseases and abortions. In 1994, they have been confirmed as a pathogen also in humans. They are gram-negative, obligatory intracellular bacteria and, unlike *Chlamydia*, are able to synthesize ATP. The clinical pictures reach from fever, hepatitis, renal dysfunction, and polyarthropathy to symptoms of the central nervous system. Doxycycline is effective against *Ehrlichia.*

Toxoplasmosis

Pathogen. The disease is caused by *Toxoplasma gondii,* a comma-shaped protozoon (Fig. 1.2, p. 7). This obligatory intracellular parasite is found in a wide range of hosts, including humans, other mammals, and birds.

Frequency. About 40–50% of adults have developed antibodies against *Toxoplasma gondii.*

Transmission. The definitive hosts are cats, which excrete oocysts with their feces for several weeks after infection. These oocysts are very resistant, may be spread even by road dust, and are taken up orally by humans. Most infections occur without having one's own cat. The disease is less often transmitted by raw or insufficiently broiled meat, especially pork.

Clinical picture. Postnatal toxoplasmosis is a relatively common though benign infection. It largely runs its course without symptoms, or with mild flulike symptoms at most.

Some infected persons (30–40%) have lymph node swellings that persist over weeks and months. It is not uncommon that a tentative diagnosis is first established by the pathologist based on histological findings.

In isolated cases, the disease may drag on over weeks and months with subfebrile temperatures, weakness, and fatigue.

Serological follow-ups have shown that IgM antibodies often persist for up to one or several years, thus indicating a chronic infection. Despite antibiotic treatment, early healing does not always occur.

The infection primarily takes place in the lymphatic tissue, but it may also cause benign myocarditis, chorioretinitis, and even encephalitis.

A child with toxoplasmosis (due to infection of the fetus rather than the embryo) may develop the following diseases:

- systemic infections: hepatitis, myocarditis, encephalitis
- damages following encephalitis: sclerosis, hydrocephalus, and chorioretinitis.

After years or decades, a latent infection may be reactivated in some persons by bursting of the cysts. This is particularly noticed in the retina because it causes impaired vision. However, the brain or the heart may be affected as well.

It is not known whether these reactivated infections are due to prenatal or postnatal infections.

Toxoplasmosis and Pregnancy

(Table 8.**7**)

Infection with *Toxoplasma gondii* during pregnancy is feared because the child may become infected in utero. Years later, congenital infections—unlike postnatal infections—lead to sequelae (e.g., chorioretinitis). The risk of infecting the child exists only during primary infection of the pregnant mother. The risk can only be determined through screening, since the clinical picture of the infection is mild and its course is not characteristic. In Germany, screening during pregnancy is voluntary because of the limited risk, and for other reasons as well, and is covered by health care insurance only if there is a risk for the child.

Serological screening of the mother is medically indicated in the following cases:

- lymph node swelling
- unexplained flulike symptoms, especially when antibodies against *Toxoplasma gondii* are absent.

Risk for the child. If the primary infection—which causes parasitemia—takes place during pregnancy, it may lead to infection of the fetus. Initially, foci of infection form in the fetal membranes or in the placenta, from where the pathogen breaks into the fetal circulation only later, thus causing an infection.

This explains why treatment administered long after the infection of the mother may still lower the risk for the fetus. In some cases, however, treatment comes too late, and the infection leads to damages to the child.

Exact figures regarding the incidence of primary toxoplasma infections during pregnancy are not available. According to estimates, one may expect 0.1 % of all pregnant women to have a primary toxoplasmosis infection (Table 8.**8**). On average, infection of the fetus takes place in 35 % of women affected. Frequency of transmission increases during the pregnancy, while the rate of damage decreases (Fig. 8.**19**). Unfortunately, there are no reliable data on the frequency of damages, especially those that are severe and irreparable.

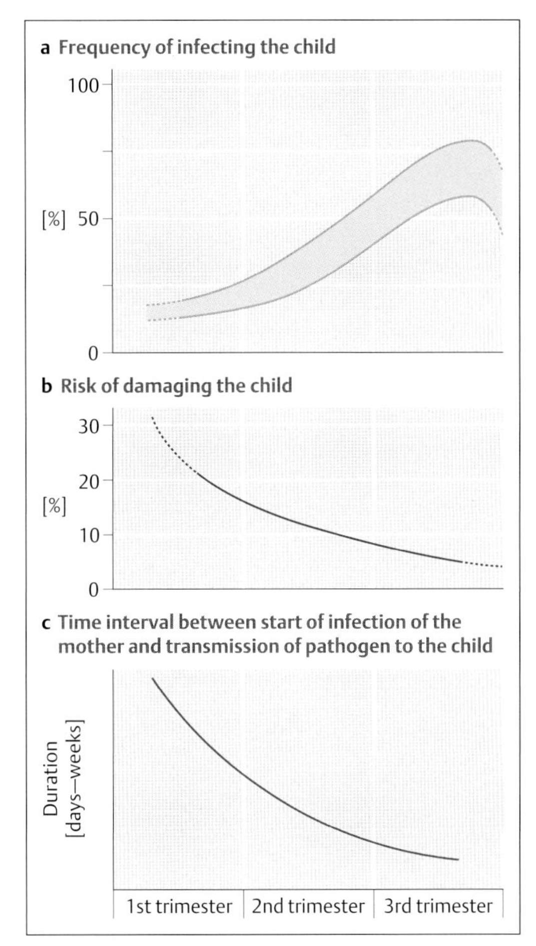

Fig. 8.**19** Toxoplasmosis during pregnancy. The risk for the child to become infected increases during the course of the pregnancy (a), while the risk of damage decreases during the course of the pregnancy (b). Even if the infection has been present in the mother for an extended period (i. e., antibodies are already detectable), an infection of the child can still be prevented by antibiotic therapy because the pathogen is transmitted to the child only after days or weeks (c).

Results of Studies on Toxoplasmosis During Pregnancy

- In a European multicenter study (*Foulon* et al., 1999), 64 (44%) out of 144 pregnant women with fresh toxoplasmosis gave birth to infected children. Of these children, 19 (13 %) exhibited severe damages, including:
  - three stillbirths
  - three children with hydrocephalus
  - two children with neurological damages
  - one child with severely impaired vision.

Therapy. The usual treatment with spiramycin reduced the sequelae but did not prevent transmission. Infected children were treated with antibiotics for up to one year.

Table 8.7 Toxoplasmosis during pregnancy—an overview

Parameter	
Pathogen	*Toxoplasma gondii*
Risk for the child	First infection of the mother during pregnancy ▶ Hydrocephalus ▶ Ocular toxoplasmosis (the most common damage to the child, usually leading to visual field defects many years later)
Routine diagnostics	Serology ▶ IgM antibody detection: florid infection ▶ IgA antibody detection: of questionable significance
Special diagnostics	Detection of pathogen DNA by means of PCR (e. g., in the amniotic fluid)
Problem	1–3 % of pregnant women with antibodies have also toxoplasmosis-specific IgM antibodies, about 90 % of which are the result of chronic-persistent infection, i. e., there is no risk for the child (hematogenous transmission is not possible)
Diagnostics	▶ Simple IgG antibody test at the start of the pregnancy (at the latest) ▶ If IgG negative (about 60 %): titer checks during weeks 24 and 36–38 of pregnancy ▶ If IgG positive (about 40 %): determination of IgM antibodies ▶ If IgM negative (about 37 %): no risk; results are recorded in maternity passport ▶ If IgM positive (about 3 %): florid infection; now it is important to determine whether the infection has started before or during the pregnancy ▶ First possibility: quantitative titer check after two to four weeks ▶ Second possibility: additional tests in special laboratory ▶ Third possibility: PCR of amniotic fluid (approx. during the 20th week of pregnancy) to see if the child is infected. If PCR is positive, treatment should be extended by at least four weeks, or until birth.
Treatment	Before the 16th week of pregnancy: spiramycin (2 g/day) for four weeks. From the 16th week on: sulfadiazine (3–4 g/day) for four weeks + pyrimethamine (25 mg/day) + folic acid. Every treatment with spiramycin must be followed by treatment with a sulfadiazine with placental permeability. The blood count should be checked at least every two weeks during treatment with folic acid inhibitors.

Table 8.8 Toxoplasmosis: estimated risks of infection and damage in 700 000 births per year

Number of cases	Risk of toxoplasmosis during pregnancy
385 000	Seronegative pregnant women (55 %)
7 000	Florid infection during pregnancy, i. e., positive tests for toxoplasmosis-specific IgM antibodies
700	Seroconversion (primary infection of the mother) during pregnancy (0.1 % of all pregnancies)
250	Congenital infection of the child (35 % of primary infection of the mother) (0.03 % of all pregnancies)
35	Severe damage to the child (14 % of cases). This does not include damages that become apparent only after years or decades (0.005 % of all pregnancies)
20–30	Reported cases of congenital toxoplasmosis during recent years

- A screening study in Norway (Jenum et al., 1998) involved 35 940 pregnant women, of which 47 (0.17 %) had a primary infection during pregnancy. Eleven children (23 %) showed congenital infection, but only one infant (0.03 % of all pregnancies) was found to be clinically affected after one year.

In the majority of cases, the infected children show no symptoms at birth, and a congenital toxoplasmosis infection is recognized only after years or decades, for example, when a focus in the retina is reactivated.

In isolated cases, however, severe infection of the CNS occurs already in utero, and this may lead to hydrocephalus. Sclerosis in the brain indicates a previous encephalitis due to toxoplasmosis.

Diagnosis. *Serology* (Fig. 8.**20**) plays an important role in the diagnosis:

- direct agglutination (DA) test: this is a very reasonable screening procedure
- CFT (hardly used anymore): titers of more than 1 : 20 indicate a florid infection
- immunofluorescence test (IFT): used to detect previous toxoplasmosis infections; this test has replaced the Sabin–Feldman test (SFT)

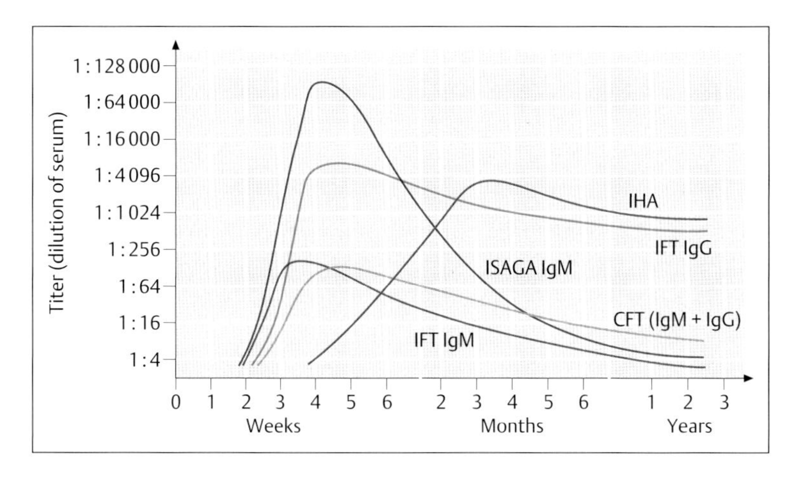

Fig. 8.**20** Diagnostic tests for toxoplasmosis of the mother. Titer level and detectability of IgM antibodies depend on the kind of test used. However, the production of hemagglutinizing antibodies (indirect hemagglutination, IHA) is slow, and a high titer indicates an infection that occurred some time ago. If no serum is available from the time before the infection, the actual infection can only be deduced from the course of the disease and from the ratios of the various test results to one another.

- indirect hemagglutination assay (IHA): titers are low initially but may rise from 1 : 10 to 1 : 4000 in the following weeks
- IgM IFT: used after separation of IgM antibodies
- IgM ISAGA (immunosorbent agglutination assay): a very sensitive test, yielding high titers
- western blot.

Detection of pathogen:

- PCR for direct pathogen detection, especially during prenatal diagnosis
- culture of *Toxoplasma* is extremely difficult; it is therefore rarely offered.

Timely antibiotic treatment of the mother lowers the risk of fetal infection—and therefore also the risk of damages to the child—by a factor of three. Screening is used to recognize primary infection during pregnancy. Due to the lack of symptoms, or due to uncharacteristic symptoms if clinical signs do occur, screening is the only way of recognizing a dangerous situation for the child.

Practical approach. The first serological examination should take place as soon as possible, preferably even before the start of the pregnancy. This examination is carried out with a cost-effective test, such as the direct agglutination test.

If antibodies are detected, a further test for detection or exclusion of IgM antibodies should follow. This test will turn out positive in 1–3 % of all pregnant women. Additional tests should be used to clarify how long the florid *Toxoplasma* infection already exists.

If the examination has been carried out very early in the pregnancy (sixth to eighth weeks), it is assumed that these antibody titers have already existed prior to the pregnancy. This assumption is confirmed if a second serological test after four weeks shows that there has been no further titer rise.

If, however, the second blood sample does yield a higher titer, this may indicate a relatively fresh *Toxoplasma* infection that needs to be treated.

If antibodies against *Toxoplasma* are absent at the first examination, the pregnancy is susceptible and toxoplasmosis may occur during the pregnancy.

In order to recognize such an infection, at least two additional serological examinations are required, for example, during the 24th week and during the 36th to 38th weeks of pregnancy. This is the only way of recognizing a *Toxoplasma* infection that occurred during pregnancy. The risk for the child may then be lowered by appropriate treatment.

Serious problems of interpretation arise when the first serological examination is carried out during advanced pregnancy (e. g., in the 20th week). Once IgM antibodies are detected, it is no longer possible to decide with certainty whether the infection already existed prior to the pregnancy or occurred only during the pregnancy. Here, testing the amniotic fluid may help (prenatal diagnostics).

Every serological examination during pregnancy should be recorded in the maternity passport in order to avoid repeat examinations and to ensure timely follow-up examinations of pregnant women who are susceptible.

Prenatal diagnostics. In unclear cases one should limit the risk for the child by attempting to detect the pathogen or IgM antibodies in the fetus. Two options are available:

- detection of the pathogen by means of PCR in the amniotic fluid (16th to 22nd weeks) or by means of chorionic villus sampling (CVS)
- detection of IgM and IgA antibodies in the fetal blood following cordocentesis. By adding EDTA to some of the blood samples, it may be

Table 8.**9** Toxoplasmosis treatment during pregnancy

Monotherapy* with a drug that does not pass the placenta (up to the 14th week of pregnancy)	Spiramycin (2–3 g or 3 × 3 million IU/day), **for four weeks**
Combination therapy with drugs that do pass the placenta (from weeks 14–16 onward)	Sulfadiazine (3–4 g/day), pyrimethamine (25 mg/day; 50 mg on the first day), folic acid (5–10 mg/day), **for four weeks; if there is evidence of fetal infection, then eight weeks or until birth**
Alternatives	Co-Trimoxazol, clindamycin

* Every monotherapy should be followed by combination therapy with drugs that pass the placenta.

possible to detect the pathogen by means of PCR also in the fetal blood.

Any decisions as to whether to treat at all, or how to design the treatment during pregnancy, should be discussed in detail with the parents. Because the risk is limited, particularly if the serology is unclear, there are always patients who do not want to be treated—and others who definitely ask for treatment.

Therapy. In the absence of pregnancy, treatment of toxoplasmosis is only required if there are clear clinical symptoms.

The following cases call for treatment:

- every primary infection, i. e., one occurring the first time during pregnancy (seroconversion, i. e., the serology shifts from negative to positive)
- florid infection (detection of IgM antibodies) where a start during pregnancy cannot be ruled out
- confirmed infection of the fetus (prenatal diagnostics)
- congenital infection of the newborn.

There is still disagreement on which might be the right time for treating toxoplasmosis during early pregnancy. In the past, late treatment has been recommended as toxoplasmosis causes fetopathy and infection of the fetus occurs only after the 16th week of pregnancy.

Meanwhile, however, this has been contradicted by a number of cases in which fetal damages have been observed earlier.

For this reason, the current recommendation is to start treatment as early as possible. However, it is essential to confirm that one is really dealing with a primary infection during pregnancy rather than a persistent infection that is still florid.

There is no agreement on the total duration of treatment either. The trend is to treat over several months until birth if there is evidence of fetal infection (Table 8.**9**).

Malaria

During pregnancy, the susceptibility to infections with *Plasmodium falciparum* is increased. The frequency and severity of the disease depend also on the state of acquired protective immunity. The increased susceptibility during pregnancy is probably due to sequestration of *Plasmodium* in the placenta and a mild depression of the immune system during pregnancy.

Malaria is one of the most common infectious diseases worldwide. The number of malaria cases imported to Germany lies between 800 and 1000 per year, with a lethality of 2.4%. Over 80% of cases originate from Africa.

In case of fever during pregnancy and any risk indicated by the patient's history, such as a stay in malaria-prone areas, malaria should be excluded by examination of the blood (thick blood film).

Therapy. Therapeutic drugs against malaria:

- quinine for initial treatment of cerebral and complicated tropical malaria (malaria falciparum)
- chloroquine for prophylaxis (permitted during pregnancy) and for treatment of tertian and quartan malaria
- mefloquine for prophylaxis (1 tablet per week) and for treatment (3–4 tablets per day)
- proguanil for prophylaxis in combination with other drugs
- doxycycline for prophylaxis
- atovaquone
- atovaquone/proguanil (Malarone).

Mefloquine has a long half-life of about 20 days, making it possible to use single-dose or one-day intake for treatment and once-per-week intake for prophylaxis.

Experience during pregnancy. Chloroquine is permitted, for there has been long-time experience with this drug. Unfortunately, it is no longer very effective due to the development of

Table 8.10 Diseases caused by group A streptococci

- Puerperal sepsis (p. 218)
- Tonsillitis/pharyngitis
- Scarlet fever
- Erysipelas, an edematous inflammation in lymphatic spaces of the skin
- Phlegmon, a diffuse suppuration affecting also the subcutaneous tissue
- Impetigo contagiosa, an infection of only the epidermis, with vesicle formation; occurs especially in children from poor social environments (Fig. 7.29, p. 81)
- Vulvitis and vaginitis (pp. 78, 120)
- Fasciitis

resistance in the case of malaria falciparum in Africa. All other drugs are contraindicated during pregnancy. The risk for the child is low, however, and any use of these drugs does not justify termination of the pregnancy. If the risk of malaria is very high, both risks should be carefully considered and, in case of doubt, prophylaxis (after the 12th week of pregnancy) should be carried out (see also p. 216).

Treatment with mefloquine has been reported to increase the rate of stillbirths by a factor of four or five, but it did not increase the frequency of malformation or neurological dysfunctions.

Infections Caused by Group A Streptococci

Group A streptococci belong to the most dangerous bacteria in the genital region, and especially so during pregnancy. They cause a large number of diseases (Table 8.10). The clinical pictures differ considerably and reach from local skin infections to deadly sepsis.

Pharyngitis/Tonsillitis

This is the most common disease caused by group A streptococci, with about one million patients per year in Germany. Colonization of the nasopharyngeal cavity is even more common. Streptococci of group A can be cultured from the pharynx of 5(–10)% of children and also of adults. The pathogen spreads repeatedly from this region. Depending on the site of infection, elimination of the pathogen is not always possible.

Erysipelas (See p. 81)

Pyoderma (See impetigo contagiosa, p. 81)

Scarlet Fever

Scarlet fever is a special form of the far more common pharyngitis caused by group A streptococci.

Pathogen. Scarlet fever is caused by group A streptococcal strains that are infected by a bacteriophage producing erythrogenic toxin. Five different erythrogenic toxins are known, which means that scarlet fever may affect a person more than once.

Incubation time and infectivity. The incubation time is short with only three to five days, and excretion (i. e., infectiousness) starts already 24 hours before the exanthema appears.

Clinical picture. The erythrogenic toxin causes a diffuse skin erythema that pales upon pressure. The color of the skin resembles that of a boiled lobster. The oral triangle, the palms of the hands, and the soles of the feet remain free of exanthema. The tongue appears strawberrylike due to the intensely reddened papillae and white coating.

Risks for mother and child. Occurrence of scarlet fever in the surroundings of a pregnant woman is always a cause for concern. However, scarlet fever is rare in pregnant women. The risks of damage to the fetus or severe infection of the mother during pregnancy are low. Only very few patients are known in which the mother experienced a severe infection during pregnancy. The danger to the child, but even more so the danger to the mother, starts with the rupture of the fetal membranes or during delivery.

Direct damage to the child caused by scarlet fever streptococci is unknown. Nevertheless, every detection of group A streptococcus during pregnancy should be taken seriously, and the mother should be treated with antibiotics.

Diagnosis:

- *Clinical picture.* Exanthema, erythema, pyoderma, fever.
- *Culture. Detection* of β-hemolysin group A streptococci from the throat and vagina.
- *Laboratory parameters.* Leukocytosis, C-reactive protein.
- *Serology.* While meaningless for the acute infection, it is important for sequelae, such as rheumatic fever (antistreptolysin O titer).

There is no antibody response, or only a minor one, if the infection is quickly treated with penicillin.

Therapy. Group A streptococci are sensitive to many antibiotics. Penicillins, cephalosporins, as well as macrolides and clindamycin are effective, while quinolones are less effective.

Oral treatment:

- amoxicillin (3 × 750–1000 mg per day)
- cefuroxime (2 × 500 mg per day).

The recommended duration of treatment is 10 days.

General prophylaxis during pregnancy:

- If scarlet fever (or another infection caused by group A streptococci) is present in the surroundings of a pregnant woman, swabs should be taken from the throat and vagina. In case the pregnant woman turns out to be colonized, antibiotics should be administered for 10 days. It is essential that the vaginal swab is repeated immediately prior to delivery to avoid infection during childbed via the puerperal uterus.
- In case of vaginitis (or even just leukorrhea in the discharge) during pregnancy, a swab should be taken for bacteriology at least once.
- In case of exanthema, the possibility of infection due to group A streptococci should be considered.
- In case of pyoderma, one should attempt to detect the pathogen and make sure the pregnant women is treated with oral antibiotics.
- Antibiotic prophylaxis is indicated in case of cesarean section or other surgical interventions.

Pertussis (Whooping Cough)

Pathogen. The disease is caused by the bacterium *Bordetella pertussis*, which produces the pertussis toxin.

Clinical picture. The disease begins as a fluelike infection (catarrhal stage, days 7 to 14 after infection). At this point, the infected person is highly contagious. During the subsequent stage (paroxysmal stage, which may last for weeks), there is hardly any infectiousness.

The characteristic coughing bouts with dyspnea and subsequent deep inhalation are not caused by the pathogen itself but rather by the pertussis toxin. Hence, they can no longer be influenced. Superinfection with bronchopneumonia is possible.

Risk for the child. Direct damages to the child are unknown. The paroxysmal stage may lead to premature delivery.

Diagnosis. Diagnosis is established by isolating the pathogen from the nasopharynx in special culture media and by direct fluorescence test.

Detection of *Bordetella* antibodies is possible and can lead to the diagnosis even at the paroxysmal stage.

Therapy (adults). Treatment makes only sense during the early phase and should last for 10–14 days.

- ampicillin (i. v., 3 × 2 g per day)
- amoxicillin (orally, 3 × 1 g per day)
- erythromycin (orally, 4 × 500 mg per day)
- azithromycin (orally, 1.5 g once).

Prevention. If there is a risk of infection, the pregnant woman may receive antibiotic prophylaxis (see therapy). Vaccination with the P antigen (Pac Mérieux) is recommended for children.

Salmonella Infection (Salmonellosis)

Forms of the disease. We distinguish between generalized salmonellosis (typhoid fever and paratyphoid fever, which are serious systemic illnesses) and localized salmonellosis (enteric fever due to a local intestinal infection). The latter form (gastroenteritis) is far more common and occasionally also seen during pregnancy.

Transmission. The pathogen, *Salmonella enterica*, is spread through smear infection by clinically healthy carriers (about 0.1–0.2% of the population) or by food.

Risk for the child. Although risks for the pregnancy are not anticipated, precaution is indicated during delivery to prevent infection of the child, since it may take a more severe course in the infant.

Diagnosis. Diagnosis is established by isolating the pathogen from the stool. Almost 2000 serologically different types of *Salmonella* are known.

Prophylaxis. If the pregnant woman has a confirmed salmonellosis, or diarrhea, the stool should be examined for pathogenic bacteria immediately before delivery. If the mother is still excreting salmonellae, contamination of the child via the stool should be avoided, if possible. So far, there is still no satisfactory answer as to whether the newborn might be at risk during birth if the mother is ill or is a carrier. The routinely recommended hygienic measures are far easier to observe during childbed than during vaginal birth. Close monitoring of the newborn and early treatment of the newborn will probably suffice. Cesarean section is only justified if the child is at high risk. Mother and child should not be separated; breast-feeding is the best prophylaxis for the child as mother's milk is the best probiotic food. Fairly good results have been obtained by treating the salmonella-excreting mother with probiotic bacterial suspensions containing lactobacilli.

Infections Caused by *Campylobacter fetus* and *C. jejuni*

Pathogen and clinical picture. These pathogens are common in animals. Thanks to continuous improvements in the methods of detection, they are now more frequently discovered in cases of diarrhea and febrile infections. These pathogens—especially *Campylobacter jejuni*—have become more important in recent years. Bacteremia is not uncommon and may reach the fetus by the hematogenous route.

Transmission. Infection occurs by means of infected animals or contaminated foods.

Diagnosis. Isolation of the pathogen from blood cultures, amniotic fluid, or the cervix.

Risk for the child. Systemic infection of the mother may result in the following:

- septic abortion
- sepsis causing premature birth
- sepsis causing fetal death.

Several cases of sepsis have been reported in which intrauterine infection and fetal death were caused also by *Campylobacter fetus*.

Therapy:

- erythromycin, 4 × 500 mg per day
- aminopenicillins (e.g., ampicillin, amoxicillin)
- metronidazole or other 5-nitroimidazoles
- azithromycin
- clindamycin.

Q Fever

This is a zoonosis caused by *Coxiella burnetii* of the family *Rickettsiaceae*, which multiplies only inside host cells and which is highly resistant to environmental factors. The pathogen is occasionally transmitted from sheep or other domestic animals to humans and through inhalation of contaminated dust, causing headache, fever, muscle pain, and other symptoms. Detection is difficult and requires special culture media.

Importance during pregnancy. Infections of the placenta have been described, and abortions, stillbirths, and premature delivery have been reported. Direct damages to the child are unknown. In Germany, the disease is rare due to the surveillance of domestic livestock. It therefore hardly plays a role, and minor outbreaks are often spectacular events. They should be considered in cases of unclear febrile diseases after contact with animals.

Infections Caused by Group B Streptococci

Group B streptococci are important only during pregnancy. They are often found as a harmless colonizing germ in the vagina. They constitute one of the main causes of neonatal morbidity and mortality. We distinguish between early-onset and late-onset streptococcal diseases of the child.

Since the problem has been recognized in the 1970 s, the rate of invasive infection has been reduced through consistent prophylaxis from two to three per 1000 live-born newborns to 1.5 initially and then to 0.5 during the last 10 years.

Pathogen. Group B streptococci (GBS) according to *Lancefield*, also called *Streptococcus agalactiae*, belong to the genus *Streptococcus* of the family *Streptococcaceae*, which are gram-positive cocci. Four different serotypes (polysaccharide antigens) and subtypes (protein antigens) are known.

Until 35 years ago, these bacteria have been regarded as harmless saprophytes. We now know that group B streptococci belong to the most common pathogens of serious infections in newborns.

Occurrence and frequency. Group B streptococci are part of the normal intestinal flora in 20–30% of adults. The bacteria of the intestinal flora cannot be eliminated from the body. In women, they reach the vagina and also the bladder from the

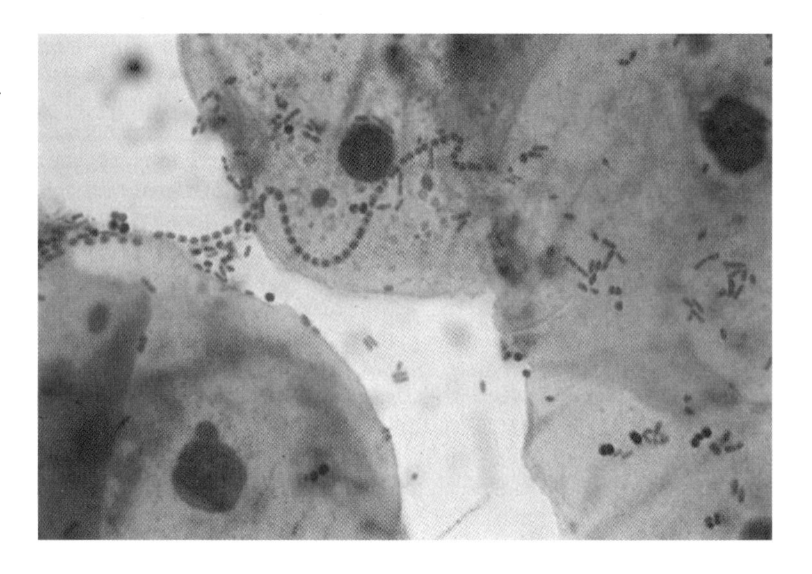

Fig. 8.**21** Streptococci of group B in the vagina. Wet mount in 0.1 % methylene blue solution, viewed under oil with a 100× objective. Occurrence of such long chains of streptococci is rare. Usually, one finds two, three, or four bacteria close together. Frequently, other bacteria are found as well. The diagnosis can only be established by means of microbiological tests.

anus. In 10–30 % of pregnant women, group B streptococci are detected in the vagina (culture on special media). Their concentration in the vagina varies. They may occur at low numbers together with lactobacilli without being recognized microscopically, or alone at high concentration (Fig. 8.**21**). They do not cause inflammatory reactions in the vagina; like almost all intestinal bacteria, they only colonize the vagina. Detection of group B streptococci in the urine is regarded as a massive colonization, posing an increased risk of transmission to the newborn.

Transmission to the child. The child usually becomes infected in the birth canal. In special cases, group B streptococci may also pass through the intact fetal membranes and infect the child in utero. High concentration of bacteria, inhalation during delivery, and also immaturity of the child increase the risk of infection. Without prophylaxis, 1–2 % of the children from colonized mothers fall ill.

Disease of the mother. Group B streptococci do not seem to pose a risk for the mother herself, since they rarely cause definite illness. Detection of group B streptococci in connection with endometritis or peritonitis leads one to suspect them as occasional pathogens. As they often colonize the vagina, their detection in neighboring inflamed areas does not necessarily identify them as the cause of the infection. Even if frequently detected in connection with vaginitis (e. g., plasma cell vaginitis), this does not indicate that they are the cause of vaginitis; it rather reflects the frequent colonization by group B streptococci, which are the more numerous the more disturbed the vaginal flora.

Risk for the child. The highest risk is posed by high bacterial numbers, inhalation by the child during the phase of expulsion, and immaturity.

There are two forms of these perinatal and neonatal infections: *early-onset* disease, which is acquired during birth and occurs within the first 24–48 hours, and *late-onset* disease, which probably results from nosocomial infection and manifests itself only eight to 10 days after birth.

The more dangerous form is the early-onset disease; it runs a quick course, beginning with relatively uncharacteristic symptoms, such as disturbed pulmonary adaptation, expiratory grunts, poor tonus, bradycardia, signs of cyanosis, attacks of apnea, and sucking weakness. They result in rapid wasting of the child and development of pneumonia and sepsis.

Forms of infection:

- respiratory distress syndrome (RDS)
- pneumonia (80–90 % of these children)
- meningitis/sepsis
- intrauterine death of the child.

Until now, a connection between premature rupture of fetal membranes and vaginal colonization by group B streptococci has not been demonstrated.

Diagnosis:

Mother: swabs from the vagina and rectum, collected during the 35th to 38th weeks of pregnancy or prior to delivery and transported in transport medium:

- culture on selective media, with findings recorded in the maternity passport
- rapid tests for serologic detection of GBS (less sensitive)

- serology (low antibody titers seem to increase the risk for the child).

Child: detection of pathogen after birth:
- microscopy of gastric secretion (quick testing method)
- rapid tests for serological detection of GBS in gastric secretion or swab
- culture on selective media.

Therapy:
Prophylactic treatment of the pregnant woman if group B streptococci have been detected:
- Systemic antibiotics (CDC recommendation):
  - during delivery: penicillin G (i. v., five million IU initially, then 2.5 million IU every four hours until birth), ampicillin (i. v., 2 g initially, then 1 g every four hours)
  - with low risk of allergy: cephalosporin of the second generation (2 g initially, then 1 g every eight hours)
  - with high risk of allergy: erythromycin (500 mg every six hours), clindamycin (900 mg every eight hours).
- If the pregnant women shows symptoms (e. g., premature labor, cervical thinning and dilatation, or early premature rupture of fetal membranes, fever), antibiotic treatment (e. g., amoxicillin orally or i. v.) is recommended. Prior to treatment, it is important to examine a native preparation by microscopy and to collect a swab for bacteriology.
- Reduction of group B streptococci during pregnancy or prior to delivery:
  - acidification of the vagina for several weeks (e. g., daily vaginal vitamin C tablets)
  - hexetidine or dequalinium chloride for one week
  - amoxicillin (3 × 1 g per day for five days).

Prophylactic care of the child:
- close clinical monitoring
- search for pathogen in gastric secretion and swab
- early transfer of the child to a children's hospital if there are the slightest distinctive features
- postnatal chemoprophylaxis is not required for the normal child if the mother received prophylactic treatment
- generous antibody treatment if the child is immature
- possibly antibiotic treatment if the fetal membranes rupture prematurely (> 12 hours) and the child is immature.

Recommendations for Prophylaxis (According to the CDC Recommendations in 2002)

These recommendations are based on the prenatal screening of all pregnant women for group B streptococci.

Between the 35th and 37th weeks of pregnancy, vaginal and rectal swabs are taken for the detection of GBS on selective media. During delivery chemoprophylaxis is administered to:
- all pregnant women with GBS detection during the 35th and 37th weeks of pregnancy
- all pregnant women with GBS in the urine at any time during pregnancy
- all pregnant women with invasive infection of the child during early pregnancy
- all pregnant women without known GBS diagnosis, until the GBS test becomes negative
- in case of imminent premature delivery prior to the 37th week of pregnancy.

Remark: There are now several recommendations as to how to proceed in case of GBS detection during pregnancy. Nevertheless, it is still being debated whether every pregnant woman with GBS should receive prophylactic treatment. By microscopic assessment of the vaginal flora, the obstetrician can very well distinguish between low and high degrees of colonization. A microbiological result of very few GBS during normal birth is hardly associated with an increased risk of infection. Unfortunately, there are no studies on this subject. The concentration of GBS in the vagina can be reduced, or their presence even eliminated, through local measures. The options are long-term acidification (vaginal vitamin C delayed release tablets), possibly in combination with disinfectants, and simultaneous reduction of anal microbes through preventive anal and vulvar care using ointments containing lavender oil.

Bacterial Vaginosis

Surprisingly, severe disturbance of the vaginal flora hardly interferes with conception. During pregnancy, however, the high concentration of facultative pathogens often causes infection of the pregnancy (chorioamnionitis) and premature delivery. In addition, puerperal infections occur far more frequently. One should therefore aim at normalization of the vaginal flora during pregnancy.

Pathogens and frequency. The pathogens include *Gardnerella vaginalis* and various bacteria of the intestinal flora, especially anaerobes. Since bacterial vaginosis has received more attention, it has become less common and is now only found in about 5% of pregnant women.

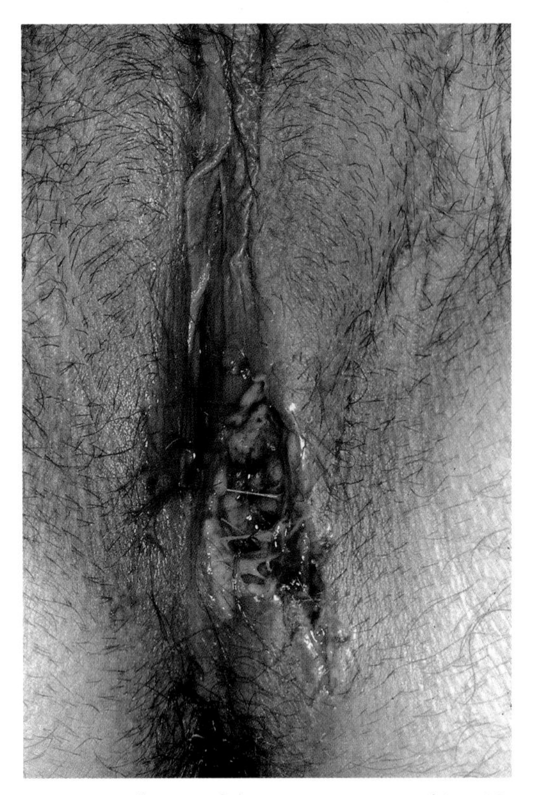

Fig. 8.22 Infection of the episiotomy wound in a 23-year old patient, at day 6 after surgery.

Clinical picture. The discharge is thin, creamy, and white. It has an unpleasant fishy odor and a pH value of about 5.0. Finding typical clue cells when examining the discharge under the microscope makes it easier to diagnose this disturbance.

In some women, the vaginal flora normalizes during the pregnancy due to increasing estrogen concentrations and a decreased frequency of intercourse.

Because of the high concentration of facultative pathogens, these women show a five times higher incidence of late abortion, premature delivery, and postpartum ascending infections, infection of the episiotomy wound (Fig. 8.**22**), puerperal endometritis, and peritonitis after cesarean section than women with a normal lactobacillus flora.

Therapy and prophylaxis. As long as bacterial vaginosis is only a local problem, topical treatment is appropriate. Acidification of the vagina with vitamin C (0.5–1 delayed-release tablet per day) early during pregnancy is usually sufficient. Other options are single-dose topical treatment with 500 mg metronidazole or, if pathogenic anaerobic bacteria are present, topical treatment with disinfectants (dequalinium chloride, hexetidine).

Oral treatment is always necessary when there is a possibility that the fetal membranes or the uterus become infected. Premature labor, increased inflammatory parameters, cervical thinning, funnel formation at the internal orifice of the uterus, prolapse of the amniotic sac, and pain are indications to be taken seriously (see also Prophylaxis of Late Abortion and Premature Delivery, p. 211).

Escherichia coli and Other Intestinal Pathogens

In addition to group B streptococci, *E. coli* is one of the most important pathogens of neonatal infections. In addition, *E. coli* is an important cause of late abortion and premature delivery. Detection of high concentrations of *E. coli* and other intestinal bacteria in pregnant women who are at high risk should therefore be taken seriously. High risk factors include: history of late abortion, premature delivery, premature labor, tendency to premature delivery, and premature rupture of fetal membranes, especially if the child is immature.

Therapy. At the stage of vaginal flora disturbance, topical treatment by acidification or disinfection may be attempted, followed by acidification in combination with anal and vulvar skin care using ointments containing lavender oil.

Otherwise, amoxicillin orally is indicated—or, even better, cephalosporin because some *E. coli* strains are resistant against amoxicillin (an antibiogram is therefore important). In case of antibiotic treatment, simultaneous acidification of the vagina is essential to promote the growth of lactobacilli, which is otherwise inhibited by the antibiotic.

In case of rupture of fetal membranes and immaturity of the child, detection of *E. coli* should be taken as seriously as a detection of group B streptococci, and an effective antibiotic should be administered. Possibly, the pregnancy has to be terminated.

The presence of other *Enterobacteriaceae*, such as *Klebsiella pneumoniae*, during pregnancy and after rupture of the fetal membranes should also be taken seriously (see Table 8.**12**, p. 216).

Infections Leading to Late Abortion, Miscarriage, and Premature Delivery

In Germany, about 5–7% of pregnancies end in premature delivery prior to the 38th week, and 1% end prior to the 32nd week. In clinical centers, the numbers are even higher. There are no data on the frequency of late abortions. Currently, at least one-half of all complications can be

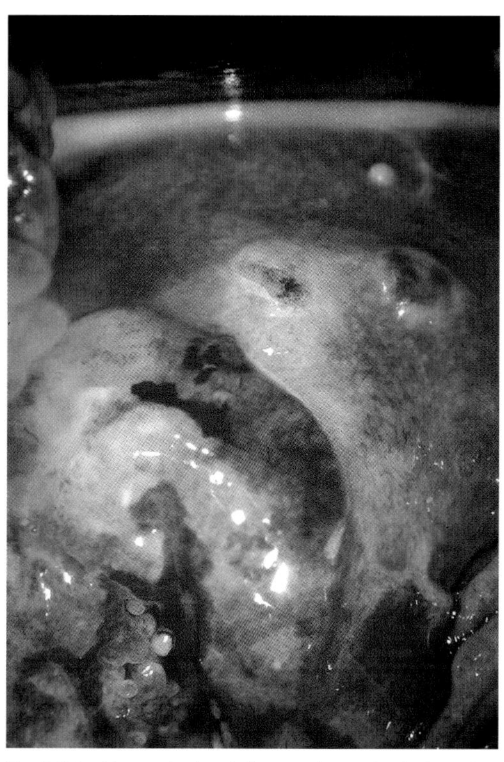

Fig. 8.**23** Hyperplasia of the portio vaginalis in a 26-year-old patient during the 22nd week of pregnancy.

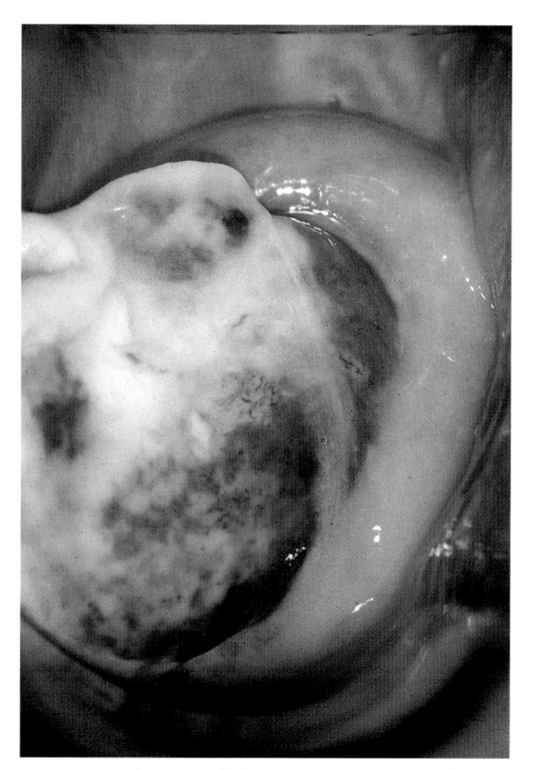

Fig. 8.**24** A large, slightly necrotic cervical polyp in a 25-year-old patient during the 6th week of pregnancy.

traced back to infections. Hematogenous infections with known pathogens (e. g., *Listeria*, *Campylobacter jejuni*) are only rarely detected. Pathogens causing cervicitis, such as gonococci or chlamydiae, are also rarely found in this situation. Most of these infections are caused by apparently harmless intestinal bacteria ascending from the vagina. The risk of repeated infections is relatively high, namely, 60 %.

The cervix plays an important role in the development of ascending infections. Occasionally, the cervix shows distinctive changes during pregnancy, such as pronounced hyperplasia associated with heavy leukorrhea (Fig. 8.**23**) or a large cervical polyp (Fig. 8.**24**). If a polyp becomes necrotic, it provides an excellent growth medium for bacteria.

Far more common, however, are risks in the patient's history, such as status after conization, repeated abrasions, prolapse of the amniotic sac, late abortion, miscarriage, and premature delivery. When these women come to the follow-up examination after a late abortion, miscarriage, or premature delivery, they usually show a normal vaginal flora. In women who went through several late abortions, it is not uncommon that the cervical canal is wide open (Fig. 8.**25**). Normally, the long cervix (50 mm) and its secretion provide a reasonably good barrier against pathogens ascending from the vagina.

Late abortion or premature delivery are most likely induced only when several unfavorable events coincide:

- ▶ increased numbers of intestinal bacteria in the vagina
- ▶ anaerobes degrading the protective mucus by means of proteases
- ▶ a weak lactobacillus flora (atypical lactobacilli)
- ▶ cervical incompetence (structural weakness), surgical damage to the cervix (conization, dilatation)
- ▶ locally lowered immune defenses
- ▶ stress situations
- ▶ severe mental stress.

Table 8.**11** shows our own study on the role of the vaginal flora.

If there is an infection prior to the extrauterine viability of the child, the pregnancy ends in late abortion. In most of these cases, this is caused by infection with intestinal bacteria, i. e., the body's own flora. It is difficult to predict which of these bacteria will cause an infection. Uterine contractions start as soon as the amniotic cavity and the fetus become infected, and it is not uncommon that this leads to prolapse of the amniotic sac and finally to expulsion of the fetus—otherwise the mother would be in danger.

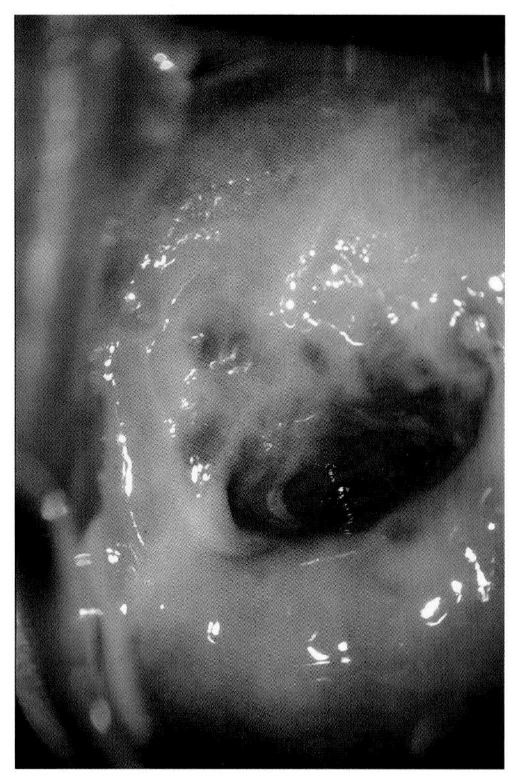

Fig. 8.**25** Condition of a 27-year-old patient after four late miscarriages, showing a gaping cervical canal.

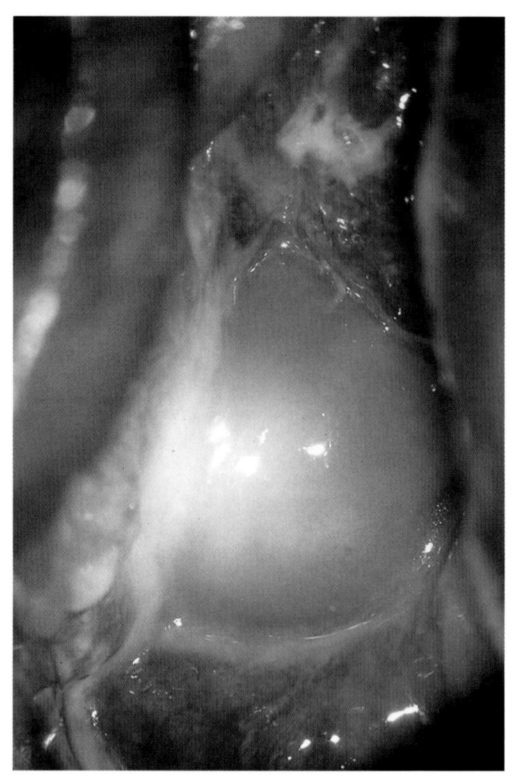

Fig. 8.**26** Prolapse of the amniotic sac in a 26-year-old patient during the 24th week of pregnancy with twins.

Table 8.**11** Relationship between the vaginal flora and premature deliveries (excluding late miscarriages) (Study at the University Women's Hospital, Freiburg, Germany, in 1985. Cases are grouped according to the microscopic evaluation of Gram-stained preparations at the time of admission to the delivery room)

	Number of women	**Delivery prior to week 37 of pregnancy**
Total number of pregnant women	1031 (100 %)	45 (4 %)
– lactobacilli	731 (72 %)	14 (2 %)
– mixed flora	154 (15 %)	20 (13 %)
– massive disturbance/bacterial vaginosis	138 (13 %)	11 (8 %)

There has been the hope that close bacterial monitoring in connection with determining the inflammatory parameters might lead to early recognition of a risk of infection or the start of an infection, thus preventing late miscarriage or premature delivery. Unfortunately, these expectations have not been met so far. This may be due to the initial local confinement of the infection, but also to the limitations of bacteriology. It is known that some pathogens are not detected during routine bacteriology because they are unstable and, in part, difficult to culture. Hence, it makes more sense to strive for general improvement of the vaginal flora early in the pregnancy.

The source of undesired bacteria in the vagina is usually the woman's own anal region. For anatomical reasons, the anal region is difficult to clean and care for. For the average patient, this is unknown territory. As the region is difficult to inspect visually, any assessment of its condition is left to the sense of touch. This unfavorable situation explains the frequent dissemination of bacteria.

Prolapse of the amniotic sac without infection of the amniotic cavity (Fig. 8.**26**) does not necessarily lead to immediate premature delivery; it may still persist for weeks.

By contrast, if the amniotic cavity becomes infected, expulsion of the fetus can no longer be prevented—not even with antibiotics. Fig. 8.**27** shows prolapse of the amniotic sac during the 18th week of pregnancy in a patient who already had two late miscarriages. The amniotic sac contains plenty of leukocytic sediment as a sign of infection of the amniotic cavity. Inflammatory

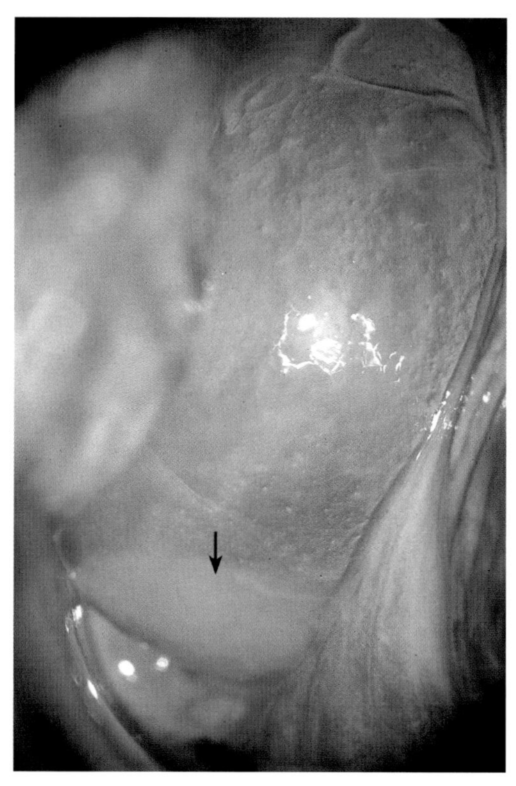

Fig. 8.**27** Prolapse of the amniotic sac with infected amniotic cavity (leukocyte sediment, arrow) during the third late miscarriage (18th week of pregnancy) in a 23-year-old patient.

Fig. 8.**28** Patient with a history of two late miscarriages, now with prophylactic cerclage in the 19th week of pregnancy.

parameters of the mother (leukocytes in the blood, CRP) were not increased, and the vaginal flora was only slightly disturbed, consisting of lactobacilli and some intestinal flora (*E. coli*). Histopathology confirmed the presence of chorioamnionitis and massive pneumonia of the fetus.

Prophylaxis of Late Miscarriage and Premature Delivery

The following conditions, in the order of their importance, are risk factors for late miscarriage, miscarriage, and premature delivery:

- ▶ the patient's history (status after late miscarriages, miscarriage, or previous premature deliveries)
- ▶ infections
- ▶ cervical changes
- ▶ disturbed vaginal flora
- ▶ stress, anxiety.

Some of these risk factors can be eliminated or, at least, reduced.

The intensity of therapeutic measures depends on the patient's history and current condition. For women who already had several late abortions, the risk of repeating the event is more than 60 %.

Out of 55 of such women, the following approach was unsuccessful only in two women (renewed loss of the child):

- ▶ intensive care with full personal involvement of the physician
- ▶ long-term improvement of the vaginal flora (daily application of vaginal vitamin C delayed-release tablets)
- ▶ cerclage during the 14th week of pregnancy (Fig. 8.**28**); even total closure of the cervical os is possible
- ▶ regular controls using the speculum
- ▶ assessment of the vaginal flora (pH value, microscopy, microbiology in the case of leukorrhea, contractions, or cervical thinning)
- ▶ cervical measurements by ultrasound (length, assessment of inner cervical os: funnel formation)
- ▶ prophylactic administration of antibiotics for cerclage (and then again at one week prior to the date of the previous late abortion) in case of pathogens, increased inflammatory parameters, or uterine contractions
- ▶ sedation by early administration of oral magnesium; elimination of stressful situations
- ▶ consistent anal and vulvar skin care by daily application of ointments containing lavender oil in order to reduce pathogens in the anovulvar region.

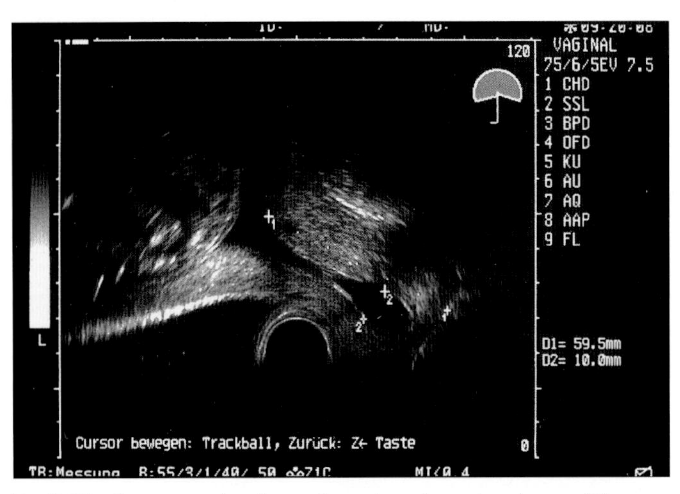

Fig. 8.**29** Sonogram showing an hourglass-shaped prolapse of the amniotic sac after therapeutic cerclage during the 24th week of pregnancy in a patient with a history of three late miscarriages.

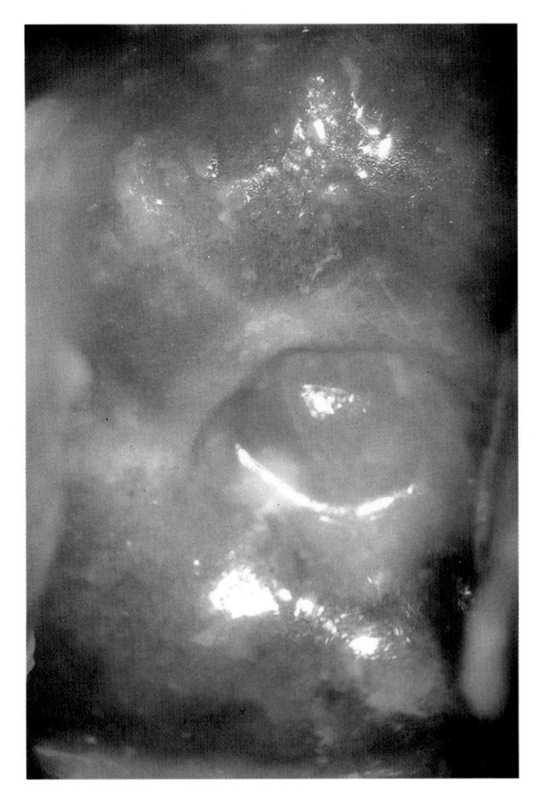

Fig. 8.**30** The same patient as in Fig. 8.**29** with the small amniotic sac visible. The pregnancy was terminated by cesarean section during the 28th week of pregnancy.

Prognosis is less promising if therapeutic cerclage is only applied when the amniotic sac is already visible deep in the cervical canal. In the pregnancy shown in the sonogram from the 24th week (Fig. 8.**29**), the cervix was held together in the proximal region by the thread of the cerclage. However, elongation of the hourglass-shaped amniotic sac dilated the distal cervix, and the amniotic sac became visible in the cervical canal (Fig. 8.**30**).

In pregnant women with a lower risk, simple improvement of the vaginal flora with vaginal vitamin C delayed release tablets may suffice. Some women feel better after insertion of a supportive cerclage pessary (Fig. 8.**31**). The individual measures taken depend on the risk, the options available, and the cooperation of the patient.

Premature Rupture of the Fetal Membranes and Infection

Premature rupture of the amniotic sac is caused by loosening of the fetal membranes and increased internal pressure. Both may occur because of inflammation due to infection. How stable the membranes sometimes are, is demonstrated by patients in which a prolapse of the amniotic sac lasted for weeks (see Fig. 8.**26**, p. 210). Detection of local infections is difficult and therefore not always successful.

The fact that bacteria actually pass through the fetal membranes has been demonstrated in studies involving the culture of pathogens from the amniotic fluid following abdominal puncture of the amniotic cavity. Bacteria can sometimes also be cultured from smears taken from between the fetal membranes (Fig. 8.**32**), especially if premature delivery is associated with signs of infection.

However, not in all cases of ruptured fetal membranes with immature child can pathogens be cultured or clues for an infectious cause be detected. This may be a strictly technical problem; chorioamnionitis is initially a local process, and the affected sites of the membranes are not always examined.

Clinical picture. Pregnant women often show only few symptoms before premature rupture of the fetal membranes. Only some of them report premature labor just before the rupture. In addition, fever is rarely present. Occasionally, increased discharge or a stressful event is reported.

Pathogens. For pathogens that cause severe in-

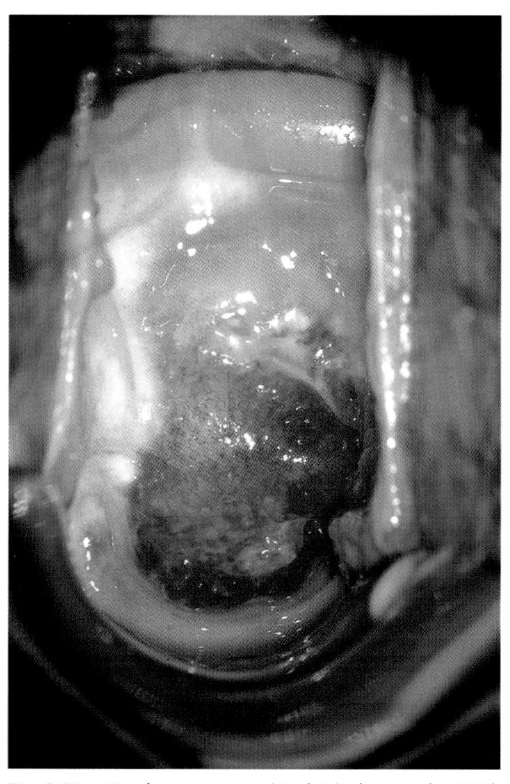

Fig. 8.**31** Cerclage-pessary (Arabin) during the 29th week of pregnancy in a 29-year-old patient with a history of two miscarriages.

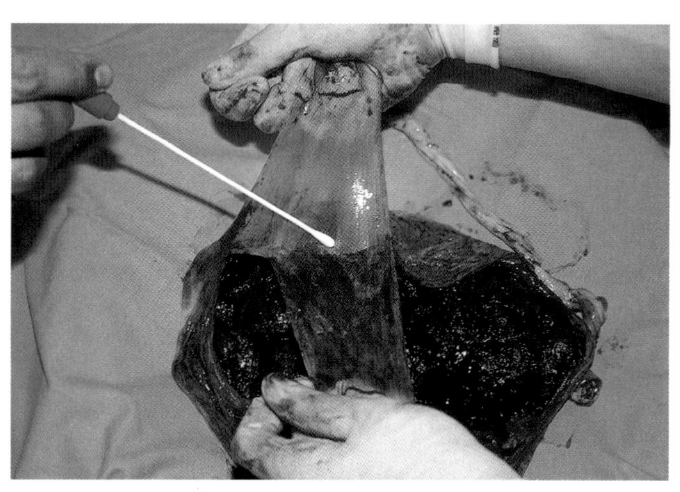

Fig. 8.**32** A smear is taken from between the fetal membranes for post partum detection of bacteria that may have passed through the fetal membranes.

flammatory reactions, such as gonococci and trichomonads, a connection has been confirmed through prospective studies—which makes sense. Chlamydiae cause only mild inflammatory reactions (cervicitis, endometritis) and, in addition, occur only in low numbers. Nevertheless, they are able to induce premature delivery. Chlamydiae play only a very minor role in premature delivery, as shown by the fact that compulsory screening and treatment in case of chlamydia detection did not change the rate of premature delivery.

In cases of the far more commonly occurring disturbances of the vaginal flora through bacteria from the intestinal flora (bacterial vaginosis, which does not cause inflammatory reactions in the vagina and cervix), the connection with premature delivery is far more difficult to recognize. Here, mechanisms of prostaglandin induction are assumed to be involved.

Diagnosis when the child is immature:

- use of the speculum; detection of amniotic fluid with flakes of vernix caseosa by means of pH value (Fig. 6.**3**, p. 59)
- clinical evaluation of cervix, discharge, and uterus
- microbiology
- assessment of the cervix by means of ultrasound
- laboratory parameters are usually normal.

Early signs of imminent rupture of the fetal membranes:

- cervical thinning with funnel formation
- premature uterine contractions
- increased levels of interleukin-6 and interleukin-8 in the cervix and in the amniotic fluid (not yet a routine test).

The actual premature rupture of the membranes is preceded by local membrane damage leading to the discharge of fetal fibronectin. It has now become possible to detect this event in the cervical secretion by fetal fibronectin immunoassay.

Therapy when the child is immature. After rupture of the membranes, the vaginal flora changes—slowly if the lactobacillus flora is normal, rapidly if the flora is disturbed, and very rapidly if chorioamnionitis had induced the rupture of membranes—and infection of the amnion follows. Whether or not delivery can be delayed for a few days depends on the week of pregnancy and the condition of the child:

- sedation
- arrest of uterine contractions (tocolysis)
- if lactobacillus flora is microbiologically normal, one may initially do without antibiotics
- antibiotics are given whenever the vaginal flora is disturbed or findings are unclear, initially for five days, e. g., amoxicillin, ampicillin/sulbactam (Unasyn), other antibiotics (cephalosporin) depending on the microbiological and clinical findings
- acidification of the vagina to inhibit growth of intestinal bacteria in this region
- if premature delivery is imminent, fetal pulmonary maturity is promoted with cortisone.

Close bacteriological monitoring by repeated determination of inflammatory parameters in the blood allows one to recognize dangerous situations for mother and child.

Selection of pathogens that can no longer be controlled with very effective antibiotics, such as meropenem, is promoted by continuous administration of antibiotics. Interval therapy or alternating antibiotics—always with simultaneous support of the lactobacillus flora through vaginal vitamin C—will slow down the development of resistances.

Amniotic Infection Syndrome (AIS)

Initially, inflammation of the fetal membranes is a local process. It is called chorioamnionitis if there are uterine contractions, fever, and increased inflammatory parameters. In the presence of clinical symptoms, delivery can only be delayed for a short time even with antibiotics. As it is not possible to treat the child adequately in utero, the pregnancy will have to be terminated, often by cesarean section—provided the week of pregnancy does permit this.

Clinical picture. The full picture of amniotic infection syndrome—with placentitis, amnionitis, deciduitis, infection of the umbilical cord, and infection of the child—is fortunately very rare. In most cases, one is dealing with chorioamnionitis with mild fever and moderately increased inflammatory parameters.

Risk for the child. The main risk for the child is immaturity. Only some of the children show signs of infection after birth. Because the risk of infecting the child cannot be excluded, children receive prophylactic antibiotics the more often, the younger they are.

Pathogens. Any bacteria of the vaginal flora may be involved, above all *E. coli* and other intestinal bacteria. Highly pathogenic bacteria, such as group A streptococci, are rarely involved, but should be taken very seriously if they are. In addition, *Staphylococcus aureus* is more than just a facultative pathogen.

Risk factors:

- premature rupture of fetal membranes
- premature uterine contractions
- bacterial vaginosis
- disturbed vaginal flora
- pathogens, such as *Listeria*, gonococci, group A streptococci, *Staphylococcus aureus*
- high numbers of other facultative pathogens, such as group B streptococci, *Escherichia coli*, and *Haemophilus influenzae.*

Decisive factors for the prognosis of the child include the week of pregnancy and early recognition and treatment of the infection.

Diagnosis:

- leukocytic discharge (> 80 leukocytes per field of view at a magnification of 400×)
- pathogen detection in the cervical smear or amniotic fluid
- temperature of the mother
- increased heart frequency of the child
- leukocytosis of the mother
- increase of CRP in the serum of the mother
- histology of fetal membranes (final confirmation of the infection).

Induction of labor and therapy. Both depend on the week of pregnancy. Immediate delivery should be initiated if the child is fairly mature. If vaginal delivery is not possible, cesarean section should be performed. If treatment with antibiotics has not yet been started or has not been necessary, it should be postponed until after the umbilical cord has been cut in order to give the pediatrician a chance to carry out bacteriological tests prior to therapy. Of course, in particularly severe cases, one will not make allowances for this but starts immediately with antibiotic therapy. In most patients, however, the infection will not be that advanced, and diagnostic tests should be considered.

Cesarean section does not worsen the amniotic infection syndrome. However, it is important to carry out an adequate antibiotic treatment that covers the most important possible pathogens.

Close follow-ups of mother and child are essential.

Fever During Pregnancy

Fever during pregnancy should always be taken very seriously as it may be caused by a number of severe infections that may threaten mother and child.

Diagnosis:
- *blood culture* to exclude listeriosis, sepsis due to *Campylobacter fetus*, sepsis in general
- *urinalysis* to exclude pyelonephritis
- *physical examination* of the pregnant woman: the uterus is tender to pressure in case of chorioamnionitis
- use of speculum to obtain bacteriological smear from the cervix (bacteria and chlamydiae)
- *microscopic examination* of the vaginal flora (leukorrhea may indicate a local process)
- *laboratory tests* including CRP, leukocytes in the blood; thrombocyte determination and differential blood counts to exclude viral infection
- *serological examination* to exclude primary infection with cytomegalovirus
- exclusion of malaria when taking the patient's history.

Clinical picture and therapy. Antibiotic therapy with ampicillin (3 × 2 g), if the fever persists and a viral infection has been virtually excluded. Use other appropriate treatments, if other pathogens have been detected or other diagnoses apply.

In case of persistent fever, the antibiotic is switched from the third day on to cephalosporin of the second or third generation and, possibly, metronidazole is added.

Fever during pregnancy is feared because it may induce labor. One should always keep in mind that chorioamnionitis may endanger the child and that the appropriate diagnostic tests need to be carried out repeatedly.

Trichomoniasis During Pregnancy

Trichomonads may occasionally occur during pregnancy (Fig. 8.**33**). This should be considered whenever vaginitis is associated with discharge and high leukocyte numbers. An appropriate wet mount with NaCl solution should be prepared.

Therapy consists of metronidazole or tinidazole (2 g, orally), also for the partner. There are no concerns against this treatment after the 14th week of pregnancy. Topical therapeutics, such as disinfectants, are preferred as a precaution during early pregnancy.

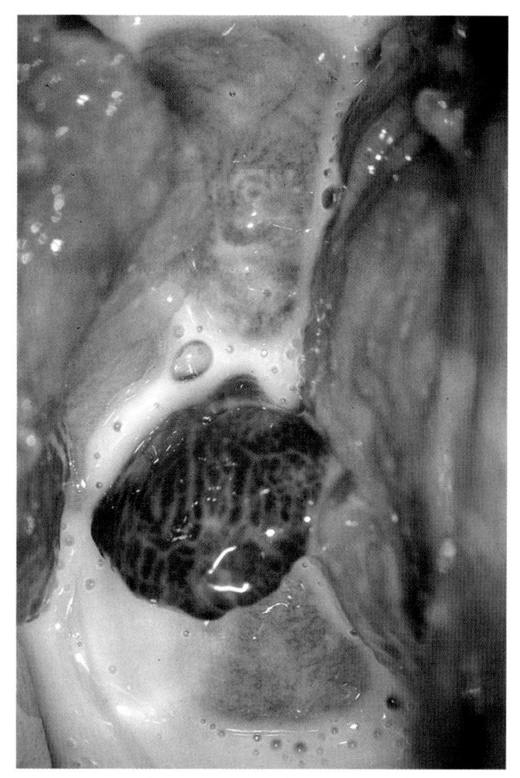

Fig. 8.**33** Trichomoniasis and cervical polyp in a 24-year-old patient during the 20th week of pregnancy.

Tuberculosis During Pregnancy

(see p. 166)

Pregnancy and Risk of Infections in Tropical Countries

Apart from diarrhea, infections that may be acquired on journeys to tropical countries include primarily malaria, hepatitis A, and dengue fever.

Malaria

Pregnant women are especially endangered by malaria, since the disease takes a more severe course due to the mild immunosuppression during pregnancy. The dangerous period extends over two months after giving birth.

The main risk for the child is mortality, premature delivery, underweight, and retardation. The child is largely endangered by the mother's anemia and poor condition, less often by transmission of plasmodia through the placenta.

Clinical picture. The infection begins with flulike symptoms, such as headache, pain in the limbs, tiredness. These are followed by repeated febrile attacks of up to 40 °C associated with cold spells and shaking chills. With the more dangerous form, malaria tropica (*Plasmodium falciparum*), the febrile attacks take a more irregular course.

Diagnosis. A thick blood film is required for detection of plasmodia in erythrocytes (Giemsa staining performed in special laboratories). Concentration methods and rapid tests are now also available.

Therapy. Chloroquine or, in case of resistance, mefloquine, possibly together with atovaquone plus proguanil (Malarone).

There is no contraindication for mefloquine during pregnancy.

Malaria prophylaxis. Because of the limited chemoprophylaxis, exposure prophylaxis is of special importance for pregnant women (no staying outdoors at dusk and during the night, proper clothing, mosquito nets, etc.).

- *Suppression prophylaxis:* the drug does not prevent hepatic schizogony and must still be taken until four weeks after leaving the malaria area:
  - chloroquine, only for Central America
  - mefloquine is the drug of choice from the 14th week of pregnancy onward
  - doxycycline (as an alternative) should not be used after the 14th week of pregnancy.
- *Causal prophylaxis:* the drug needs only to be taken for up to seven days after leaving the malaria area:
  - atovaquone/proguanil (Malarone); there is no experience with this drug during pregnancy. If the risk is low, prophylaxis may be foregone and a malaria drug may be taken in therapeutic doses (see p. 202). Infants and children are particularly endangered by malaria. If one cannot avoid the journey to malaria areas, chloroquine, mefloquine, and proguanil may be used. Breast-fed children need their own prophylaxis as only insufficient amounts of these drugs pass into the mother's milk.

In general, a journey to areas with high risk of infection and resistant strains should be avoided during pregnancy, if possible.

Hepatitis A

In countries with a high incidence of hepatitis A, contraction of the disease through smear infection is possible. There are no known risks for the child. Vaccination prior to the start of the journey is recommended in case of susceptibility (serostatus).

Dengue Fever

This is a febrile exanthematous disease caused by a virus belonging to the group of flaviviruses (other flaviviruses include the hepatitis C virus and the pathogen of yellow fever). The risk for the child lies mainly in the severity of the disease of the mother. There is very little indication that the disease increases the incidence of premature births or intrauterine deaths.

Table 8.**12** Detection and evaluation of bacteria (and other pathogens) in the vagina

Pathogens Always treatment	**Facultative pathogens** Treatment if symptoms are present or counts are high	**Apathogenic microbes** No treatment
– Group A streptococci – Group G streptococci – Gonococci – *Staphylococcus aureus* – *Chlamydia trachomatis* – Trichomonads **To be treated or considered during pregnancy:** – *Candida albicans** – *E. coli* – Group B streptococci – *Klebsiella pneumoniae* – *Haemophilus influenzae* – Pneumococci – Mycoplasmas	– *E. coli* (various strains) – *Staphylococcus epidermidis* – Group B streptococci – Group D streptococci (enterococci) – *Pseudomonas aeruginosa* – *Proteus mirabilis* – Mycoplasmas – *Gardnerella vaginalis* – Anaerobes (*Bacteroides*, peptococci, *Porphyromonas*, *Prevotella*, fusobacteria, etc.) – *Acinetobacter* – *Citrobacter* – *Candida albicans**	– Lactobacilli – *Candida glabrata** – *Saccharomyces cerevisiae** (baker or brewer yeast) – *Geotrichum candidum** – *Rhodotorula rubra**

* Fungus

9 Peripartal and Puerperal Infections

Infections During Childbed

Infections during childbed are relatively common. This is due to the large wound surfaces in the uterus (the site of the placenta), the wounds caused by episiotomy and cesarean section, and the lactating breasts. Nevertheless, the body is surprisingly well equipped to cope with these risks, and the best defense is mainly provided by the high blood flow in these regions.

A dangerous situation arises only when highly pathogenic bacteria invade the open uterus. Here, group A streptococci are particularly dreaded. They are the only bacteria that quickly cause fulminant infections, overwhelming the body in a very short time. Women carrying the undetected pathogen in the vagina at the time of delivery are especially endangered. Transmission of pathogens by the obstetrician or personnel is possible, but this is more the exception.

Far more common are infections due to *Staphylococcus aureus*. This pathogen is normally found on the patient's skin and may occur in the vagina as well. It is the primary pathogen of wound infection, abscess-forming infections, and above all, puerperal mastitis. Sepsis due to *Staphylococcus aureus* takes a slower course than that caused by group A streptococci, thus giving the body more time to develop symptoms and warning signs that make one think of an infection.

Another large group of pathogens consists of aerobic intestinal bacteria, such as *Escherichia coli*, *Klebsiella*, and many more. They become dangerous when large numbers are introduced into the uterus, tissue, or abdominal cavity, when local conditions favor their multiplication, or when the body's defenses are weakened. The same applies also to anaerobic bacteria. More than 20 years ago, anaerobes occasionally caused severe infections; until that time, they were hardly known to cause diseases and were therefore not considered when deciding on the therapy.

Infections during childbed include:

- puerperal sepsis
- endometritis
- peritonitis (ascending infection, intestinal injury)
- infection of the episiotomy wound
- infection of the suprapubic incision
- abscess-forming infection between the intestine and the genitals after intestinal injury (suture error, tear)
- ascending *Chlamydia* infection
- urinary tract infection
- puerperal mastitis.

Ascending Infections after Delivery

Promoting Factors

The genital tract is especially susceptible to bacterial infections immediately after delivery, and so are abdominal wounds. The following factors promote such infections: the altered and slightly suppressed immune system during pregnancy, the wide opening of the uterine cavity—making it easier for pathogens to be introduced in large numbers from the vagina by manipulation during delivery—combined with tissue trauma while giving birth.

The fact that severe infections are relatively rare after delivery is partly explained by the heavy blood flow to the genitals at that time, thus providing plenty of humoral and cellular defenses.

Factors that promote infection are listed below. No single factor is responsible for the occurrence of an infection; it is more likely that several factors have to come together. The presence of one or more of these factors should prompt the obstetrician to pay special attention.

Risks of infection:

- pathogenic bacteria (group A streptococci, *Staphylococcus aureus*, and others)
- high numbers of other bacteria (e. g., bacterial vaginosis)
- prolonged labor combined with many examinations
- injuries (tears of cervix and vagina)
- episiotomy
- vaginal delivery including surgical intervention (vacuum, forceps, manual detachment of placenta)
- cesarean section
- premature rupture of fetal membranes

- diabetes mellitus
- immune suppression
- anemia.

Puerperal Sepsis (see also p. 156)

Until the time of Semmelweiss (1818–1865), the primary pathogens involved in the lethal course of infections after delivery have been group A streptococci. During the worst puerperal fever epidemic, one in every four mothers died of this infection. In 1847, Semmelweiss published his results on the cause of puerperal fever, but they were ignored for many years—as so often is the case in the history of medicine.

The pathogen's port of entrance is usually the uterus, but it may also be the episiotomy wound or the suprapubic incision. In the vast majority of patients, the pathogen resides in the vagina at the time of delivery. After delivery, it rapidly spreads from here over the entire uterus and into the blood, and thus to all organs of the body.

Pathogens. *Streptococcus pyogenes*, streptococci of serogroup A.

Epidemiology. Unfortunately, no data are available in Germany on the frequency of puerperal sepsis or infections caused by group A streptococci during pregnancy and childbed. Only deaths during puerperal sepsis are notifiable. Probably, not all of the postpartum deaths caused by group A streptococci are officially recorded because the pathogen is not yet known at the time of death, or because samples for bacteriology have not been collected—or only after antibiotic treatment.

The frequency of group A streptococcal infection during childbed is mostly unknown, since patients with fever are far more often treated with antibiotics than swabs are taken for microbiology. The media only report on rare spectacular cases with legal battles in the courts. As a result, the public seems to believe that puerperal infection due to group A streptococci are a rare event. This is not the case. Fortunately, a lethal outcome of puerperal sepsis is a rare event.

Based on official death statistics, figures from our own department, a large survey in German clinics, and a dissertation, I have estimated that there are at least 200 infections due to group A streptococci, about 10–20 cases of puerperal sepsis, and 0.5–1 cases of death per 100000 pregnancies.

According to one survey, group A streptococci were detected in 39 out of 97 patients with puerperal sepsis. Of the 39 patients infected, 13 died. Of 35 patients in whom other bacteria had been detected, five patients died, and of 23 patients without any bacteria detected, or without any information available, only one patient died.

Clinical picture. One of the most typical signs of a beginning puerperal sepsis is that the patient is very ill in the absence of any recognizable cause. Symptoms like fever and increased pulse rate are not very typical, since these are also present with many other infections.

More characteristic are respiratory problems, diffuse pain, in most patients the absence of guarding (due to the stretched abdominal wall), diarrhea, hypothermia, leukopenia, and the absence of any cause for the poor general health of the patient. Fever may be absent, especially if the infection appeared suddenly and took an unfavorable course.

Pain in the lower abdomen or in the region of the symphysis should not be taken for symphysiolysis, unless infection has been excluded.

A sore throat may indicate the beginning of an infection caused by group A streptococci. Sore throats or flulike infections in the patient's surroundings should increase awareness regarding a possible risk.

A full-blown sepsis is always associated with massive respiratory insufficiency, since inflammatory damage to the endothelium makes gas exchange hardly possible.

Unfortunately, the uterine pain described in textbooks is not a reliable sign, although it should be taken seriously if present.

The full picture of puerperal sepsis is fortunately very rare. At an advanced stage of sepsis, lethality is still around 20% even today. The endotoxins quickly cause disseminated intravascular coagulopathy (DIC), thus leading to multiorgan failures.

A common complication is fasciitis associated with tissue necrosis (Fig. 9.**1**). Here, tissues die because of inflammatory damage to the endothelium. This may lead to partial or complete amputation of limbs.

Differential diagnosis. The above-mentioned condition should be distinguished from the very rare case of **necrotic fasciitis.** This is a progressive, severe, necrotic inflammation of deep tissue layers after surgical intervention or manipulation. Initially, the skin area shows only a mild redness. A typical pathogen is not known. Various pathogens seem to be involved (synergism), particularly anaerobes. Unknown immunological processes may play an important role.

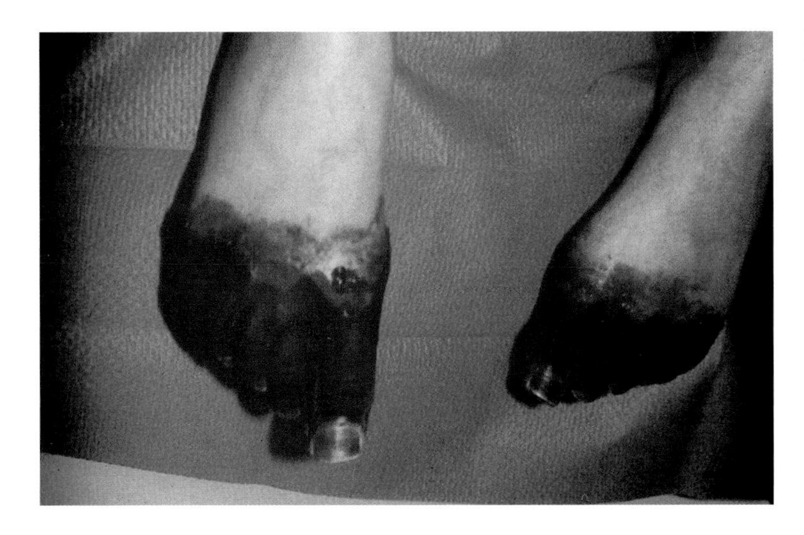

Fig. 9.**1** Necrosis of both forefeet in a 26-year-old patient with severe puerperal sepsis.

Therapeutic approach. High doses of broad-spectrum antibiotics and surgical abrasion of the necrotic tissue, and high doses of cortisone, if necessary.

Diagnosis. If only few laboratory tests are carried out, the dangerous course of sepsis cannot be recognized in time. Just taking the temperature and ordering a general blood count are therefore totally inadequate for the early recognition of sepsis. CRP is the only reliable laboratory parameter, and the test is meanwhile available in every country. An increase by a factor of 30–100, associated with seemingly normal or decreasing leukocyte values, indicates a dangerous situation, namely, sepsis and septic shock. The decrease in thrombocytes occurs relatively late and is therefore not a good warning sign:

- clinical signs of disease, poor condition of the patient
- hypotension, systolic pressure $\leq$80 mmHg
- tachypnea > 25/min
- tachycardia > 120/min
- conspicuous blood count
- markedly increased CRP
- differential blood count shows shift to the left
- microbiological swab from the vagina/uterus, possibly also from the suprapubic incision or episiotomy; pathogens are detected after 24–48 hours, at the earliest
- prior to the first administration of antibiotics, blood should be collected for cultures, even if there is no fever
- pathological parameters for liver, kidney, and coagulation.

Detection of bacteria in blood cultures is the best evidence for sepsis. However, blood cultures must have been collected before the first administration of antibiotics. Sensitive bacteria are no longer detectable in the blood once antibiotic therapy has been started, although—in the case of sepsis—the pathogen has already established itself in the organs because of bacteremia.

Therapy. Still the most effective measure against puerperal sepsis is early administration of antibiotics. Successful treatment during the early phase depends on the type of antibiotic.

The drug of first choice in case of group A streptococci is penicillin. As the pathogen is not known at the beginning, treatment is initially based on the severity of the disease. In case of a mild early form of infection, broad-spectrum penicillins like Augmentin and Unasyn are sufficient. Otherwise, cephalosporin of the second or third generations should be administered together with metronidazole.

Fluoroquinolones or even Co-Trimoxazole are not very effective against group A streptococci; they are therefore contraindicated.

High doses of penicillin with clindamycin are recommended for cases of confirmed puerperal sepsis due to group A streptococci.

If antibiotic administration comes too late, even the most effective broad-spectrum antibiotic, such as meropenem, will only inhibit multiplication of the pathogen. Antibiotics have no effect on the inflammation triggered by the pathogen's toxins and the body's mediators. Attempts at preventing the immune response to bacterial endotoxins or at strengthening the body's immune system have so far been unsuccessful. So far, anti-inflammatory agents and TNF antagonists did not yield the success one had hoped for.

How to avoid puerperal sepsis:

- every detection of group A streptococci during pregnancy should be taken seriously and treated accordingly
- in case of vaginitis or leukorrhea, a swab for microbiological examination should be taken prior to delivery
- any infections caused by group A streptococci in the surroundings of the pregnant woman should be taken seriously
- antibiotic prophylaxis in case of cesarean section
- the possibility of a postpartum infection should always be considered
- determination of CRP if the patient is in poor condition
- in case of severe postpartum pain, repeat administration of pain killers is only permitted in combination with a laboratory diagnosis (CRP)
- a swab for microbiological examination should be taken from the uterus prior to administration of antibiotics
- if the patient is in poor condition, one should consider an infection rather than wait for fever to develop
- in case of postpartum diarrhea, one should first consider peritonitis and sepsis, and only then intestinal infection
- if the patient's condition is poor, generous antibiotic treatment is advised.

Endometritis and Wound Infection

Endometritis

Endomyometritis is a rare form of endometritis in which the inflammation involves the uterine muscles in addition to the mucosa (see p. 146). Characteristic symptoms are pain, fever, discharge, and bleeding. Depending on the pathogen, endometritis may occur suddenly, namely, a few hours after delivery in case of group A streptococci, one to three days after delivery in case of *Staphylococcus aureus* and *Enterobacteriaceae*, three to five days after delivery in case of anaerobes, and very late after four to six weeks in case of chlamydia.

Clinical picture. The symptoms reach from odorous discharge or bleeding to severe pain and fever. Upon clinical examination, the site of inflammation turns out to be the uterus.

The most common form is moderate endometritis caused by anaerobic bacteria. Its earliest appearance is 48 hours after delivery. The temperature is moderate, and symptoms are usually limited. The lochia has decreased and has a foul-smelling odor. The uterus is soft and slightly painful, and the fundus is located higher than it should be according to the number of days after delivery.

Bleeding is the main symptom in case of late-onset endometritis (e. g., due to chlamydia).

Diagnosis:

- clinical examination
- ultrasound to exclude congestion and pregnancy remnants
- laboratory parameters (CRP and blood count) to recognize the severity of inflammation
- swab for microbiology.

If the fever does not abate soon, this may indicate an infection caused by *Staphylococcus aureus*, possibly with abscess formation.

Therapy. The type of treatment depends on the clinical picture and the inflammatory parameters, above all, on the CRP. Since CRP values increase with every tissue trauma, a certain increase is also observed after normal delivery or cesarean section. On the second day, for example, the value may be temporarily increased 10-fold or more in the absence of any severe infection. However, any further increase during the following days or values between 20–100 times the normal value should be regarded as warning signs, and the administration of antibiotics should not be postponed further.

In mild cases without pathogens, the administration of drugs causing uterine contraction may initially suffice. If these drugs do not lead to quick normalization, antibiotics are indicated, such as broad-spectrum penicillins or cephalosporins; depending on the severity, also metronidazole right away.

Differential diagnosis. Although endometritis is the most common cause of fever after vaginal delivery, other causes should be considered as well, such as urinary tract infection, infection of the episiotomy wound, respiratory infection, inflammation caused by an infected venous catheter, mastitis, and viral infections.

Late-onset Endometritis Caused by Chlamydia

The extremely late onset of symptoms is characteristic for chlamydial endometritis. In most patients, symptoms appear only four to six weeks after delivery (see p. 133) due to the slow multiplication of chlamydia. The symptoms are usually minor, with bleeding being the main symptom.

Ovarian Vein Thrombophlebitis

Pathogens:

- anaerobic bacteria:
  - *Bacteroides* species
  - peptococci
  - peptostreptococci
- *Escherichia coli*
- *Staphylococcus aureus*
- *Proteus* species.

Frequency and pathogenesis. Puerperal ovarian vein thrombophlebitis is a severe complication associated with infection of the small pelvis. It is not at all an uncommon event (incidence: 0.05–0.1 %).

It may be the result of sepsis, or the initial focus of it. In the majority of patients, it affects the right ovarian vein.

It is frequently not diagnosed and then only recognized during laparotomy performed when peritonitis or appendicitis are suspected.

Clinical picture:

- fever
- pain in the lower abdomen
- soft uterus, sensitive to pressure
- odorous lochia.

Special risks:

- sepsis
- septic shock
- pulmonary embolism.

Diagnosis:

- detection of pathogen in the uterus or in the lochial secretion
- pain upon palpation, cylindrical resistance in the right adnexal region
- ultrasound
- computed tomography
- possibly phlebography (not during the acute septic process).

Therapy. Although it is difficult to establish a diagnosis without laparotomy, one should first try conservative treatment with antibiotics and heparin. Only if this is not successful and there is the danger of further exacerbation, laparotomy should be performed—which usually results in loss of the uterus. The earlier the treatment is initiated, the higher the chance that the uterus may be saved:

- antibiotics: cephalosporin together with 1 g metronidazole per day
- heparin perfusion
- laparotomy with extirpation of the adnexa and, possibly, the uterus.

Infections After Cesarean Section

Pathogens. Here, too, the most dreaded pathogens include group A streptococci, followed by *Staphylococcus aureus*, *Enterobacteriaceae*, anaerobic bacteria, and also *Gardnerella vaginalis.* The latter pathogen is difficult to detect, and in many publications it is hardly considered an infection-causing pathogen.

Frequency, pathogenesis, and therapy. Infections are 10 times more frequent after cesarean section than after vaginal delivery. The severe tissue trauma, combined with hematoma formation and stimulation by suture material, promotes the growth of cutaneous and vaginal pathogens introduced into the surgical areas of uterus, peritoneal cavity, and abdominal wall during surgical manipulation.

Depending on the evaluation of inflammatory parameters and on the group of patients, the incidence of infection without antibiotic prophylaxis after cesarean section ranges from 10–40 %.

Severe life-threatening infections are rare; their incidence is below 1 % even without antibiotic prophylaxis. The incidence of moderately severe infections associated with endometritis, disturbed wound healing, etc., is between 5–10 %.

All other infections are mild and can quickly be eliminated by early antibiotic treatment.

Despite the frequency of bacterial imbalances in the vagina (about 10 % of all pregnant women are affected), there have been only very few patients where this has led to severe abscess-forming infections.

Peritonitis

(See also p. 155)

In most patients, early surgical intervention with sufficient drainage and broad-spectrum antibiotic therapy will prevent loss of the uterus.

During the puerperal period, guarding is largely absent though it is usually a sign associated with peritonitis.

Disturbed Wound Healing

Pathogens. The primary cause of disturbed wound healing is *Staphylococcus aureus* (80–90 % of cases). Various species of *Streptococcus*, *Enterobacteriaceae* (especially *Escherichia coli*), and anaerobic bacteria may occasionally also be detected in case of disturbed wound healing in the abdominal wall.

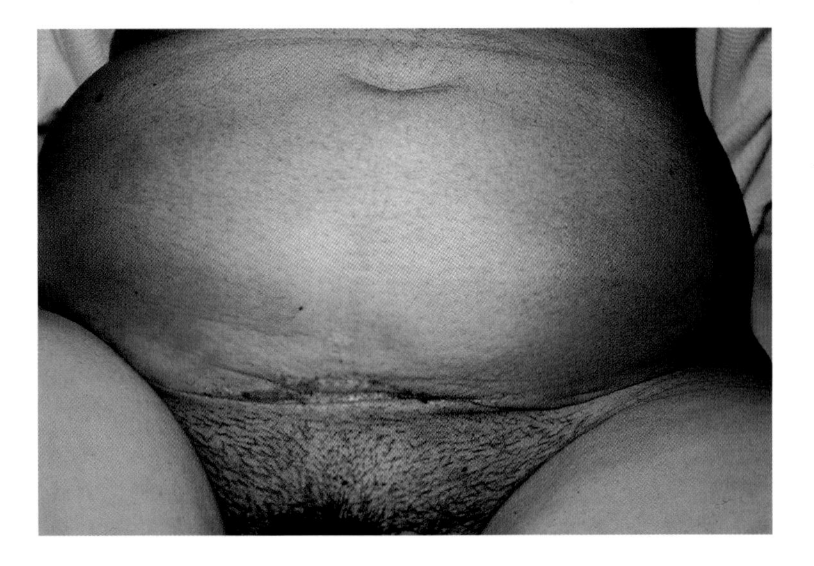

Fig. 9.**2** Wound infection of the suprapubic incision, caused by Staphylococcus aureus after cesarean section in a 22-year-old patient.

Frequency: About 5 % (0–15 %) without antibiotic prophylaxis, and 1–2 % with antibiotic prophylaxis.

Clinical picture. Redness of the abdominal wall (Fig. 9.**2**), pain in the suprapubic incision, and drainage of a secretion that is initially serous and later putrid. Fever may occur, though this is not necessarily the case.

Diagnosis. If the patient has fever, swabs from the cervical canal and also from the dehiscent suprapubic incision should be examined. Monitoring a febrile patient after cesarean section should include laboratory parameters like CRP, hemoglobin, leukocytes, and thrombocytes.

A rise in leukocyte numbers, even in the absence of fever, indicates an infection or abscess formation in the surgical area.

If the incision is red without dehiscence, it may be opened with the blunt cotton end of the swab in order to collect material for pathogen isolation.

Occasionally, the clinical and gynecological findings are difficult to evaluate. Resistances are not always identified unambiguously, and the surgical area itself is very sensitive during the first days.

Fever after cesarean section is not uncommon and is not always the sign of an advanced infection.

Therapy. The type of treatment depends on the patient's clinical condition and on the inflammatory parameters. If the CRP is increased 20 times and if there is fever early after surgery, antibiotic treatment needs to start immediately. The antibiotic selected should always be effective against group A streptococci and *Staphylococcus aureus*. Apart from that, antibiotic therapy should start on the second day of fever at the latest. It is essential to use a broad spectrum antibiotic that is β-lactamase resistant and also effective against most anaerobes, because of the multitude of possible pathogens.

In the most severe cases of infection, therapy should immediately start with combinations of antibiotics. If involvement of anaerobic bacteria is suspected, timely administration of 5-nitroimidazoles will prevent the infection from turning into a long-lasting, abscess-forming process.

Due to the heavy blood flow to the uterus after delivery, antibiotics reach high concentrations here. Hence, conservative treatment may be attempted first. If this does not lead to rapid improvement, early relaparotomy is advised.

Miscarriage with Fever

Miscarriage due to infection or fever is usually called septic miscarriage. In most cases, however, these are only local infections of the uterus. Nevertheless, these infections may easily turn into sepsis if the bacteria are highly pathogenic and the treatment inadequate. Because of the large port of entry, as is the puerperal uterus, early antibiotic therapy is particularly important. For pathogen detection and further treatment, a similar approach as with endometritis or puerperal sepsis is recommended.

Table 9.1 Risks of infection for the newborn

Infection	Measure
Herpes labialis	Only disinfection of the hands is required, caution if the mouth is infected
Chickenpox of the mother in the peripartal period	The child receives VZV-specific immune globulin, observation of child
Hepatitis B	Breast-feeding is permitted after vaccination
Hepatitis C	Breast-feeding should only be restricted when the viral load is high
Mastitis	Breast-feeding is generally permitted, but special attention is advised
CMV infection	Breast-feeding is permitted if the child is mature
HIV infection	No breast-feeding
Tuberculosis	Separation of mother and child only in case of open tuberculosis
Gastroenteritis	Breast-feeding is permitted after disinfection of the hands

Pathogen detection and therapy:

- blood cultures
- cervical swab for bacteriological cultures
- antibiotic treatment
- abrasion
- histology of abortion material (fetus), using special staining methods.

Late Miscarriage Without Fever

When looking for a cause of late abortion without fever, intense diagnostic procedures usually do not yield any results. One may therefore restrict the search to a few measures. A swab from the cervical canal may provide an explanation if special pathogens, such as *Listeria*, are detected; the risk of having another miscarriage due to this pathogen in the future is very low. Detection of intestinal bacteria is of no consequence now; however, these bacteria need to be considered during the next pregnancy. Histology should be performed in any case, because an explanation for the miscarriage may be discovered in individual patients.

Risk of Infection for the Newborn

There are almost no situations where it seems necessary to separate mother and child because of an infection, and there are only a few situations in which one should advise against breast-feeding (Table 9.1).

Water Birth and Risk of Infection

When keeping to the rules of hygiene, the risk for mother, child, and personnel is so low that infections are no argument against delivery under water.

Theoretically, infections may be transmitted from the mother to the child, from the mother to the obstetric team, and from the water to the child:

- risks originating from the mother: HIV, hepatitis
- risks originating from the water: inadequately cleaned bathtubs, bacterial colonization of the water-supply line with counts of more than 10^5/mL.

Water birth is not permitted if the mother has the following infections:

- HIV infection
- hepatitis (any hepatitis virus)
- gonorrhea
- staphyloderma (*Staphylococcus aureus*)
- pyoderma (group A streptococci)
- florid genital herpes
- other florid infections.

10 Inflammation of the Breast

Mastitis

Mastitis is a mostly unilateral inflammation of the mammary gland, associated with redness, pain, and fever (Fig. 10.**1**). In addition to puerperal mastitis, which is well known during childbed, and nonpuperperal mastitis, which occurs independently of pregnancy and breast-feeding, there are a number of rare infections and inflammations of the breast that, in part, only affect the skin and its appendages.

Puerperal Mastitis

Pathogen. *Staphylococcus aureus* is the pathogen in 95 % of patients. Rarely is any other pathogen detected, such as *Staphylococcus epidermidis*, *Streptococcus* species, *Proteus* species, *Escherichia coli*, *Klebsiella*, and very rarely anaerobes or even *Pseudomonas aeruginosa*. It is questionable whether the latter bacteria are actually involved in causing the inflammation.

Frequency. About 1 % of all puerpera suffer from mastitis. This figure may be higher or lower depending on whether retention of the milk is already classified as mastitis, or only the full-blown clinical picture with high fever or even abscess formation.

Transmission. In most cases, the pathogen is transmitted by the child's mouth, which during the first days of life becomes increasingly colonized with microbes from the child's surroundings. The infection is promoted through milk retention and formation of cracks in the region around the nipple.

It is very common that the milk becomes contaminated with the above-mentioned pathogens, although germ counts are usually in the lower range ($< 10^4$/mL). In about 80 % of all breast-fed children, *Staphylococcus aureus* can be detected in the oral cavity after a week.

Retention of milk promotes intense microbial multiplication, thus causing clinically manifest mastitis in isolated cases.

Hematogenous infections with the above-mentioned pathogens are rare.

Clinical picture. The clinical picture may vary from a mild painful redness (Fig. 10.**2**) to a highly febrile, very painful inflammation of the breast. Only in rare cases are both breasts affected (Fig. 10.**3**):

- mostly moderate inflammation, rarely causing severe malaise
- shaking chills and fever above 39 °C are common
- a mostly unilateral reddening associated with pain, hyperthermia, and induration.

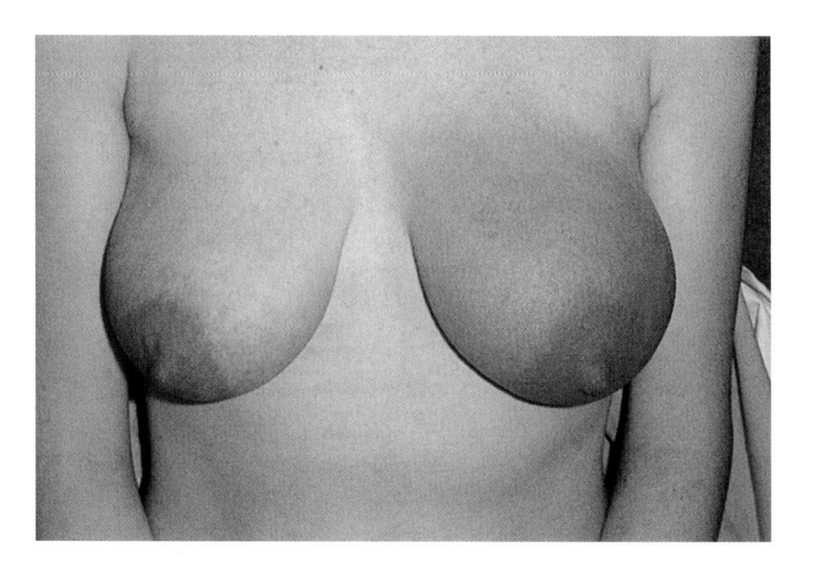

Fig. 10.**1** Acute puerperal mastitis in a 21-year-old patient three weeks after delivery.

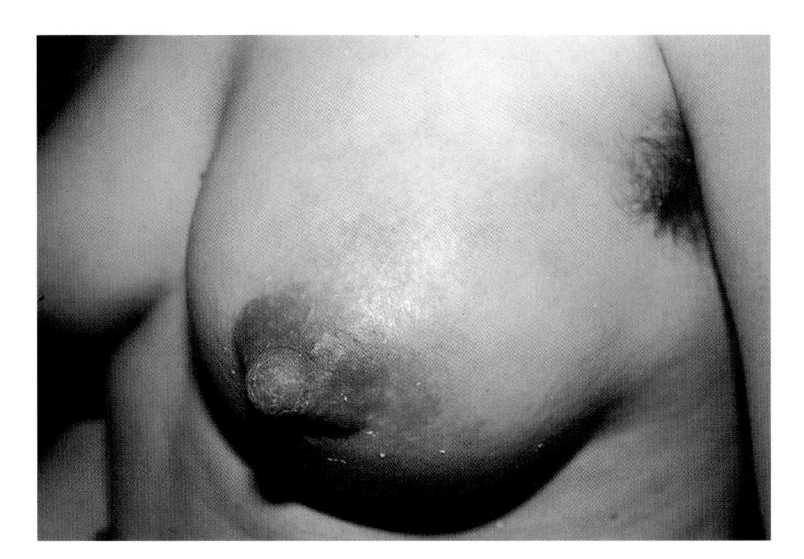

Fig. 10.**2** Puerperal mastitis in a 28-year-old patient.

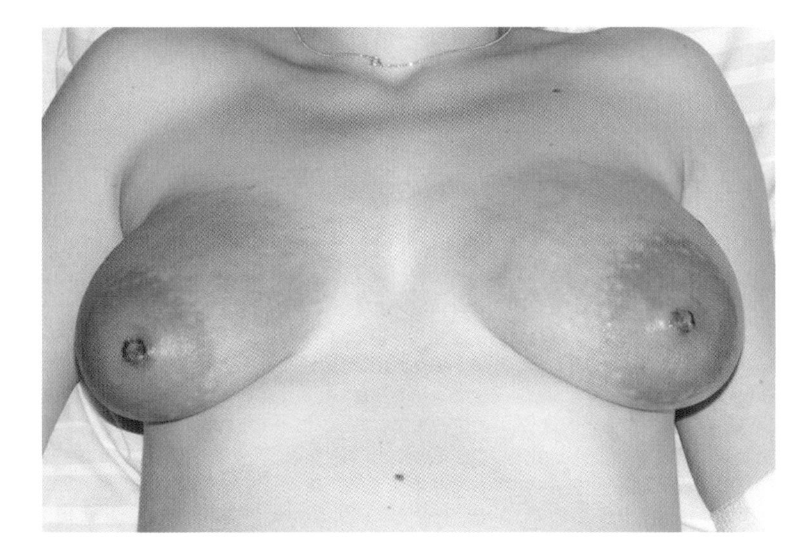

Fig. 10.**3** Puerperal mastitis in a 20-year-old patient three weeks after delivery. Conspicuous signs are the bilateral inflammation and the mammillae with yellow crusts *(Staphylococcus aureus)*.

Therapy. As in many areas of medicine, the recommendations are changing here.

Before the era of antibiotics, only topical treatment with alcohol packs and breast binding were available. Later, antibiotics have been added. With the introduction of prolactin inhibitors, it was initially hoped that one might rely completely on their effectiveness. Meanwhile, timely administration of antibiotics is regaining more importance. This clearly shows that there is a certain therapeutic range, especially because there is no clear dividing line between painful milk retention and infection.

Practical approach:

- drainage of the breast; the safest way to do this is with an electric milk pump (prescription)
- physical measures, such as a well-fitted nursing bra, breast binding, and cooling
- prolactin inhibitors, such as bromocriptine and lisuride, quickly lead to relaxation and reabsorption, while inflammatory signs are reduced; low doses prevent weaning
- early administration of antibiotics—penicillinase-resistant penicillins, such as oxacillin and flucloxacillin, or better right away cephalosporins of the second generation, such as cefotiam (i. v.) or cefuroxime axetil (orally)—shortens the time of infection, while breast-feeding is hardly affected. In severe cases with fever, cephalosporin of the second generation should always be given immediately. In mild cases, healing may be achieved with Co-Trimoxazole. Clindamycin or a macrolide antibiotic are also an option

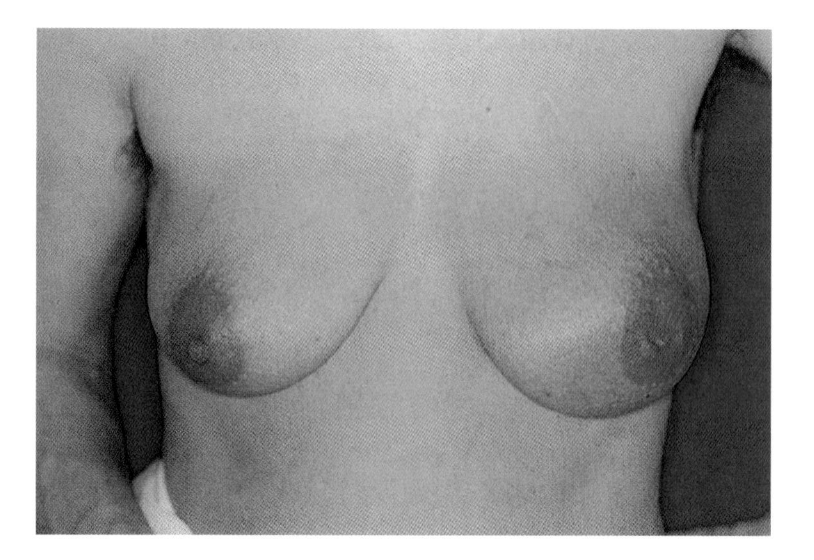

Fig. 10.**4** Nonpuerperal mastitis in a 36-year-old patient, with diffuse redness and swelling of the breast and a retracted mammillae.

- close clinical monitoring
- in severe cases, admission to a hospital.

Many women with mastitis wish to continue breast-feeding, and there is nothing that advises against it. The dose and duration of any prolactin inhibitor need to be adjusted so that the flow of milk does not stop completely.

Antibiotics should only be administered as long as symptoms are present.

Abscess-forming Mastitis

If treatment is too late or inadequate, the inflammation may advance to a point where conservative measures no longer bring healing or an abscess has already formed.

Blood flow to the breast can be improved by red light, which promotes healing or necrolysis of the focus of inflammation.

If an abscess is detected, the pus needs to be drained. This is now increasingly performed by puncturing the abscess cavity under ultrasonic guidance and antibiotic treatment. Good results have been reported with this method.

In the past, when effective antibiotics were not available, the right approach was surgery. This involved perimamillary incision, blunt opening of the abscess cavities, and counterincision in the submammary fold followed by drainage and daily rinsing. Today, this approach is being increasingly abandoned, although the cosmetic results have been surprisingly good.

Therapeutic options:

- antibiotics + puncture of the abscess cavities (may be performed repeatedly)
- antibiotics + incision of the abscess cavity
- antibiotics + incision of the abscess cavity + drainage
- antibiotics + incision of the abscess cavity + counterincision + drainage.

Mastitis and Breast-feeding

Surprisingly, uptake of mother's milk rich in staphylococci only rarely causes infection of the child. Feeding at the diseased breast should only be interrupted for safety reasons during the acute phase of infection, namely, when high bacterial counts ($> 10^5$/mL) are detected.

Experience has shown that many women who continued breast-feeding despite clear signs of inflammation have hardly ever infected their child. It is therefore not wise to forbid breast-feeding in general; there is now an increasing tendency toward continuation of breast-feeding.

Careful observation and monitoring of the child are nevertheless advised.

In addition, one should keep in mind that high counts of *Staphylococcus aureus* are already detected in the mother's milk in the majority of women with preclinical inflammation.

Nonpuerperal Mastitis

In the majority of patients, nonpuerperal mastitis is localized (Figs. 10.**4**, 10.**5**) yet long lasting, protracting in some patients over many years in a chronic recurrent form.

Pathogens. It is not known whether there really is such a thing as nonbacterial mastitis or mastitis without a pathogen (viruses and parasites are also possible causes). The lack of pathogen detection is by no means evidence that microbes are not involved.

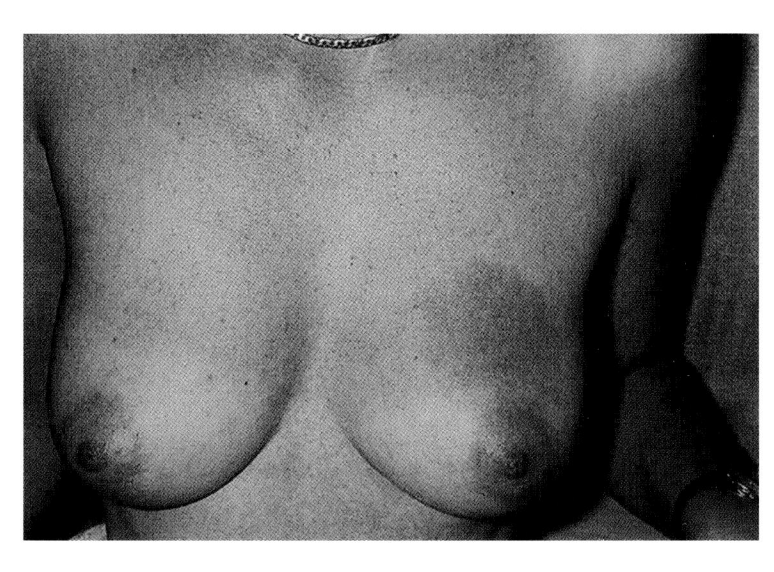

Fig. 10.**5** Nonpuerperal mastitis in a 26-year-old patient, with a circumscribed area of redness.

Frequently detected pathogens:
- *Staphylococcus aureus* (40–50 %)
- coagulase-negative staphylococci, which belong to the flora of the skin (40 %)
- anaerobe bacteria (10–20 %)
- *Escherichia coli* (< 5 %)
- *Streptococcus* species (< 5 %)
- *Proteus mirabilis* (< 5 %).

Cultures often reveal several microbes. Due to the low counts, it is sometimes difficult to decide whether a certain type of microbes represents only a contaminating germ or a pathogen involved in the inflammation.

Frequency and age distribution. Nonpuerperal mastitis affects 0.1–1 % of gynecological patients. The age distribution corresponds roughly to that of puerperal mastitis, i. e., most patients are between 20 and 35 years old.

Clinical picture and pathogenesis. The inflammation is mostly localized and near the mammilla. It comes and goes, being partly associated with necrolysis, external drainage of a small abscess cavity, and fistula formation.

The inflammation is caused by secretory congestion of the efferent glandular ducts near the mammilla. This, in turn, is due to squamous cell metaplasia with keratinization and increasingly scarlike lesions resulting from previous episodes of inflammation.

Therapy:
- prolactin inhibitors (continuous use over weeks or months)
- systemic administration of antibiotics, depending on the pathogen
- surgical approach, with distal cone-shaped milk-duct resection promising the best results; nevertheless, relapses are common.

Tuberculous Mastitis

This form of mastitis is 10–100 times more common in women from Africa and Asia (India, Thailand). In Germany, it is a rare event and therefore difficult to diagnose.

Diagnosis:
- histology
- microbiology (PCR)
- tuberculin skin test.

Other Forms of Inflammation and Differential Diagnosis

Inflammatory Mammary Carcinoma

The patient's history, the course of the disease, and the clinical picture may indicate an inflammatory mammary carcinoma. Redness of the skin, minor pain or no pain at all, diffuse hardening of the breast, and the lack of response to antibiotics are characteristic signs.

This is especially true during pregnancy or after delivery, when the carcinoma often looks like a mild mastitis that hardly needs any treatment. A carcinoma is suspected when the entire breast is firm, hardly painful, and only slightly reddened (Fig. 10.**6**).

Diagnosis:
- mammography is difficult to evaluate and therefore not very convincing

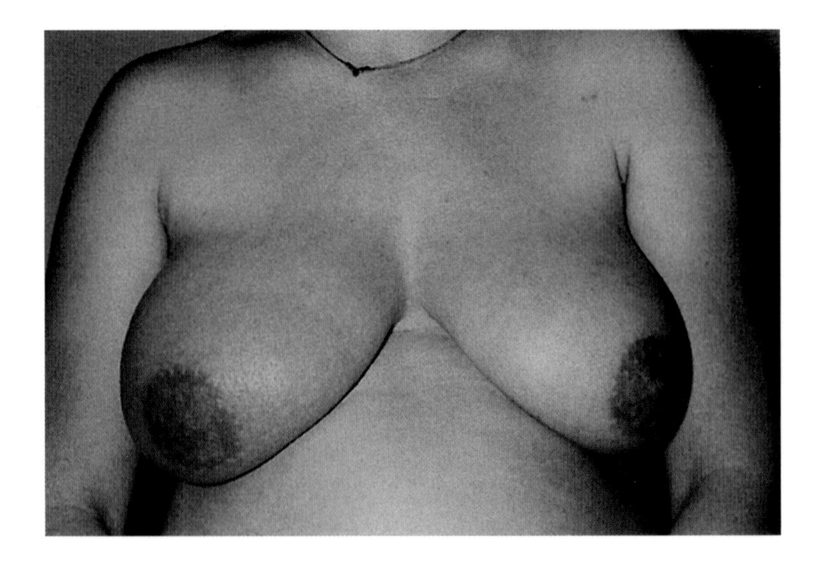

Fig. 10.**6** Inflammatory mammary carcinoma in a 23-year-old patient in the 27th week of pregnancy. Cesarean section in the 34th week of pregnancy. The patient died two years later despite treatment.

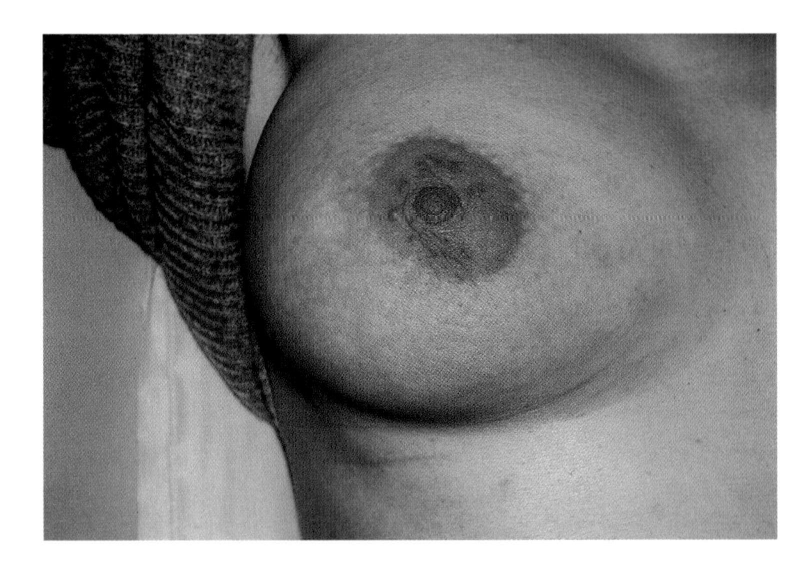

Fig. 10.**7** Erythema of the breast in a 25-year-old patient during the 12th week of pregnancy.

- mammasonography has good chances for providing a clue
- fine-needle biopsy is highly convincing
- exploratory excision confirms the diagnosis.

Erythema of the Breast

A rare disorder, occurring predominantly during pregnancy.

Clinical picture. Redness and hyperthermia of the skin in the lower half of the breast (Fig. 10.**7**), usually bilateral, with only little pain. No lumps in the breast.

Diagnosis:

- palpation
- CRP (exclusion test)
- sonography.

Therapy. No treatment, soothing measures, support of the breast by a well-fitted bra.

Erysipelas of the Breast

The clear demarcation of a painful redness of the skin is indicative of erysipelas (Fig. 10.**8**). Routine detection of the pathogen (group A streptococci) is not possible. Diagnosis is established clinically

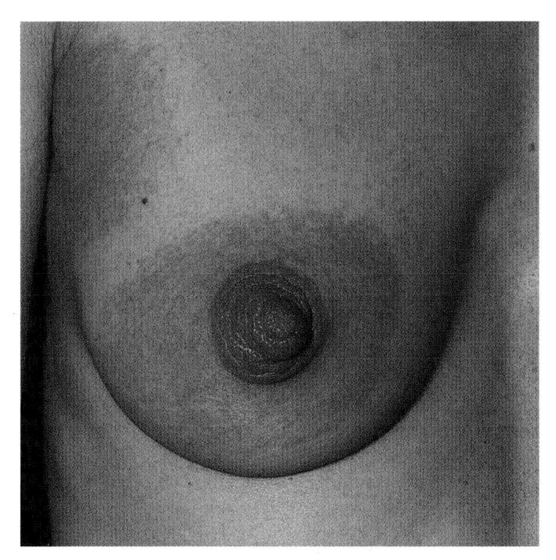

Fig. 10.**8** Erysipelas of the right breast (group A streptococci) in a 36-year-old patient without a known risk factor.

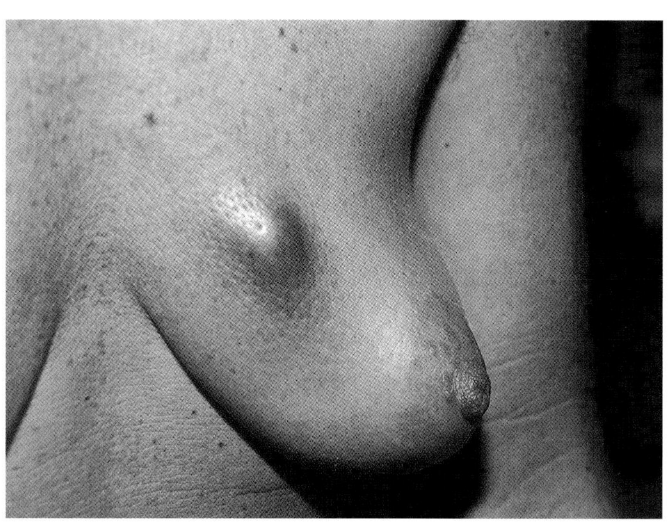

Fig. 10.**9** Granulomatous mastitis in a 65-year-old patient. The lesion caused by biopsy healed only after cortisone treatment.

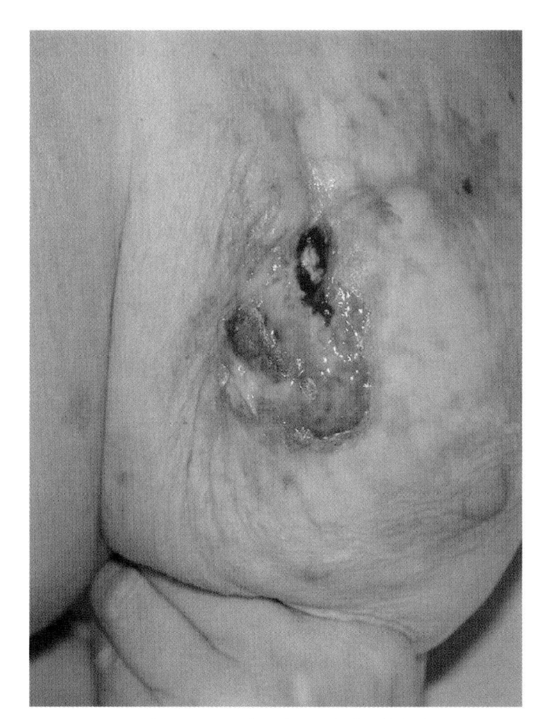

Fig. 10.**10** Abscess in the skin of the left breast of a 45-year-old patient.

and confirmed by the good response to penicillins (10 days).

Furuncle of the Breast

Rare localization of an abscess caused by *Staphylococcus aureus*, originating from sebaceous glands and hair follicles (Fig. 10.**9**).

Granulomatous Mastitis

This rare disease is characterized by the lack of wound healing after a biopsy (Fig. 10.**10**) or breast surgery, usually because mammary carcinoma has been suspected. The typical finding is that repeated biopsies do not reveal any clues for a malignancy, only for inflammation, and that antibiotics do not lead to healing either. Healing is only achieved by systemic treatment with high doses of cortisone.

Dermatitis of the Mammillae

Staphylococcus aureus infection of skin lesions caused by a chafing bra or continuous rubbing may lead to a painful inflammation (Fig. 10.**11**) that is usually bilateral. The inflammation may become chronic if treatment is delayed, thus making the diagnosis more difficult due to additional skin lesions.

Diagnosis. Microbiological cultures from a swab taken with a moist cotton probe.

Therapy. Polyvidone–iodine (PVP–I) ointment.
If healing does not come soon:
- antibiotic over eight days, such as cefuroxime axetil (3 × 500 mg per day)
- possibly cortisone ointment or cream over several days
- avoidance of skin lesions.

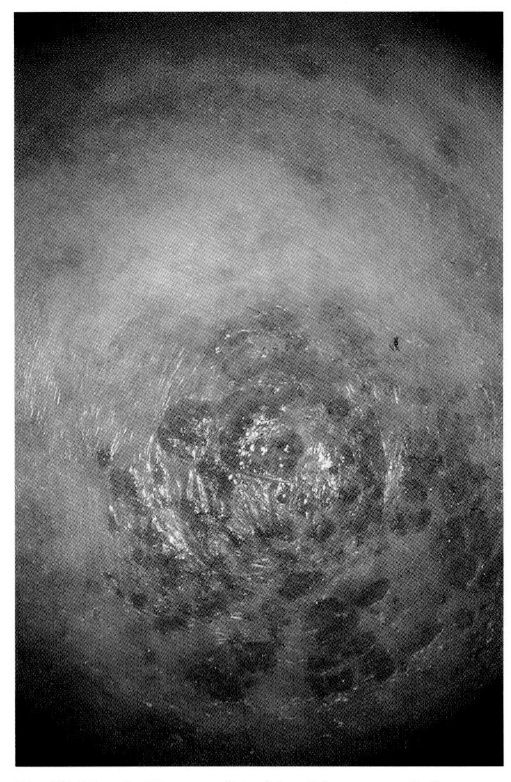

Fig. 10.**11** A 12-year-old girl with severe inflammation of both mammillae due to *Staphylococcus aureus*; condition after several topical and systemic treatment attempts.

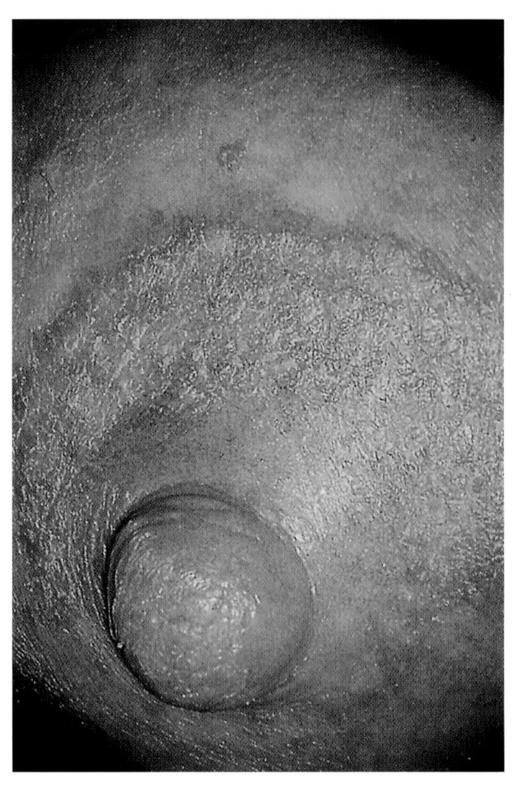

Fig. 10.**12** Postpartum candidiasis of the mammilla in a 30-year-old breast-feeding patient.

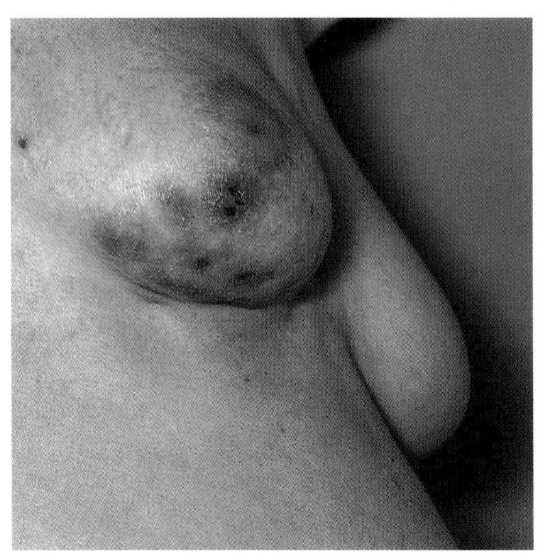

Fig. 10.**13** Chronic mastitis during the 28th week of pregnancy in a 32-year-old patient with sarcoidosis. Treatment was initially with antibiotics in the absence of pathogen detection, later with prednisone; only then did the condition improve.

Candidiasis of the Mammillae

Candida infection of the nipple and its areola (Fig. 10.**12**) during the breast-feeding period is a rare event.

Clinical picture. Redness with dry scaling and a burning or itching sensation.

Diagnosis. Fungal culture from a swab taken with a moist cotton probe.

Therapy. Topical antimycotic, such as clotrimazole.

Chronic Mastitis During Pregnancy with Sarcoidosis

When mastitis does not heal under antibiotic treatment, one should always consider other causes of the inflammation. Apart from malignancy, which needs to be excluded by a biopsy, several immune diseases should be taken into consideration. In a pregnant patient with sarcoidosis (benign lymphogranulomatosis), the

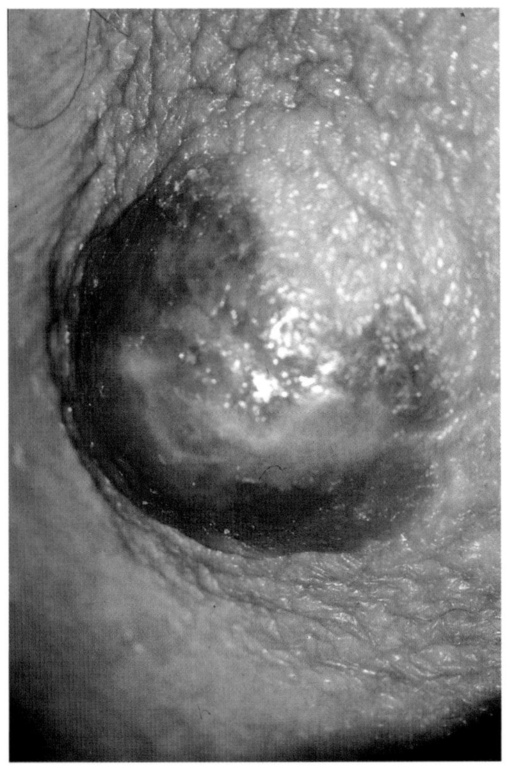

Fig. 10.**14** Chronic inflammation of the mammilla in a 52-year-old patient; the biopsy revealed Paget disease.

mastitis with multiple spontaneous perforation sites (Fig. 10.**13**) did not heal despite several weeks of antibiotic treatment. The condition only improved under subsequent treatment with prednisone.

Chronic Redness of the Mammilla

If a suspected inflammation of the mammilla does not heal, especially when it is unilateral, one should always take a biopsy. The cause may be Paget disease (Fig. 10.**14**).

11 Sexually Transmitted Infections

Definition and Forms

These infections include the four classic venereal diseases, which have been notifiable in the past, as well as the many other infections caused by pathogens transmitted through close mucosal contact during sexual activity.

The only data available on the frequency of these diseases are those for the four notifiable infections. These diseases had to be reported because they lead to serious sequelae, which can now be avoided by antibiotic treatment.

Venereal diseases are those leading to symptoms of the genitals, and they are acquired through sexual activity. Of course, they include many more diseases than the four classic ones. Because of the negative connotation, the term "venereal disease (VD)" is rarely used today and has been replaced by "sexually transmitted disease (STD)."

Here, we will discuss only those STDs in more detail that have not yet been described elsewhere in this book.

Table 11.**1** provides an overview of various infections.

Gonorrhea

Gonorrhea (p. 138) is the most common of formerly notifiable sexually transmitted diseases in Europe. The incidence in gynecological patients lies between 0.05–0.5 %, depending on the patient group and the clinic.

Syphilis (Lues)

Syphilis (p. 100) is certainly the most serious of sexually transmitted diseases. In Europe, the incidence is less than three reported cases per 100 000 people. Only a third of these are women.

Lymphogranuloma venereum (LGV)

Pathogen. *Chlamydia trachomatis*, serotypes L_1–L_3.

Frequency. Lymphogranuloma venereum is very rare in temperate climates. The incidence is one reported case per one million people.

Table 11.**1** Sexually and nonsexually transmitted infections and differential diagnosis of various dermatoses

1. Classic venereal diseases	– gonorrhea, syphilis, lymphogranuloma venereum, chancroid
2. Other sexually transmitted diseases of the genitals	– trichomoniasis, chlamydial (serum group D–K infection), primary genital herpes, acuminate condyloma (papillomaviruses), phthiriasis (pubic lice), granuloma inguinale
3. Pathogens/infections that may be sexually transmitted	– *Candida albicans*, bacterial vaginosis, *Gardnerella vaginalis*, *Mobiluncus*, *Bacteroides* species, group A streptococci, scabies (mites), molluscum contagiosum
4. Infections that are mostly sexually transmitted but cause disease in other organs	– AIDS (HIV), hepatitis B, possibly hepatitis C*, cytomegalic inclusion disease
5. Infections of the genitals without sexual transmission	– recurrent genital herpes, erysipelas (group A streptococci), erythrasma (*Corynebacterium minutissimum*), folliculitis (staphylococci), schistosomiasis
6. Differential diagnosis of diseases that should be considered	– allergic contact eczema, drug exanthema, Behçet syndrome, dermatitis herpetiformis (Duhring disease), Stevens–Johnson syndrome, lichen planus of the mucosae, mycosis fungoides, pityriasis rosea, psoriasis, lichen sclerosus, lichen simplex chronicus

* A rare infection.

Incubation time. Six to 14 days, or longer.

Pathogenesis and clinical picture. The disease is characterized by a local vesicular lesion that quickly ulcerates and heals. This is followed by painful enlargement of the inguinal lymph nodes, which is associated with necrolysis, redness, and increasing pus formation in the infected area. Fever, malaise, and pain in the joints may occur. Anorexia, vomiting, and back pain are also observed occasionally.

The infection causes chronic purulent lymphangitis, thus leading to the obstruction of lymph vessels. This results in severe edema with ulceration, fistula formation, and finally elephantiasis of the leg or affected region.

Diagnosis:
- clinical picture
- *serology:* Frei test, CFR, ELISA, fluorescence test (cross-reaction with other *Chlamydia* species)
- *culture:* available only in very few centers around the world.

Therapy. Doxycycline (200 mg per day) and other antibiotics effective against chlamydial infections (see p. 137). Surgery is required at a late stage.

Chancroid (Venereal Ulcer)

Pathogen. *Haemophilus ducreyi.*

Frequency. Chancroid is slightly more common, with a frequency of four cases per one million people, but it is still so rare that a physician will hardly see this disease during his or her lifetime.

Due to ulceration and leukorrhea, chancroid is a cofactor in the transmission of HIV in Africa and Asia.

Incubation time. Three to seven days.

Pathogenesis and clinical picture. Small painful papules appear, which quickly disintegrate and turn into ulcers with ragged, undermined borders. The ulcers are flat and soft, painful, and surrounded by a red border. They vary in size and may become confluent. Gangrenous erosion may lead to considerable tissue destruction. The inguinal lymph nodes are also affected, become larger, and finally form abscesses. Possible sequelae are urethral stricture and urethral fistulae.

Diagnosis:
- clinical picture
- culture of *Haemophilus ducreyi*
- microscopic detection of bacteria arranged in a fishnetlike pattern.

As with all sexually transmitted diseases, additional serology for syphilis should be carried out immediately as well as four to 12 weeks after infection. This is important because syphilis may coexist with chancroid and cause severe sequelae if left untreated.

Therapy:
- erythromycin (4 × 500 mg per day orally, for seven days)
- fluoroquinolones (e. g., ciprofloxacin 2 × 500 mg per day orally, for three days)
- azithromycin (1 × 1 g orally)
- ceftriaxone (1 × 250 mg i.m.).

Granuloma Inguinale

Granuloma inguinale, also called granuloma venereum, is a very rare sexually transmitted disease and hardly occurs in Europe.

This is a chronic granulomatous disease of the genital region. It is probably caused by a rod-shaped bacterium called *Calymmatobacterium granulomatis.* The disease begins as a single node, spreads slowly but steadily, and finally covers the entire genitals. There are ulcerating and verrucous forms. The healing process is slow and leads to scar formation.

Diagnosis:
- clinical picture without pathogen detection (exclusion diagnosis)
- Giemsa staining of smear preparations reveals capsulated bacteria (Donovan bodies) in leukocytes.

Therapy:
- doxycycline (200 mg per day, for two weeks)
- erythromycin (4 × 500 mg per day, for two to four weeks)
- Co-Trimoxazole (2 × 500 mg per day, for two weeks)
- azithromycin (1 × 1 g per week, for four weeks).

12 Helminthic Infections

Worm Species and Their Frequencies

Occasionally, a gynecologist is confronted with worms crawling about in the anal region or on the vulva. These are usually pinworms (*Enterobius [Oxyuris] vermicularis*), also called oxyurids. They are the most common worms in temperate climates and belong to the nematodes, which cause about 90% of all helminthic diseases.

Less common in temperate climates are cestodes, which cause about 9% of helminthic diseases.

Trematodes cause only 1% of helminthic diseases in temperate climates.

Pinworms (Oxyurids)

Pathogen, transmission, and clinical picture. The pinworm *Enterobius (Oxyuris) vermicularis* is the most common worm species in temperate climates. Pinworms are 3–12 mm long and cause anal itching (Fig. 12.**1**). They are transmitted by the fecal–oral route. Scratching of the itching area leads to oral uptake of the eggs deposited in the perianal region. The worms live in the ileocecum and may remain for decades as commensal parasites with the affected person. Fertile females migrate down the colon and migrate from the rectum to the outside where they deposit masses of eggs in the perianal region.

Infestation of the genitals is very rare, but it may lead to oxyuriasis of the fallopian tubes. The clinical picture is adnexitis that does not respond to antibiotics. The diagnosis is usually established by chance through histology.

Diagnosis. Pinworm infestation is diagnosed by identification of tiny worms in the stool. When searching intensely under the colposcope, the worms are also found in the perianal or vulvar region (Fig. 12.**2**). Perianal detection is accomplished by attaching an adhesive tape to the anal region, pulling it off, and mounting it on a slide that is then investigated for eggs under the microscope (Fig. 12.**3**).

In rare cases, oxyurid eggs may also be observed in cytological smears.

Therapy:

- mebendazole (Vermox), 1 × 100 mg per day for three days (the single-dose treatment of the past has been abandoned because resistance may develop)
- pyrantel pamoate (Antiminth), a single dose of 10 mg/kg body weight
- pyrvinium embonate (Molevac); it gives the stool a red color and is only effective against oxyurids.

Single dose treatment leads to discharge of the pinworms. Additional hygienic measures are required (hand washing, washing laundry in boiling water) to avoid reinfection through eggs.

Treatment of worm infestation during **pregnancy** may be required only occasionally, since transmission between humans takes place only via mature pinworms. Single dose treatment should be administered just before delivery. There are no special risks for the child because the drug is hardly resorbed.

Other Worm Species in Temperate Climates

Roundworm (*Ascaris lumbricoides*)

This nematode reaches a length of 15–40 cm. Ascarids may or may not cause nonspecific symptoms, such as nausea, malaise, weight loss, and other complaints.

Whipworm (*Trichuris trichiura*)

This nematode is 3–5 cm long.

Transmission. Both nematode species are transmitted by eating raw lettuce or strawberries that have been fertilized with liquid manure.

Tapeworms

The beef tapeworm *(Taenia saginata)* is the most common cestode in Europe. It is transmitted by

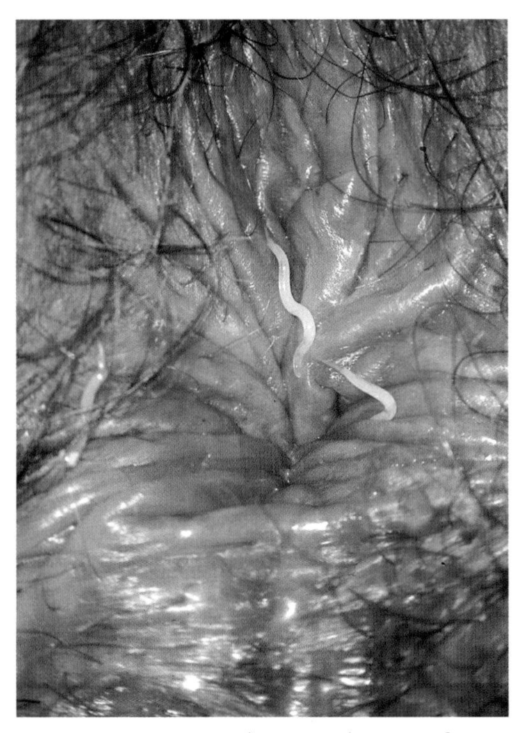

Fig. 12.**1** Pinworms in the perianal region of a 38-year-old patient.

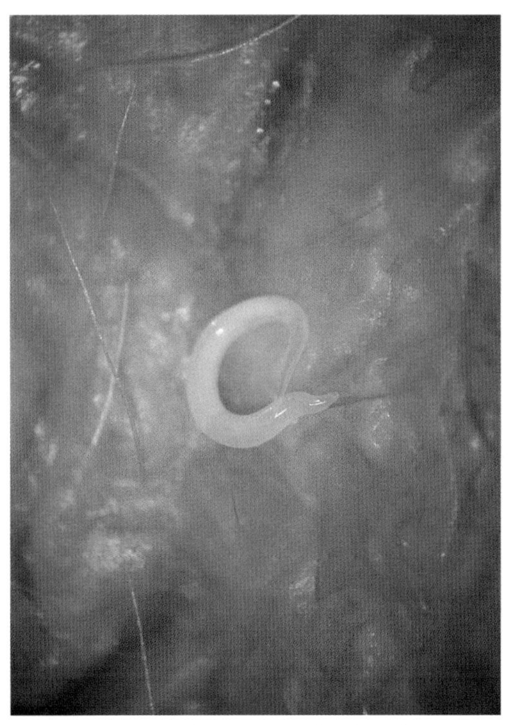

Fig. 12.**2** Pinworm in the perineal region of a 54-year-old patient with lichen sclerosus, chronic itching, and rhagades.

eating raw or insufficiently roasted beef that contains the larval form (cysticercus).

Diagnosis. Identification of a helminthic disease is usually based on the microscopic detection of eggs in the stool. In the presence of a tapeworm, segments of the worm (proglottids) may be found in the feces as well. Eosinophilia of the blood count or an increase in IgE antibodies may indicate an infection with worms.

Therapy. There are several anthelmintic preparations on the market. They have a wide spectrum of activity and are effective against the majority of worm species, for example:

- mebendazole (Vermox), 1 × 100 mg per day for three days (the single-dose treatment of the past has been abandoned because resistance may develop)
- pyrantel pamoate (Antiminth), a single dose of 10 mg/kg body weight
- albendazole (Albenza).

In case of pinworm and roundworm infestation, single-dose treatment (or better, three days of treatment) is sufficient. Treatment of whipworm infestation requires experimenting with varying anthelmintics.

The best treatment of the beef tapeworm is niclosamide (Yomesan).

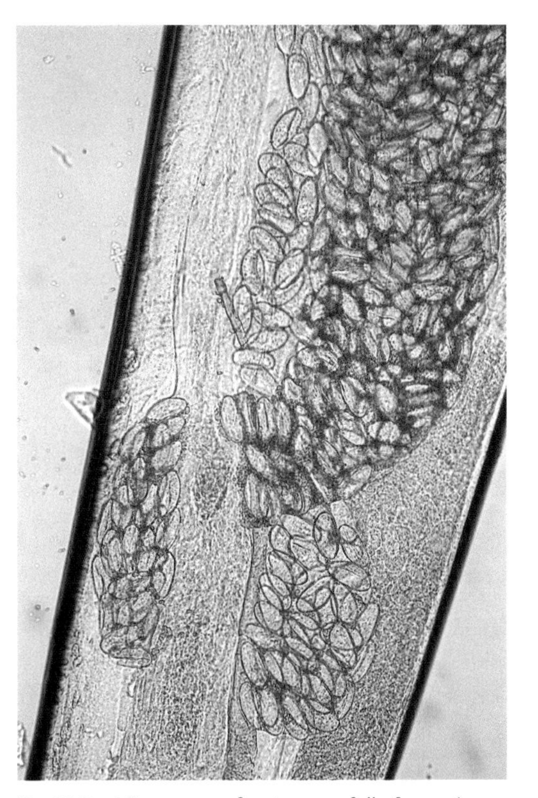

Fig. 12.**3** Microscopy of a pinworm full of eggs (magnification 400×).

Fig. 12.**4** Schistosomiasis of the vulva in a 30-year-old patient, one year after taking a bath in Lake Malawi.

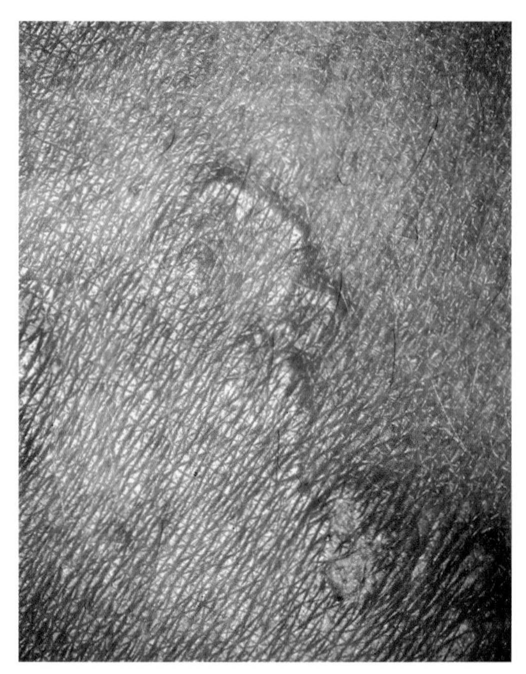

Fig. 12.**6** Cutaneous larva migrans (creeping eruption) in a 32-year-old patient after a stay in India where she had contact with dogs at the beach.

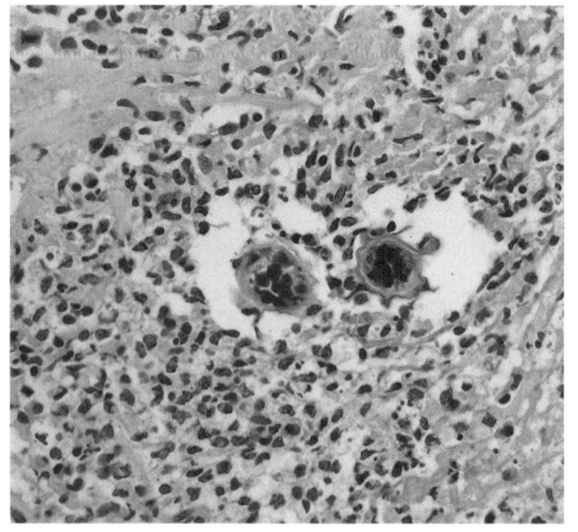

Fig. 12.**5** The same patient as in Fig. 12.**4**, histology of the biopsy leading to the detection of *Schistosoma hematobium.*

Worm Infections Acquired in the Tropics

Schistosomiasis

This is one of the most common tropical diseases. It is caused by trematodes of the genus *Schistosoma*, which are widely distributed in Africa. Occasionally, *Schistosoma hematobium* is picked up during a vacation in southern Africa. Treatment is essential; otherwise, there will be serious sequelae in the genitourinary tract (urinary schistosomiasis).

An unusual case with *Schistosoma* infestation of the vulva was observed in our clinic (Fig. 12.**4**). Changes in the vulvar region appeared only one year after a stay in Malawi. Serological examination of the entire tourist party revealed that all participants had been infected. They were immediately treated.

Diagnosis:

- direct detection of eggs in the feces and urine (successful after 10 weeks, at the earliest)
- serology (carried out in a tropical institute)
- eosinophilia
- biopsy with detection of the pathogen (Fig. 12.**5**).

Therapy. Praziquantel (Biltricide), a single dose of 40 mg/kg body weight.

Strongyloidiasis/Cutaneous Larva Migrans

The strongyloid threadworm (*Strongyloides [Anguillula] stercoralis*) is a small intestinal nematode (2–3 mm long). Its larvae burrow into the skin, thus creating characteristic subcutaneous channels (Fig. 12.**6**). Here, too, eosinophilia is a typical sign of infestation. The infection is treated with ivermectin (Stromectol, 200 mg/kg body weight).

13 Infections of Other Body Regions

Pneumonia

The main pathogens are pneumococci. They are widely distributed, and every second person carries them in the nasopharyngeal space without having symptoms.

Pneumococcal infections are particularly dangerous for splenectomized patients, the elderly, or other individuals with a weak immune system. The lethality of pneumococcal bacteremia is 30%, or even 50% in persons over 60. Vaccination will especially benefit those at high risk.

The most common pathogens of pneumonia are listed in Table 13.**1**.

Appendicitis

This is a common bacterial infection of the vermiform appendix, which is promoted by obstructing events. Occasionally, it is difficult to distinguish it from adnexal processes by differential diagnosis. It should therefore always be considered if there is pain on the right side of the lower abdomen. On the other hand, a gynecological examination should take place before appendectomy is performed in a young woman. Pain upon abrupt release of steady pressure (rebound tenderness) at McBurney point is characteristic for appendicitis, whereas pelvic inflammatory disease is almost always associated with cervicitis and purulent cervical secretion. Clear, threadable cervical secretion and normal inflammatory parameters indicate more a follicular cyst, rupture of an ovarian follicle, or something else. Examination by ultrasound will help to establish a diagnosis.

Appendicitis during pregnancy is fairly rare, yet it is sometimes very difficult to diagnose because of the upward shift of the appendix due to the enlarged uterus.

Arthritis

Some pathogens of genital infection cause arthritis as a late sequela. The most important pathogens of arthritis include:

- gonococci
- *Chlamydia trachomatis* (D-K) and *Chlamydia pneumoniae*
- *Borrelia*
- parvovirus B19 virus (erythema infectiosum)
- *Yersinia* and *Campylobacter.*

It is recommended that serological diagnosis and, if necessary, antibiotic treatment should precede any expensive diagnostic procedures (arthroscopy) or therapeutic measures (intra-articular injections).

Table 13.**1** Pathogens of pneumonia

Pathogens	Drugs of first choice	Drugs of second choice
Streptococcus pneumoniae (pneumococci)	Cephalosporins (2nd/3rd generations)	Macrolides
Haemophilus influenzae	Amoxicillin	Cephalosporins
Moraxella catarrhalis	Ampicillin + β-lactamase inhibitor	Cefuroxime
Staphylococci	Cephalosporins (2nd/3rd generations)	Fluoroquinolones
Klebsiella pneumoniae	Cephalosporins (2nd/3rd generations)	
Enterobacteriaceae	Carbapenems	
Pathogens of atypical pneumonia include:		
Chlamydia pneumoniae	Azithromycin	Doxycycline
Mycoplasmas	Azithromycin	Doxycycline
Legionella	Azithromycin	Macrolides

14 Self-inflicted Infections

Munchausen Syndrome

Occasionally, one may see patients with diseases, including recurrent infections, for which there is initially no explanation and which do not fit easily into common clinical experience. There is often a discrepancy between the relatively good condition of the patient and the symptoms. The clinical pictures include recurrent abscess formation, skin lesions, fever, pathogen detection in the blood, and other findings. Frequently, these patients come from a medical background. It takes a lot of experience to recognize the underlying cause and usually a very long time before such factitious infections are uncovered. Although this is a rare diagnosis, it is nevertheless not so rare that one is not confronted with such a patient at some time or other. Careful observation and a cautious approach to the patient's problems are advised.

Examples of factitious infections:

- factitious mastitis
- factitious vulvitis (Figs. 14.**1**, 14.**2**)
- factitious sepsis
- wound infection.

The possibility of artificial infection by the patient herself should be considered with every chronic infection that, for no obvious reason, does not heal and repeatedly reoccurs with varying pathogens being involved.

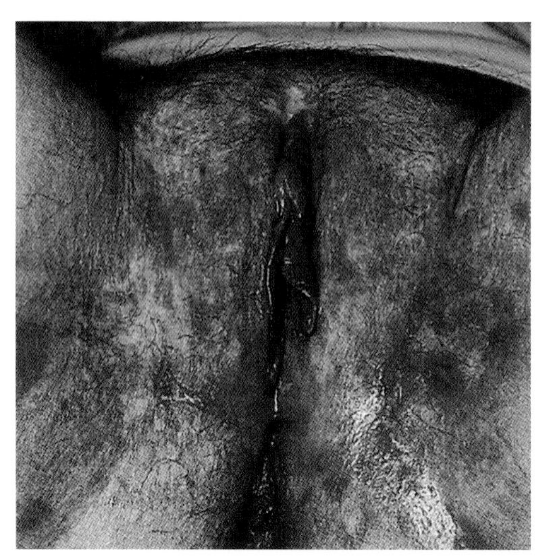

Fig. 14.**1** Factitious vulvitis in a 60-year-old patient. self-inflicted injuries with detection of *Staphylococcus aureus*, caused by pinching of the vulvar skin. Similar injuries also in the face.

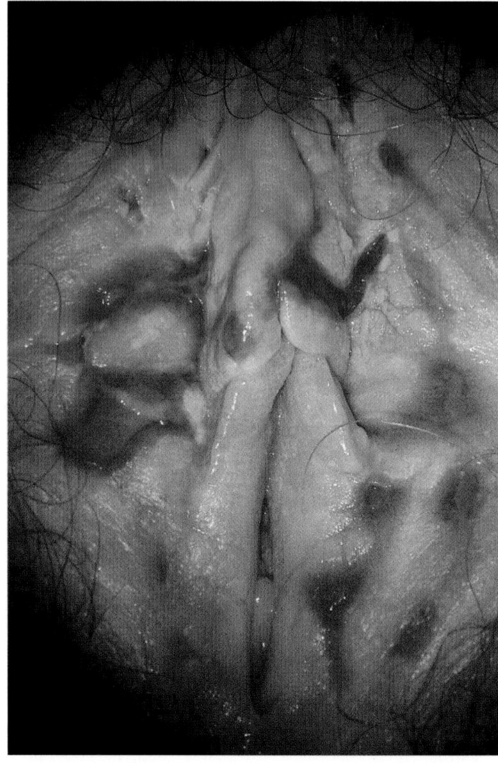

Fig. 14.**2** Factitious vulvitis in a 14-year-old girl, persisting over the last six months. The diagnosis was established based on the denial of pain and on the fact that healing occurred after an extensive interview.

15 Prevention of Infections

Infection Risks and Countermeasures

The risk of infection associated with invasive procedures, such as venipuncture, bladder catheter, surgical interventions, delivery, depends on the virulence of the pathogen (both obligatory or facultative pathogens) and on the germ count, in particular.

The majority of infections after surgical intervention are caused by facultative pathogens originating from the patient herself. These pathogens are normally present at low counts in the external genital region and on the skin of every person.

Whether or not this will lead to an infection depends primarily on how many germs are introduced into the wound, on the growth conditions the germs find there, and on the response of the body's immune system.

By using prophylactic procedures with respect to nursing or hygiene, and also by antibiotic prophylaxis, the number of bacteria can be kept so low that the infection risk remains low as well.

No single method can achieve complete absence of germs in regions of the skin, intestines, and genitals—only a reduction in the number of germs. As far as that goes, the various procedures of disinfection, catheter hygiene, and wound care will have to supplement antibiotic prophylaxis and therapy.

Venipuncture and Maintenance of a Venous Catheter

Disinfection of the skin. The skin needs to be disinfected *chemically* and *mechanically*. High-proof alcohol solutions are commonly used to degrease the skin and inactivate bacteria. Since spores are able to survive in 70% alcohol, mixtures of 60% isopropyl alcohol and antiseptics like phenylphenol have gained acceptance.

Just spraying the skin area with disinfectant is not good enough. The commercially available spray pumps should only serve to moisten the swab, which is then used for rubbing the disinfectant into the skin.

Every time an indwelling catheter is put in place, the disinfectant needs to be applied several times (for two to four minutes), since the inactivation of bacteria depends on the time of application.

Since the body is able to deal with low numbers of bacteria introduced, this is not so important during the usual collection of blood from immunocompetent patients.

However, the situation is quite different when applying an **indwelling (intravenous) catheter**. These plastic catheters may become contaminated with coagulase-negative staphylococci, especially *Staphylococcus epidermidis*. Less common is a contamination with *Candida* or *Enterobacteriaceae*, such as *Pseudomonas aeruginosa*.

Especially coagulase-negative staphylococci are able to adhere to the polymer surface of the catheter, where they multiply and produce an extracellular mucous substance, thus protecting themselves against immune defenses and antibiotics. The bacteremia originating from the catheter tip may then lead to chronic sepsis (catheter sepsis).

A peripheral venous catheter should therefore only be applied after careful disinfection and under aseptic conditions. It should not stay in place for longer than 24–48 hours, at the most.

Central venous catheters, which are supposed to remain for several days, must be applied with special care and under strictly aseptic conditions with surgical covering.

Any venous catheter put in place in an emergency should be changed after 12 hours, at the latest.

Disinfection Prior to Surgical Interventions

There is no ideal disinfectant for the mucosa. So far, polyvidone–iodine proved to be the most suitable agent. It is marketed in alcoholic form for the disinfection of skin. This normal solution should be diluted when used for disinfection of the vagina. The time of application should be at least five minutes. Chlorohexidine is another effective antiseptic.

One should keep in mind that all disinfection procedures reduce only the amount of germs on the surface, and that a considerable number of microbes will recolonize the skin within a short time (hours).

The removal of hairs before surgical interventions has to take place immediately before the surgery. This is achieved either by wet shaving or a hair removal cream. Shaving of the surgical area on the day before surgery is not permitted as this would increase the number of germs and, hence, the risk of infection.

Wound Drainage

After abdominal or vaginal hysterectomy, the vaginal stump should not be closed completely. Insertion of a T-tube for 24 hours permits the drainage of wound secretion without increasing the risk of ascending microbes. The insertion of a gauze strip (tamponade) promotes the multiplication of germs more than insertion of a drainage tube.

The tamponade should not remain in place for more than 24 hours, preferably less.

Any subfascial Redon drainage should stay in place as short as possible, normally not longer than 24 hours, preferably less.

If the drainage needs to remain for a longer period in the abdominal cavity or in the tissue, the drainage opening should be carefully covered with sterile material, and it should be repeatedly disinfected. It is also important to make sure that there is no backflow of secretion. At the first signs of an infection, early antibiotic treatment with a drug effective against staphylococci is advised, and the drainage tube should be removed soon.

Wound Care

After vaginal hysterectomy and vaginoplasty, it is not uncommon that the high numbers of bacteria present in the vagina lead to superficial infection of the wound area, which is further promoted by necrotic tissue and wound secretion. Early rinsing of the wound with a 1:100 dilution of the polyvidone–iodine solution reduces the number of germs and promotes healing.

Sitting baths are largely obsolete and only suitable for superficial wounds. Because of the macerating effect, the duration of a sitting bath should be short. Astringent bath additives, such as tanning agents (Tannolact), yield better results.

Skin infections (e. g., at the suprapubic incision) should be opened early and, depending on the pathogen, rinsed once or twice daily with polyvidone–iodine (*Staphylococcus aureus*) or with hydrogen peroxide (anaerobic bacteria).

The germ-reducing effect of these procedures lasts only for a few hours.

Urinary Diversion

Ascending infections due to an indwelling transurethral catheter are very common. After eight days, about 70–90% of catheterized women exhibit bacteriuria. This may turn into symptomatic cystitis and may also cause bacteria to ascend further. If urinary diversion is supposed to last for more than three days, one should always attempt suprapubic catheterization. The rate of bacteriuria is much lower here, namely, only about 20% after five days. Even after 10 days, the rate increases only to about 30% if the site of the cutaneous incision is being cared for properly.

Approach:

- careful disinfection of the urethra prior to catheterization
- transurethral catheters should stay in place as short as possible; in case of simple interventions, they should be removed once the anesthesia subsides—after 24 hours, at the latest
- if a longer stay is required, suprapubic catheterization is advised
- closed diversion systems, which do not lead to reflux of urine, should be used.

Prophylaxis of Bacterial Infections

The introduction of antibiotic prophylaxis for patients undergoing hysterectomy and cesarean section has reduced the infection risk by a factor of three to four.

Objective for antibiotic prophylaxis. Whether or not antibiotic prophylaxis should be used depends also on the frequency of infections in the individual clinic.

When deciding whether or not to use antibiotics for preventing infections, one should be guided by the type of intervention as well as the patient's condition. Patients who suffer from several systemic diseases—such as diabetes mellitus, obesity, and suspected immunodeficiency (age, cancer, AIDS, condition after transplantation)—should always receive antibiotics even if the intervention is minor.

In principle, it is safer to use antibiotic prophylaxis. Of course, it may not prevent all infections, particularly not late infections.

In addition to preventing the more common but mild infections, which nevertheless may bother the patient, the main purpose is to reduce the rare but serious infectious complications that occasionally lead to death and occur almost exclusively in patients who have undergone surgery without antibiotic prophylaxis. These cases then tend to be called "fateful events."

The **type** of the antibiotic used as well as the duration of prophylaxis are of secondary importance, the purpose of prophylaxis being to reduce the germs in the surgical area to such an extent that no infection will occur in the deeper regions.

The antibiotic used does not need to be effective against all potential microbes, since it is frequently the synergism between aerobic and anaerobic microbes that leads to wound infection and, finally, sepsis.

Thus, a considerable reduction in postoperative infections has also been achieved by using substances effective only against aerobes, or those effective only against anaerobes.

The **duration** of prophylaxis is also of secondary importance. In today's view, a high level of antibiotic at the time of surgery is all that is required. Antibiotic prophylaxis for more than 24 hours, or even for three or five days, has been abandoned because it does not yield better results and, apart from higher costs, carries the risk of microbial selection.

Likewise, the half-life of the antibiotic used is of secondary importance. Nevertheless, there is a slight difference in the frequency of, for example, urinary tract infections. The rate is lower for an antibiotic with a long half-life (e. g., ceftriaxone) than for an antibiotic with a comparable spectrum but a half-life of only one hour (e. g., cefotiam).

If the surgery takes longer than three to four hours, single-dose antibiotics with longer half-lives seem to be better, especially when one is not only looking for wound infections but also for postoperative pneumonia and other infections that should definitely be regarded as infectious complications caused by surgery. Postoperative pneumonia develops when the pathogen has been introduced during intubation and when postoperative ventilation during the first days after surgery has been poor.

As most gynecological interventions last only one to three hours, administering a single dose of an antibiotic with a short half-life (one hour) will suffice in most cases. If the intervention takes more time, one may administer a second dose or shift to an antibiotic with a longer half-life. Slow instillation of the antibiotic during the entire intervention is also possible, thus ensuring a high antibiotic level for as long as necessary.

Indications:

- vaginal hysterectomy with vaginoplasty
- abdominal hysterectomy
- extensive oncological abdominal surgery
- cesarean section (antibiotic can be administered after cutting the umbilical cord)
- surgical vaginal delivery in the presence of a disturbed vaginal flora
- patients with a valvular defect are at risk of endocarditis due to bacteria introduced during normal spontaneous delivery or surgical interventions
- patients with plastic implants are at risk as staphylococci are able to adhere to the implant
- spontaneous delivery by women who have already lost a child due to infection with group B streptococci during a previous delivery.

Also in women undergoing so-called clean interventions, in which the vaginal region is not touched (e. g., intervention in the adnexal region or in the breast region), wound infections of the skin—which are found in about 5% of these patients—can be largely prevented by single-dose antibiotic prophylaxis.

Single-dose antibiotic prophylaxis does not cause a selection of germs. If antibiotics are used that are well tolerated and have a low rate of adverse effects, the benefits greatly outweigh the risks.

Immunoprophylaxis of Viral Infections

The best prophylaxis against viral infections is vaccination with live attenuated pathogens (p. 243). However, this is no longer possible during pregnancy. Here, temporary immunity may be achieved as a preventive measure by administering specific immune globulins before exposure, or even a short time after exposure. The effect depends on the amount of antibodies applied and the time of application, with the protection being the greater the earlier the immune globulin is administered (for details, see individual infections).

Chemoprophylaxis of Viral Infections

Chemoprophylaxis plays a role especially during pregnancy. It is presently used in case of HIV infection (see p. 178). It is recommended for certain forms of genital herpes, otherwise only for very frequently recurring genital herpes (suppression therapy).

Approach in the Event of Professional Exposure to HIV

(Postexposure Prophylaxis, PEP)

Risk. The risk of infection is about 0.3% in the event of stabs or cuts, and about 0.03% in case of contamination of injured skin, the eyes, or the mouth.

Emergency procedures:

- stimulation of blood flow in case of injury, then disinfection (e.g., with an ethanol–propanol solution)
- intensive rinsing with water in the event of mucosal contact, possibly with diluted polyvidone–iodine solution.

Chemoprophylaxis (if possible, within two to 72 hours):

- risk assessment, depending on the type of injury and the viral load of the patient
- chemotherapy is recommended in case of deep injury, and also when the puncture needle is long and the viral load high
- chemotherapy should be offered in case of superficial injury, stab with surgical needle, or mucosal contact
- no chemotherapy in case of contact with intact skin, or mucosal contact with urine or saliva.

Drugs. Combivir (cidovuline/lamivudine) 2 × 1 tablet + Kaletra (lopinavir/ritonavir) 2 × 3 capsules for 28 days.

Further measures:

- collection of blood for documentation of the initial status
- documentation of the accident
- report of accident to company and insurance
- close medical follow-up with laboratory tests and virology.

Ocular Prophylaxis in Newborns

Pathogen. The child may pick up a whole series of pathogens from the mother when passing through the birth canal, with the eyes being particularly susceptible. Especially dreaded is infection with *gonococci*, since it may lead to blindness of the newborn. Far more common is infection with *Chlamydia trachomatis*, which affects about 1% of all newborns. Other pathogens, such as staphylococci (especially *Staphylococcus aureus*), streptococci, and *Haemophilus influenzae*, may also lead to eye infection of the newborn.

At present, the role of eye infections caused by other pathogens transmitted during birth is largely unknown.

It should be possible to reduce any risk by paying more attention to the vaginal flora during the pregnancy and by initiating timely sanitation, if necessary.

Prophylaxis. *Credé prophylaxis* with *0.5–1% silver nitrate solution* has been introduced over 100 years ago for preventing gonococcal conjunctivitis. It is also fairly effective against *Staphylococcus aureus*, but only moderately effective against *Chlamydia*. For this reason, some experts recommend ocular prophylaxis with *1% tetracycline solution* or *0.5% erythromycin solution*. The disadvantage of these treatments is their low effectiveness against staphylococci and *Enterobacteriaceae*. They are usually fairly effective against gonococci.

In general, Credé prophylaxis for preventing gonococcal conjunctivitis is no longer justified in many countries since gonococcal infections during pregnancy have become rare (estimated frequency: < 0.05%).

Gonorrhea is easy to treat these days. In most patients, a single antibiotic dose suffices to treat the mother. It is therefore simply no longer in keeping with the times to administer gonococcal prophylaxis to 99.9% of newborns who do not need it, while overlooking the gonorrhea of the mother because this disease has not been considered.

Only in isolated cases should Credé ocular prophylaxis still be administered, namely, when the social conditions are poor, proper prenatal care has not been provided, and the follow-up care of the newborn is not guaranteed.

Likewise, ocular prophylaxis for preventing chlamydial conjunctivitis does not solve the problem of transmitting a chlamydial infection to the child, because the child's lungs and genitals may be affected in addition to the eyes. The risk of neonatal infection is only eliminated and chronic neonatal infection is only prevented if the chlamydial cervicitis of the mother is recognized and treated before delivery.

Tuberculosis Vaccination of Newborns

Tuberculosis and, hence, the risk for newborns to contract tuberculosis have become so rare that vaccination is no longer recommended

Even some years ago, newborns were still receiving upon discharge from the clinic a live attenuated vaccine (Bacillus Calmette–Guérin

Table 15.1 Vaccination during pregnancy

	Live vaccine (attenuated microbe)	Inactivated vaccine (killed microbe) or toxoid vaccine (toxin of microbe)
1. Permitted	Poliomyelitis	Poliomyelitis Tetanus Influenza
2. Permitted under certain conditions	Yellow fever (only at official vaccination office) Typhoid fever, oral (Typhoral L, Vivotif Berna)	Rabies Hepatitis B Hepatitis A Cholera Central European encephalitis (CEE)
3. Not permitted	Rubella, measles, mumps, tuberculosis, smallpox, chickenpox	

strain, BCG) by strictly intracutaneous injection of 10^5 bacteria into the thigh. Vaccination reaction was expected after about six weeks. Severe complications have been very rare; as with all live vaccinations, complications may occur in case of immunodeficiency.

Nevertheless, newborns with an increased risk due to their surroundings should still be vaccinated even today.

Vaccination of adults who have an increased risk of infection is only permitted these days after tuberculin testing with negative results.

Vaccination During Pregnancy

Prohibition or conditional permission of vaccination are just measures of precaution (Table 15.**1**). The exception is variola vaccination (smallpox), which is no longer necessary.

Even after rubella vaccination, there has been no confirmed case of bodily harm.

Hence, accidental vaccination during pregnancy should not worry the patient, and there is no reason for terminating the pregnancy.

For reasons of precaution, it is important to consider whether vaccination at this time is necessary if vaccination is only permitted under certain conditions. A low rate of adverse effects cannot be excluded for any vaccination.

During pregnancy, these adverse effects are taken seriously by the affected women because they fear for their child.

Vaccines

Relevance and Indication

Vaccination plays a decisive role in the prevention of viral infections and, therefore, also in the fight against diseases caused by viruses. So far, there are hardly any effective and well-tolerated therapeutic drugs, and these will not be available in the near future. This disadvantage is somewhat compensated by the possibility of developing effective and well-tolerated vaccines especially against viruses.

Bacteria are less suited as a vaccine material because of their size and antigenic diversity.

Only when the vaccine contains bacterial constituents—namely, toxins rendered into harmless toxoids by special treatment, as in the case of tetanus and diphtheria—is it well tolerated and effective. Even vaccination against whooping cough clearly causes fewer side effects since the introduction of acellular pertussis vaccine.

The eradication of viral diseases by vaccination is not easily achieved—with the exception of smallpox, which has been a dreaded, easily recognized disease that occurred only in humans.

Regular and continued vaccination is therefore the only chance to keep the damage caused by certain viral diseases as low as possible (Table 15.**2**).

Types of Vaccine

- Inactivated vaccine (dead viruses or bacteria, toxoids, pathogen subunits).
- Live vaccine (attenuated pathogen, which is less virulent but still able to reproduce).

Nonresponders. Not every person shows a measurable antibody response after vaccination with either live or inactivated vaccine. The response rate ranges from 5% to 10%. It is determined by the vaccine itself (e. g., instability, immunogenicity), but also by the genetic code of the individual vaccinated (e. g., the threshold for infections or reactions). Only in rare cases will a double dose of vaccine yield a better result.

Table 15.**2** Vaccination recommendations for children and adults

Vaccination of infants, children, and adolescents
according to the vaccination recommendations by the standing vaccination committee (STIKO) at the Robert Koch Institute

Vaccination age	Vaccination	Vaccination age	Vaccination
At birth	Simultaneous vaccination (active + passive) against hepatitis B if the mother is HBsAg-positive	From 13th month onward	4th diphtheria–pertussis–tetanus + 3rd hepatitis B + 3rd poliomyelitis trivalent + 3rd *Haemophilus influenzae* type b
From 3rd month onward	1st diphtheria–pertussis–tetanus–*Haemophilus influenzae* type b + 1st hepatitis B + 1st poliomyelitis trivalent	From 11th to 14th months	1st measles–mumps–rubella (live vaccine)
From 4th month onward	2nd diphtheria–pertussis–tetanus	From 6th year onward	5th tetanus–diphtheria (1st booster vaccination)
From 5th month onward	3rd diphtheria–pertussis–tetanus + 2nd hepatitis B + 2nd poliomyelitis trivalent + 2nd *Haemophilus influenzae* type b	From 9th to 17th years	6th tetanus–diphtheria (2nd booster) 4th hepatitis B (1st booster) 2nd (1st) rubella (all girls) Varicella (if no history of VZV)
		From 13th year onward	1st hepatitis B (3 injections) for all those not vaccinated

Vaccination recommendations for adults

Disease	Who should be vaccinated?	Disease	Who should be vaccinated?
Hepatitis A (3 × inactive)	Everyone, if possible, particularly when traveling to endemic countries; risk of infection (laboratory staff, infectologists, sewage workers, child care facilities); check immune status prior to vaccination	**Poliomyelitis** (m × inactive)	Everyone, particularly when traveling to endemic countries; booster vaccination every 10 years
Hepatitis B (3 × GM)	Everyone, if possible, particularly health care professionals, relatives of infectious patients; persons at sexual risk	**Influenza** (m × inactive)	Always offered to high-risk patients; everyone in case of a threatening epidemic
Tetanus (m × toxoid)	Booster vaccination every 10 years, in case of injuries already after five years	**Diphtheria** (m × toxoid)	Booster vaccination every 10 years
CEE (3 × inactive)	Persons in endemic countries, forest workers	**Tuberculosis** (1 × live)	Health care professionals (only if tuberculin test is negative, e. g., tine test)
Measles/ Mumps (1 × live)	Seronegative personnel at pediatric and child care facilities; check immune status prior to vaccination	**Rabies** (3 × inactive)	Persons with professional and recreational risks; also after exposure
Varicella (1 × live)	As with measles and mumps	**Yellow fever** (1 × live)	When traveling to endemic countries; vaccination only at official vaccination office.
Rubella (1 × live)	Women who want children, if negative or HAH titer < 16; personnel (including men) in pediatric and child care facilities; check immune status prior to vaccination	**Pneumococci** (m × toxoid)	High-risk persons with systemic diseases, persons over 60

GM, genetically modified vaccine; m, multiple administrations.

Officially recommended vaccinations*

Without age limitation	From 3rd month of life onward	From 13th month onward	High-risk groups
– Hepatitis A – Hepatitis B – Influenza – CEE – *Haemophilus influenzae* type b	– Tetanus – Diphtheria – Pertussis – Varicella – Poliomyelitis	– Measles – Mumps – Rubella	– Rabies – Tuberculosis – Pneumococci

* In Germany, the risk is carried also by the government.

Inactivated Vaccine

Advantages:
- few adverse effects
- few contraindications
- may be administered during pregnancy with some restrictions.

Disadvantages:
- repeated application is required
- effectiveness and duration of protection are lower than with live vaccines
- local reaction is possible due to the adjuvant.

Vaccines on the market. Influenza (subunits, or split virion), hepatitis A, hepatitis B, CEE, polio (IPV, inactivated poliovirus vaccine according to Salk), tetanus, diphtheria, pertussis, *Haemophilus influenzae*, pneumococci (the indications include immunodeficiency, hyposplenism or asplenia, increased exposure, persons over 60), rabies (only high-risk persons).

Some inactivated vaccines are now being produced using gene technology (hepatitis B, *Haemophilus influenzae*). The advantages include excellent tolerability, absence, or reduction of the risk of contamination with other pathogens, and cost-effective manufacturing.

Live Vaccine

At present, most vaccinations against viral diseases are carried out with live vaccines. These contain viruses that are still able to reproduce, though their virulence has been reduced. Live vaccines are applied at a low dose, thus causing a mild infection that usually leads to lifelong immunity.

Live vaccines are also available for some bacterial infections, namely, against tuberculosis (BCG vaccine), typhoid fever (Ty21 a vaccine), and cholera (CVD 103HgR vaccine).

Live vaccines may be combined. Available are, for example, measles–mumps–rubella, and measles–mumps–rubella–varicella.

Advantages:
- highly effective
- lifelong protection in most patients
- single application.

Disadvantages:
- adverse effects (weak symptoms of the disease may occur)
- contraindicated during pregnancy
- interference with other viruses is possible, although this plays a minor role
- vaccines *must be* stored in a cool place.

Vaccines on the market. Measles, mumps, rubella (also available as trivalent vaccine), varicella (Oka strain), polio (trivalent vaccine against all three types; tuberculosis (BCG), typhoid fever (Ty21 a), and cholera (CVD 103HgR).

Vaccinations have become important in gynecology; they are increasingly carried out by the gynecologist or administered upon the advice of the gynecologist.

Vaccines in progress. HPV, toxoplasmosis (recombinant protein), HIV, and herpes simplex.

Drug Interactions

Enzyme Induction

Enzyme induction may reduce the effectiveness of contraceptives in case of the following drugs:
- Analgesics:
  - phenacetin (acetophenetidin)
  - pyrazolone
  - dihydroergotamine.
- Antibiotics:
  - rifampin
  - chloramphenicol
  - nitrofurans, such as nitrofurantoin
  - ampicillin
  - phenoxymethyl penicillin
  - sulfonamides, such as sulfasalazine, Co-Trimoxazole
  - tetracyclines, such as doxycycline.
- Barbiturates and almost all anticonvulsives, antipsychotics, and tranquilizers
- Lipid-lowering drugs:
  - clofibrate
  - cholestyramine
- Ion exchangers, such as polystyrolsulfonate.

Prolongation of the Q–T interval. Many drugs (antidepressives, antihistamines, neuroleptics, antiarrhythmics, tamoxifen, etc.) and also antibiotics (penicillins, macrolides, fluoroquinolones, Co-Trimoxazole, malaria drugs, etc.) may be causing this.

Metronidazole inhibits the activity of alcohol-degrading dehydrogenases.

The damaging effect of *itraconazole* on the liver is increased by alcohol.

15

Table 15.**3** Antibiotics during pregnancy and breast-feeding

Antibiotic	Risk		Transmission to milk
	Mother	Child	
1. Permitted			
Penicillins	Allergy	Nothing is known	Yes
Cephalosporins	(Allergy)	Nothing is known	Traces
Erythromycin base	(Allergy)	Nothing is known	Yes
2. Permitted with restrictions or to be used with caution			
Aminoglycosides	Ototoxicity, nephrotoxicity	Toxic to cranial nerve III	Yes (minimal resorption)
5-Nitroimidazole (metronidazole etc.)	Theoretical risk	Nothing is known	Yes
Sulfonamides	Allergy	Bilirubin increase, hemolysis (G6PD* deficiency)	Yes
Clindamycin	Allergy, pseudomembranous colitis	Nothing is known	Traces
Nitrofurantoin	Neuropathies	Hemolysis (G6PD* deficiency)	Yes
3. Not permitted			
Tetracyclines	(Liver toxicity)	Dental discoloration 4th months of pregnancy and later	Yes (minimal resorption)
Fluoroquinolones	Allergy	Theoretical risk (cartilage damage in growing dogs)	Yes
Erythromycin estolate	Liver toxicity	Nothing is known	Yes
Co-Trimoxazol	Vasculitis	Folic acid antagonism, congenital malformations (animal experiments)	Yes
Chloramphenicol	Agranulocytosis	Gray syndrome	Yes

* Glucose-6-phosphate dehydrogenase.

Malabsorption

Changes in the intestinal flora due to oral antibiotic treatment may cause a reduction in the resorption of hormone preparations (see p. 46). Together with enzyme induction, this may weaken the effect of ovulation inhibitors. In case of prolonged antibiotic treatment (more than eight days), this special risk needs to be pointed out to the patient. Perhaps, the dose of the ovulation inhibitor needs to be doubled, or other additional precautions have to be taken.

Antibiotics During Pregnancy and Lactation Period

The risk of damaging the child through antibiotics during pregnancy is very low. Most of the concerns are of a theoretical nature (Table 15.**3**). Accidentally administered antibiotics do not justify termination of the pregnancy.

Appendix

References

Ackermann R. Erythema-migrans-Borreliose und Frühsommer-Meningoenzephalitis. Dtsch Ärztebl. 1986; 24:1765–1774.

Allan HH. Bacterial pathogens in postsurgical infections; immunocompromised and normal patients. J Obstet Gynaecol, 6, Suppl. 1. 1986:40–42.

Ayliffe GA. Surgical scrub and skin desinfection. Infect Control. 1984; 5:23–27.

Baltzer J, Geißler K, Gloning Ph, Schramm T, Haider M. Clostridien-Infektion im Wochenbett nach vorausgegangener Sectio. Geburtsh u. Frauenheilk. 1989;49: 1010–1013.

Bartlett JG. Anaerobic infections of the pelvis. Clin Obstet Gynecol. 1979;21:351–360.

Bauwens JE, Clark AM, Loeffelholz MJ, Herman SA, Stamm, WE: Diagnosis of chlamydia trachomatis urethritis in men by polymerase chain reaction assay of first-catch-urine. J Clin Microbiol. 1993:3023–3027.

Behr W. Nach Infektionen fahnden – die CRP-Bestimmung: Möglichkeiten und Grenzen. Diagn u Lab. 1989:95–106.

Beichert M. HIV in Gynäkologie und Geburtshilfe. In: HIV und AIDS, ed. Ader G, 5th ed. 2003, 50–63, Springer.

Bell TA, Stamm WE, Pin Wang S, Kuo CC, Holmes KK, Graystone JT. Chronic chlamydia trachomatis infections in infants. J Amer med Ass. 1992;267:400–402.

Ben-Abraham R, Keller N, Vered R, Harel R, Barzilay Z, Paret G. Invasive Group A Streptococcal Infections in a Large Tertiary Center: Epidemiology, Characteristics and Outcome. Infection. 2002;30/2:81–85.

Bergeron Ch, Ferenczy A, Shah K, Haghashfar Z. Multicentric human papillomavirus infections of the female genital tract: Correlation of viral types with abnormal miotic figures, colposcopic presentation, and location. Obstet and Gynecol. 1987;69:736–742.

Bergeron MG et al. Rapid Detection of group B Streptococci in pregnant women at delivery. N Engl Med. 2000;343:175–179.

Bialasiewicz A, Jahn G. Chamlydien-Infektionen. Sicherung der Diagnose über Augenbefunde. Dtsch Ärztebl. 1988;85:34–40.

Blum HE. Hepatitisviren und Leberkarzinom. Dtsch Ärztebl. 1993;90:1832–1836.

Bodmann K-F et al. Antimikrobielle Therapie der Sepsis. Empfehlungen einer Arbeitsgruppe der Paul-Ehrlich-Gesellschaft für Chemotherapie e.V. Chemoth J. 2001;10:43–54

Boege F, Schmidt-Rotte H, Scherberich JE. Harnwegsdiagnostik in der ärztlichen Praxis. Dtsch Ärztebl. 1993;90:1185–1192.

Boppana SB et al. Intrauterine transmission of cytomegalovirus to infants of women with preconceptual immunity. N Engl J Med. 2001;344:1366–1371.

Borelli S, Engst R, von Zumbusch R. Sexuell übertragbare Erkrankungen einschließlich HIV-Infektionen – AIDS. Cologne: Deutscher Ärzteverlag; 1992.

Bredt W. Mycoplasma-Infektionen in der Gynäkologie. Gynäkologe. 1985;18:138–141.

Broermann L, Heidenreich W. Malaria tropica und Schwangerschaft. Geburtsh u Frauenheilk. 1992;52: 624–626.

Brown ZA, Wald A, Morrow RA, Selke S, Zeh J, Corey L. Effect of serologic status and cesarean delivery on transmission rates of herpes simplex virus from mother to infant. JAMA. 2003;289:203–209.

Brunham RC, Binns B, Guijon F. Etiology and outcome of acute pelvic inflammatory disease. J Infect Dis. 1988; 158:510–517.

Bulling E, Schönberg A, Seeliger HP. Infektionen mit Listeria monocytogenes. Dtsch Ärztebl. 1988;85: 957–959.

Burg G, Kettelhack N. Haut und Alkohol. Dtsch Ärztebl. 2002;99:2712–2716.

Cassell, GH, Waites KB, Watson HL, Crouse DT, Harasawa R. Ureaplasma urealyticum intrauterine infection: role in prematurity and disease in newborns. Clin Microbiol Rev. 1993;6:69–87.

Catlin, BW. Gardnerella vaginalis: characteristics, clinical considerations, and controversies. Clin Microbiol Rev. 1992;5:213–237.

Cederqvist LL, Abdel-Latif N, Meyer J, Doctor L. Fetal and maternal humoral immune response to cytomegalovirus infection. Obstet and Gynecol. 1986;67: 214–216.

Chow AW, Jewesson PJ. Pharmacokinetics and safety of anti-microbial agents during pregnancy. Rev Infect Dis. 1985;73:287–313.

Christie SN, McCaughey C, McBride M, Coyle PV. Herpes simplex type 1 and genital herpes in Northern Ireland. Int J sex transm Dis. 1997:68–69.

Clad A, Flecken U, Petersen EE. Chlamydial serology in genital infections: ImmunoComb versus Ipazyme. Infection. 1993:384–389.

Clad A, Flohr F, Petersen EE. Genital isolates of chlamydia trachomatis survive 12 day antibiotic treatment in vitro due to delayed cell lysis. In: Bowie: Chlamydial infections. London: Cambridge University Press; 1990.

Clad A, Freidank H, Plünnecke J, Jung B, Petersen EE. Comparison of a new C. trachomatis IgG specific serology test with the microimmunofluorescence test (MIF). 10th ISSTDR Meeting, Helsinki, 1993:83.

Daffos F, Forestier F, Chapella-Pavlovsky M et al. Prenatal management of 746 pregnancies at risk for congenital toxoplasmosis. New Engl J Med. 1988;218:271–275.

Daschner F. Antibiotika am Krankenbett, 3rd ed. Berlin: Springer; 1986.

Desmonts G, Forestier F, Thulliez P, Daffos F, Capella-Pavlovsky M, Chartier M. Prenatal diagnosis of congenital toxoplasmosis. Lancet. 1985;II:500–503.

Dettenkofer M, Jonas D, Wiechmann C et al. Infection. 2002;30:282–285.

Diague N. et al. Increased susceptibility to malaria during the early postpartum period. N Engl J Med 2000;343:651–652.

Dietrich M, Kern P. Tropenlabor. Diagnostik für die ärztliche Praxis mit einfacher Laborausrüstung. Stuttgart: Fischer; 1983.

Dore GJ, Freeman AJ, Law M, Kalder JM. Is severe liver disease a common outcome for people with chronic hepatitis C? Gastroentero Hepatolog. 2002;17:423–430.

Dupuis O et al. Herpes simplex encephalitis in pregnancy. Obstet Gynecol. 1999;94:810–812.

Eggers HJ. Antivirale Chemotherapie. Dtsch Ärztebl. 1991;88:1882–1887.

Eiermann W, Tsutsulopulos C. Die non-puerperale Mastitis. 1987;FAC 6-2:401–405.

Elsner P, Martius J, eds. Vulvovaginitis. New York: Dekker; 1993.

Enders G. Infektionen und Impfungen in der Schwangerschaft. Munich: Urban & Schwarzenberg; 1988.

Enders, G. Röteln und Ringelröteln. In: Friese K, Kachel W, eds. Infektionskrankheiten der Schwangeren und des Neugeborenen. Berlin, Heidelberg: Springer; 1998:67–89.

Enders G, Braun R. Prä- und peripartale Übertragung des Hepatitis C-Virus. Internist. 2000;7:676–678.

Eschenbach DA. Vaginal infection. Clin Obst Gynecol. 1983;26:186.

Eschenbach DA. Lower genital tract infections, In: Galask RP, Larsen B. Infectious Disease in the Female Patient. Berlin: Springer; 1986.

Evans AA, Bortuolussi R, Issekutz TB, Stinson DA. Follow-up study of survivors of fetal and early onset neonatal listeriosis. Clin Invest Med. 1984;7:329–334.

Farley, TMM, Rosenberg MJ, Rowe PJ, Chen HJ, Meirik O. Intrauterine devices and pelvic inflammatory disease: an international perspective. Lancet. 1992;339:785–788.

Fischbach F, Petersen EE, Weissenbacher ER, Martius J, Hosmann J, Mayer H. Efficacy of Clindamycin vaginal cream versus oral metronidazole in the treatment of bacterial vaginosis. Obstetrics and Gynecology. 1993;82:405–410.

Fleischer B. Superantigene: Schock und Immunsuppression als Folge der T-Zell-Stimulation. Gelb. H. 1991;41:141–147.

Fleming AD, Ehrlich DW, Miller NA, Monif, GRG. Successful treatment of maternal septicemia due to listeria monocytogenes at 26 weeks' gestation. Obstet and Gynecol. 1985;66:52–53.

Fleming DW, Cochi SL, MacDonald KL et al. Pasteurized milk as a vehicle of infection in an outbreak of listeriosis. New Engl J Med. 1985;312:404–407.

Ford LC, Quan WL, Lagasse LD. Recommendations for the use of antibiotics in gynaecological oncology. J Obstet Gynaecol. Suppl 1. 1986:42–44.

Foulon W, Pinon JM, Stray-Pedersen B et al. Prenatal diagnosis of congenital toxoplasmosis: a multicenter evaluation of diffferent diagnostic parameters. Am J Obstet Gynecol. 1999 Oct;181(4):843–7.

Foulon W, Villena I, Stray-Pedersen B et al. Treatment of toxoplasmosis during pregnancy: a multicenter study of impact on fetal transmission and children's sequelae at age 1 year. Am J Obstet Gynecol. 1999; 180:410–5.

Friese K. Die medikamentöse Behandlung der sexuell übertragbaren Krankheiten. Gynäkologe. 1988;21:31–38.

Friese K, Schäfer A, Hof H. Infektionskrankheiten in Gynäkologie und Geburtshilfe. Springer, Berlin 2003.

Frösner GG. Hepatitis B – auch eine Partnerinfektion. Gynäkologe. 1985:18:151–155.

Galask RP, Larsen B. Infectious Diseases in the Female Patient. Berlin, New York: Springer; 1986.

Gastmeier P, Kampf G, Wischnewski N et al. Prevalence of nosocomial infections in representative German hospitals. J Hosp Infect. 1998;38:37–49.

Gaytant MA, Steegers EA et al. Seroprevalence of Herpes Simplex Virus Type 1 and Type 2 Among Pregnant Women in the Netherlands. Sexl Transm Dis. 2002;29/11:710–714.

Gerken G, Meyer zum Büschenfelde KH. Virushepatitis von A bis E. Gelb. H. 1992;32:97–106.

Gershon AA. Live attenuated varicella vaccine. Int J inf Dis. 1977;1:130–134.

Gerstner GJ, Schmid R. Infektionsprophylaxe bei vaginalen Hysterektomien mit Metronidazol. Geburtsh u Frauenheilk. 1982;42:269–272.

Gibb DM et al. Mother-to-child transmission of the Hepatitis C virus: evidence for preventable peripartum transmission. Lancet. 2000;89:904–907.

Gibbs R. Microbiology of the female genital tract. Amer J Obstet Gynecol. 1987;156:491–495.

Gibbs R. The relationship between infections and adverse pregnancy outcomes: An overview. Ann Periodontol. 2001;6:153–163.

Gilbert RE, Tookey PA. Perinatal mortality and morbidity among babies delivered in water: surveillance study and postal survery. Brit Med J. 1999;319.

Göppinger A, Ikenberg H, Birmelin G, Hilgarth M, Pfleiderer A, Hillemanns HG. CO_2-Lasertherapie und HPV-Typisierung bei CIN-Verlaufsbeobachtungen. Geburtsh u Frauenheilk. 1988;48:343–345.

Grab D, Kittelberger M, Flock F. Kindliche Entwicklung nach maternaler Ringelrötelninfektion in der Schwangerschaft. Gyn. 2002;7:299–303.

Granitzka S. Epidemiologie der Gonorrhoe. In: Sexuell übertragbare Krankheiten, Hahnenklee-Symposion. Basel: Editiones Roche; 1985.

Graystone JT. Infections caused by Chamydia pneumoniae strain TWAR. Clin Infect Dis. 1992;15:757–763.

Griffiths PD, Baboonian C. A prospective study of primary cytomegalovirus infection during pregnancy: final report. Brit J Obstet Gynaecol. 1984;91:307–315.

Groß U, Roos T, Friese F. Toxoplasmose in der Schwangerschaft. Dtsch Ärztebl. 2001;98/49:B2778–2783.

Gsell O, Krech U, Mohr W. Klinische Virologie. Munich: Urban & Schwarzenberg; 1986.

Gürtler L. AIDS: Welche Tests sichern die Diagnose? Diagn. 1987;37:157–167.

Hahn H. Physiologie und Pathologie der zellulären Immunität bei der Infektionsabwehr. In: Krasemann C. Infektiologisches Kolloquium 2: Der abwehrgeschwächte Patient. Berlin: De Gruyter; 1984:47–59.

Hahn H, Falke D, Klein P. Medizinische Mikrobiologie. Berlin, Heidelberg, New York: Springer; 1991.

Handrick W, von Eiff C. Durch Staphylococcus aureus verursachtes Toxic-shock-Syndrom. Gynäkologe. 2002;35:81–86.

Hankins GD, Cunningham FG, Luby JP, Butler SL, Stroud J, Roark M. Asymptomatic genital excretion of herpes simplex virus during early labor. Amer J Obstet Gynecol. 1984;150:100–101.

Harger JD, English DH. Selection of patients for antibiotic prophylaxis. Amer J Obstet Gynecol. 1981;141: 752–758.

Haustein UF. Pyrethrine und Pyrethroide (Permethrin) in der Behandlung von Skabies und Pediculosis. Hautarzt. 1991;41:453–455.

Haverkorn ML. A comparison of single-dose and multidose metronidazole prophylaxis for hysterectomy. J Hosp Infect. 1987;9:249–254.

Hawkins DF. Antimicrobial drugs in pregnancy and adverse effects on the fetus. J Obstet Gynaecol. Suppl. 1. 1986;6:11–24.

Heeg K, Miethke T, Wagner H. Neue Perspektiven zur Pathophysiologie der grampositiven Sepsis. Dtsch. Ärztebl. 1995; 92:A:1177–1180.

Hemmer CJ, Lafrenz M, Lademann M, Lösch R, Reisinger EC. Rechtzeitig auch an eine Infektion mit Plasmodien denken. Klinikarzt. 2003;32/6:208–213

Hemsell DL, Johnson ER, Bawdon RE et al. Ceftriaxone and Cefazolin prophylaxis for hysterectomy. Surg Gynecol Obstet. 1985;161:197–203.

Hemsell DL, Mensell PG, Heard MC, Nobles BJ. Infektionsprophylaxe nach Hysterektomie und Kaiserschnitt. FAC 6 – 2. 1987:357–363.

Hernández-Dias et al. Folic acid antagonist during pregnancy and the risk of birth defects. N Engl J Med. 2000;343:1608–14.

Hess G, Gross G. Sexuelle Übertragung der Hepatitisviren. Hautarzt. 1991;42:347–349.

Higa K, Dan K, Manabe H. Varicella-zoster virus infections during pregnancy: Hypothesis concerning the mechanisms of congenital malformations. Obstet and Gynecol. 1987;69:214–222.

Hill GB, Ayers OA. Antimicrobial susceptibilities of anaerobic bacteria isolated from female genital tract infections. Antimicrob Agents Chemother. 1985;27: 324–331.

Hirsch HA. Harnwegsinfektionen in der Schwangerschaft. Dtsch med Wschr. 1987;112:45–46.

Hirsch HA. Harnwegsinfektionen in der Gynäkologie und Geburtshilfe. FAC 6 – 2. 1987:333–338.

Hirsch HA, Niehues U. Mütterliche Morbidität nach Sectio: Einfluß von Infektionskontrolle und Antibiotikaprophylaxe. Geburtsh u Frauenheilk. 1988;48:1–7.

Hirschberger R, Schaefer K. Syndrom des toxischen Schocks. Dtsch med Wschr. 1983;108: 912–917.

Hof H, Ulbricht A, Stehle G. Listeriosis – a puzzling disease. Infection. 1992;20:290–292.

Hof H, Nichterlein T, Ulbricht A, Stehle G. Die Listeriose der Erwachsenen – eine Lebensmittelinfektion? Dtsch Ärztebl. 1993;90:262–265.

Holst E, Goffeng AR, Andersch B. Bacterial vaginosis and vaginal microorganisms in idiopathic premature labor and association with pregnancy outcome. J Clin Microbiol. 1994:176–186.

Huch R. Hepatitis C und Stillen, Empfehlung der Nationalen Stillkommission in Abstimmung mit der Gesellschaft für pädiatrische Gastroenterologie und Ernährung und der Deutschen Gesellschaft für pädiatrische Infektiologie. Gynäkol Praxis. 2002;26:31–34.

von Hugo R, Muck BR, Graeff G, Zander J. Kasuistische Beispiele lebensbedrohlicher Infektionen im Wochenbett. Geburtsh u Frauenheilk. 1982;42:666–671.

Ikenberg H. Der Stellenwert der Papillomviren und ihre Diagnostik bei der Vorsorge. Therapeutische Umschau. 2002;59:489–494.

Jenum PA, Stray-Pedersen B et al. Incidence of Toxoplasma gondii Infection in Norway. J Clin Microbiol. 1998;36:2900–2906.

Jilg W. Die aktive Schutzimpfung gegen Hepatitis A. Dtsch Ärztebl. 1992;89:2113–2114.

Jilg W. Gründe für eine generelle Impfung gegen Hepatitis B. Dtsch Ärztebl. 1996;93:2435–2439.

Jilg W. Immunisierung gegen Hepatitis A. Gelb. H. 1992;32:107–118.

Jilg W, Deinhardt F. Schutzimpfung gegen Hepatitis B. Dtsch Ärztebl. 1988;85:791–795.

Jochun M, Fritz H, Nast-Kolb D, Inthorn D. Granulozyten-Elastase als prognostischer Parameter. Dtsch Ärztebl. 1990;87:1106–1110.

Kaufhold A, Podbielski A, Kühnemund O, Lütticken R: Infektionen durch Streptococcus pyogenes: neuere Aspekte zur Diagnostik, Epidemiologie, Klinik und Therapie. Immun u Infekt. 1992;20:192–199.

Klebanoff MA. et al. Failure of metronidazole to prevent preterm delivery among pregnant women with asymptomatic Trichomonas vaginalis infection. N Engl J Med. 2001;345:487–493.

Kleinebrecht J, Fränz J, Windorfer A. Arzneimittel in der Schwangerschaft und Stillzeit. Stuttgart: Wissenschaftl. Verlagsges.; 1986.

Klinger JD. Isolation of listeria: a review of procedures and future prospects. Infection. Suppl. 2. 1988;16: 98–104.

Knothe H, Dette GA. Antibiotika in der Klinik, 2nd ed. Munich: Aesopus;1984.

Knörr K. Pränatale und perinatale Virusinfektionen aus gynäkologisch-geburtshilflicher Sicht. Geburtsh u Frauenheilk. 1983;43:701–709.

Koch MG. AIDS. Vom Molekül zur Pandemie. Heidelberg: Spektrum der Wissenschaft; 1987.

Konietzko N, Loddenkemper R (eds). Tuberkulose. Thieme, Stuttgart 1999.

Koppe JG, Loewer-Sieger DH, De Reover-Bonnet H. Results of 20-year follow-up of congenital toxoplasmosis. Lancet. 1986;I:254–255.

Korting HC. Cephalosporin-Therapie der Gonorrhoe. Basel: Karger; 1987.

Kramer A, Fritze F, Klebingat K-J, Rudolph P, Walter H. Zielsetzung und Möglichkeit der Antiseptik im Genitalbereich. Gyn. 1999;4:182–190.

Krause W, Weidner W. Sexuell übertragbare Krankheiten, 2nd ed. Stuttgart: Enke; 1988.

Krech T. Chlamydieninfektionen: Schnellerer Nachweis und gezielte Therapie. Dtsch Ärztebl. 1986;7:394–399.

Kurup M, Goldkran JW. Cervical incompetence: Elective, emergent, or urgent cerclage. Am J Obst Gynecol. 1999;181/2:240–246.

Landthaler M, Braun-Falco O. Vulvitis aus dermatologischer Sicht. FAC 6 – 2. 1987:327–331.

Ledger WJ. Infection in the Female, 2nd ed. Philadelphia: Lea & Febiger; 1986.

Ledger WJ. Diagnose und Therapie schwerer Adnexitis. FAC 6 – 2. 1987:407–415.

Lee HH, Chernesky MA, Schachter J et al. Diagnosis of Chlamydia trachomatis genitourinary infection in women by ligase chain reaction assay of urine. Lancet. 1995;345:213–216.

Lippes J. Pelvic actinomycosis: a review and preliminary look at prevalence. Am J Obstet Gynecol. 1999;180: 265–269.

von Loewenich V. Geburtshilfliches Vorgehen bei Infektionen in der Schwangerschaft (B-Streptokokken, Herpes simplex) aus der Sicht des Pädiaters. Gynäkologe. 1984;17:220.

Luthardt T. Pränatale und perinatale Virusinfektionen. In: Gsell O, Krech U, Mohr W. Klinische Virologie. Munich: Urban & Schwarzenberg;1986:263–274.

Mårdh PA, La Placa J, Ward M. Proceedings of the European Society of Chlamydia Research. Uppsala: Uppsala University Centre for STD-Research; 1992.

Mårdh PA, Moller BR, Ingerselv HJ et al. Endometritis caused by Chlamydia trachomatis. Brit J vener Dis. 1981;57:191–195.

Marre R, Mertens T, Trautmann M, Vanek E. Klinische Infektiologie. Urban & Fischer Munich 2000.

Martius G. Differentialdiagnose in Geburtshilfe und Gynäkologie, 2nd ed., Vol 1. Stuttgart: Thieme; 1987.

Martius J, Hirsch HA. Hämolysierende Streptokokken der Gruppe B in der Geburtshilfe. Gynäkol. u. Geburtsh. 1992:46–48.

McGregor JA, French JI. Chlamydia trachomatis infection during pregnancy. Amer J Obstet Gynecol. 1991;164: 1782–1789.

Mendling W. Puerperalsepsis durch Ovarialvenenthrombophlebitis. Gynäkol Prax. 1987;11:431–435.

Mendling W. Die Vulvovaginal-Kandidose. Theorie und Praxis. Berlin: Springer; 1987.

Mendling W, Bethke A. Oxyuriasis des Eileiters. Gynäkol Prax. 1986;10:711–714.

Mercer BM, Arheart KL. Antimicrobial therapy in expectant management of preterm premature rupture of the membranes. Lancet. 1995;346:1271–1279.

Mertens Th, Zippel C, Seufer R, Eggers HJ. Comparison of four different methods for detection of rubella IgM antibodies. Med Microbiol Immunol. 1983;172:181–189.

Meurer M, Braun-Falco O. Klinik, Diagnostik und Therapie der Syphilis in der Schwangerschaft und bei Neugeborenen. Geburtsh u Frauenheilk. 1987;47: 81–86.

Miller E, Fairley CK, Cohen BJ, Seng C. Immediate and long term outcome of human parvovirus B 19 infection in pregnancy. Br J Obstet Gynaecol. 1998;105: 174–178.

Modrow S. Parvovirus B 19. Dt Ärzteblatt 98 A. 2001: 1620–1624.

Modrow S. Parvovirus B19. Ein Infektionserreger mit vielen Erkrankungsbildern. Dtsch Ärztebl. 2003; 98/24:B1930–1394.

Morales WJ. The effect of chorioamnionitis on the developmental outcome of preterm infants at one year. Obstet and Gynecol. 1987;70: 183–190.

Moulder JW. Interaction of chlamydia and host cells in vitro. Microbiol Rev. 1991;55:143–190.

MSD-Manual der Diagnostik und Therapie, 3rd ed., Munich: Urban & Schwarzenberg; 1984.

Munoz N et al. Epidemiologic classification of human papillomavirus types assiciated with cervical cancer. N Engl J Med. 2003;348:518–526.

Oberpenning F, van Ophoven A, Hertle L. Chronische interstitielle Zystitis. Dtsch Ärztebl 99 A. 2002:204–208.

Oberpenning F, van Ophoven A, Hertle L. Chronische interstitielle Zystitis. Dtsch Ärztebl. 2002;99/4:B163–166.

Ortels S. Zur Bedeutung neuerer Forschungsergebnisse auf dem Gebiet der menschlichen Listeriose. Zbl Gynäkol. 1983;105:1295–1306.

Peters F. Laktation und Stillen. Bücherei des Frauenarztes, Vol. 26. Stuttgart: Enke: 1987.

Peters G. Plastikinfektionen durch Staphylokokken. Dtsch Ärztebl. 1988;85:234–239.

Peters F, Flick-Fillieés D, Diemer P. Stillberatung – auch eine Angelegenheit der Ärzteschaft. Gyn. 2000;5: 183–188.

Petersen EE, Pelz K. Diagnosis and therapy of nonspecific vaginitis. Correlation between KOH-Test, clue cells and microbiology. Scand J Infect Dis. Suppl 40. 1983:97–99.

Petersen EE, Pelz K, Isele T, Fuchs A. Die Aminkolpitis. Diagnose und Therapie. Gyn Prax. 1983;7:447–455.

Petersen EE. Anaerobic vaginosis. Lancet. 1984;II: 337–338.

Petersen EE. Bedeutung der Laktobazillen als Normalflora. Gynäkologe. 1985;18:128–130.

Petersen EE. Die Aminkolpitis. Gynäkologe. 1985;18: 131–135.

Petersen EE. Trichomoniasis. Gynäkologe. 1985;18:136–137.

Petersen EE. Herpes genitalis. Gynäkologe. 1985;18: 163–166.

Petersen EE, Sanabria de Isele T, Pelz K. Infection prophylaxis in cesarean section by a single dose of ceftriaxone. Chemioterapia. 1985;4:742–744.

Petersen EE, Sanabria de Isele T, Pelz K, Hillemanns HG. Die Aminkolpitis, nicht nur ein ästhetisches Problem: Erhöhtes Infektionsrisiko bei Geburt. Geburtsh u Frauenheilk. 1985;45:43–47.

Petersen EE, Sanabria de Isele T, Pelz K. Disturbed vaginal flora as a risk factor in pregnancy. J Obstet Gynaecol. 1986;65:16–18.

Petersen EE. Die Aminkolpitis, nicht nur ein ästhetetisches Problem. FAC 6 – 2. 1987:295–300.

Petersen EE, Schwarz U, Vaith P, Schneider H. AIDS und Frauen; Wandel der Probleme für den Frauenarzt. Geburtsh u Frauenheilk. 1990:50:15–19.

Petersen EE, Wingen F, Fairchild KL et al. Single dose pefloxacin compared with multiple dose co-trimoxazole in cystitis. J Antimicrob Chemotherapy. Suppl. B. 1990:147–152.

Petersen EE. Erkrankungen der Vulva. Stuttgart: Thieme; 1992.

Petersen EE, Clad A. Klinische Bedeutung der Papillomviren in der Gynäkologie: Gynäkologe. 1992;25: 20–25.

Petersen EE, Clemens R, Bock HL, Friese K, Hess G. Hepatitis B and C in heterosexual patients with various sexually transmitted diseases. Infection. 1992;20: 128–131.

Petersen EE. Antibiotikaprophylaxe in der Gynäkologie und Geburtshilfe. Gynäkol u Geburtsh. 1994:1–5.

Petersen EE, Clad A. Genitale Chlamydien-Infektionen. Dt Ärztebl. 1995;92: A:205–210.

Petersen EE, Clad A, Mendel R, Prillwitz J, Hintz K. Prevalence of chlamydial Infections in Germany: Screening of asymptomatic women and men by testing first void urine by Ligase chain reaction. Proceedings third meeting of the European society for chlamydial Research Vienna 11.-14. Sept. 1996: 415.

Petersen EE, Doerr HW, Gross G, Petzoldt D. Weissenbacher ER, Wutzler R. Der Herpes genitalis. Dtsch Ärztebl. 1999;96:2358–2364.

Petersen EE. Bakterielle Infektionen der Vulva. Gynäkologe. 2001;903–906.

Petersen EE. Genitalinfektionen und ihre Diagnostik. Th Umsch. 2002;59/9:447–453.

Potel J. 40 Jahre Listeriose-Forschung in Deutschland. Niedersächs Ärztebl. 1989;19:28–32.

Petzoldt D, Näher H. Immunologisch-serologische Verfahren zum Nachweis von Neisseria gonorrhoeae und Chlamydia trachomatis. In: Sexuell übertragbare Krankheiten. Hahnenklee-Symposion. Basel: Editiones Roche; 1985:135–140.

Preisner W, Berger A, Doerr HW. Therapie viraler Erkrankungen. Dt Ärztebl. 2000;A:3433–3439.

Prince AM. Die Non-A-Non-B-Hepatitis: ein ungelöstes Rätsel. Gelb. H. 1987;27:53–60.

Quentin R, Pierre F, Dubois M, Soutoul JH, Goudeau A. Frequent isolation of capnophilic bacteria in aspirate from Bartholin's gland abscesses and cysts. Europ J Clin Microbiol. 1990;9:138–147.

Reese RE, Douglas, RG. A Practical Approach to Infectious Diseases, 2nd ed. Boston: Little, Brown; 1986.

Reid R, Greenberg M, Jenson B et al. Sexually transmitted papillomaviral infections. Amer J Obstet Gynecol. 1985;156:212–222.

Remington JS, Klein JO: Infectious Disease of the Fetus and the Newborn Infant, 3rd. ed. Philadelphia: Saunders; 1990.

Remington JS, Araujo FG, Desmonts G. Recognition of different toxoplasma antigens by IgM and IgG antibodies in mothers and their congenitally infected newborns. J Infect Dis. 1985;152:1020–1024.

Richardson BA et al. Evaluation of a low dose nonxynol-9 gel for the prevention of sexually transmitted diseases. Sex Transm Dis. 2001;28:394–400.

Roggendorf M, Schwarz TF, Habermehl KO, Maass G. Parvovirus-B 19-Infektionen in der Schwangerschaft. Dtsch Ärztebl. 1988;85:2430.

Rosenthal SL, Cohen SS, Stanberry LR. Topical Microbicides. Current Status and Research Condiserations for Adolescent Girls. Sex Transm Dis. 1998;37725/7:368

Ross L, Mason P, Barnet-Lamb M, Robinson RE. Prophylactic metronidazole in patients with ruptured membranes undergoing emergency caesarean section. J Obstet Gynaecol. 1984;4:32–35.

Rother K. Antiinfektiöse Therapie mit Immunoglobulinen. Gelb. H. 1986;26:97–104.

Sanabrina de Isele T, Pelz K, Petersen EE. Das Keimspektrum bei Aminkolpitis in der Vagina und im Ejakulat. In: Sexuell übertragbare Krankheiten. Hahnenklee-Symposion. Basel: Editiones Roche; 1985:141–147.

Sauerbrei A, Wutzler P. Varicella-Zoster-Virusinfektionen während der Schwangerschaft. Dtsch Ärztebl. 1999;96:B930–933.
Sauerwein RW, Bisseling J, Horrerorts AM. Septic abortion associated with campylobacter fetus subspecies fetus infections. Case report and review of the literature. Infection. 1993;21:331–335.
Schachter J, Gschnait G. Chamydieninfektionen. Z Hautkr. 1985;60:1472–1485.
Schachter J, Sweet RL, Grossman M, Landers D, Robbie M, Bishop E. Experience with the routine use of erythromycin for chlamydial infections in pregnancy. New Engl J Med. 1986;314:276–279.
Schaefer C, Bunjes R. Medikamente in der Schwangerschaft und Stillzeit. Dtsch Ärztebl. 1990; 87:277–289.
Schäfer A, Jovaisas E, Stauber M, Löwenthal D, Koch MA. Nachweis einer diaplazentaren Übertragung von HILV-III/LAV vor der 20. Schwangerschaftswoche. Geburtsh u Frauenheilk. 1986;46:88–89.
Schäfer PA, Friese K. Maßnahmen zur Senkung des maternofetalen HIV-Transmissionsrisikos. Dtsch Ärztebl. 1996;93: A:2234–2236.
Schieve LA, Handler A, Hershow R, Persky V, Davis F. Urinary tract infection during pregnancy: its association with maternal morbidity and perinatal outcome. Am J Public Health. 1994;84,3:405–410.
Schleiermacher D, Puijalon OM. PCR-Genotypisierung von Plasmodium falciparum in der Schwangerschaft. Chemotherapie J. 2002;11:130–136.
Schlesinger P, Duray PH, Burke BA et al. Maternal-fetal transmission of the Lyme disease spirochete, Borrelia burgdorferi. Ann int Med. 1985;103:67–69.
Schleunig M. Parvovirus-B 19-Infektionen. Dtsch Ärztebl. 1996;93:B:2182–2185.
Schmidt-Wolf G, Seeliger HPR, Schrettenbrunner A. Menschliche Listeriose-Erkrankungen in der Bundesrepublik Deutschland, 1969–1985. Zbl Bakteriol I. Abt Orig A. 1987;265:472–486.
Schneider A, Wagner D. Infektionen der Frau mit genitalem humanem Papillomvirus. Dtsch Ärztebl. 1993; 90:530–532.
Schneider A, Schuhmann R, De Villiers EM, Knauf W, Gissmann L. Klinische Bedeutung der humanen Papilloma-Virus-(HPV) Infektionen im unteren Genitaltrakt. Geburtsh u Frauenheilk. 1986;46:261.
Schneider A, Hoyer H, Loth B et al. Screening for high grade cervical intraepithelial neoplasia and cancer by testing for high rish HPV, routine cytology or colposcopy. Int J Cancer. 2000;89:529–534.
Scholz H, Belohradsky BH, Heiniger U, Kreth W, Roos R. Handbuch Infektionen bei Kindern und Jugendlichen. Futuramed Munich, 3rd ed. p. 412–417.
Scholz H, Naber KG und eine Expertengruppe der Paul-Ehrlich-Gesellschaft für Chemotherapie e.V. Einteilung der Oralcephalosporine. Chemotherapie Journal. 1999;6:227–229.
Schwarz TF, Roggendorf M, Deinhardt F. Die Infektion mit dem Erreger der Ringelröteln (Humanes Parvovirus B 19) und ihr Einfluss auf die Schwangerschaft. Dtsch Ärztebl. 1987;49:3365–3368.
Schwarze R, Bauernmeister CD, Ortel S, Wichmann G. Perinatal listeriosis in Dresden 1981–1986: clinical and microbiological findings in 18 cases. Infection. 1989;17:131–138.
Searle K, Guilliard C, Enders G. Parvovirus B 19 diagnosis in pregnant women-quantification of IgG antibody levels (IU/ml) with reference to the international parvovirus B 19 standard serum. Infection. 1997;25: 32–34.
Seufert R, Casper F, Herzog RE, Bauer H. Die Mastitis tuberculosa – Eine seltene Differentialdiagnose der non-puerperalen Mastitis. Geburtsh u Frauenheilk. 1993;53:61–63.
Sheffield JS, Hollier LM, Hill JB, Stuart GS, Wendel GD. Acyclovir prophylaxis to prevent herpes simplex virus recurrence at delivery: A systematic review. Obstetrics & Gynecology 2003;102:1396–1403.
Shirts SR, Brown MS, Bobitt JR. Listeriosis and borreliosis as causes of antepartum fever. Obstet and Gynecol. 1983;62:256–260.
Simon C, Stille W. Antibiotika-Therapie in Klinik und Praxis, 8th ed. Stuttgart: Schattauer; 1993.
Simor AE, Ferro S. Campylobacter jejuni infection occuring during pregnancy. Europ J Clin Microbiol. 1990; 9:142–144.
Slattery MM, Morrison JJ. Preterm delivery. Lancet. 2002;360:1498–1498.
Spiegel CA. Bacterial vaginosis. Clin Microbiol Rev 1991;4:485–502.
Stagno S, Whitley RJ. Herpes simplex virus and varicella-zoster virus infections. (current concepts). New Engl J Med. 1985;313:1327–1330.
Stauber M, Schäfer A, Löwenthal D, Weingart B. Das AIDS-Problem bei schwangeren Frauen – eine Herausforderung an den Geburtshelfer. Geburtsh u Frauenheilk. 1986;46:201.
Striepecke E, Bollmann R. Pseudosulfurgranula (Pseudoaktinomyzesdrusen) bei Intrauterinpessar-Trägerinnen. Geburtsh u Frauenheilk. 1994;54:171–173.
Strohmeyer G, Müller R, Baumgarten R et al. Therapie der chronischen Virus-Hepatitis mit Alpha-Interferon. Dtsch Ärztebl. 1993;90:628–634.
Stüttgen G. Skabies und Läuse heute. Dtsch Ärztebl. 1992;89:956–963.
Svanborg C, Bergsten G, Fischer H et al. The innate host response protects and damages the infected urinary tract. Ann Med. 2001;33:563–570.
Sweet RL, Landers DV, Walker C, Schachter J. Chlamydia trachomatis infection and pregnancy outcome. Amer J Obstet Gynecol. 1987;156:824–833.
Tercanli S, Enders G, Holzgrewe W. Aktuelles Management bei mütterlichen Infektionen mit Röteln, Toxoplasmose, Zytomegalie, Varizellen und Parvovirus B 19 in der Schwangerschaft. Gynäkologe. 1996;29: 144–163.
Thomas E. Labour und Diagnose. 3rd ed. Marburg: Med. Verlagsges.; 1988.
Thorp JM, Hartmann E, Berkman D et al. Antibiotic therapy for the treatment of preterm labour: A review of the evidence. Am J Obstet Gynecol. 2002;186:587–592.
Tietz J-J, Mendling W. Haut- und Vaginalmykosen. Blackwell Berlin 2001.
Vogel F, Scholz H, Al-Nawas B et al. Rationaler Einsatz oraler Antibiotika bei Erwachsenen. Chemotherapie Journal. 2002;11
Vogt A. Heutiger Stand der Syphilis-Diagnostik. Gynäkologe. 1985;18:146–150.
Volkheimer G. Zur Diagnose von Wurmbefall. Diagn Labor. 1986;36:158–172.
Volkheimer G. Intestinale Helminthosen. Krankenhausarzt. 1988;61: 642–656.
Wagner D, Ikenberg H, Böhm N, Gissmann L. Identification of human papillomavirus in cervical swabs by DNA in situ hybridisation. Obstet and Gynecol. 1984;64:767–772.
Wallin KL, Wiklund F, Angström T et al. Type-specific persistence of Human Papillomavirus DNA before the development of invasive cervical cancer. N Engl J Med. 1999;342:1633–1638.
Wallon M et al. Congenital toxoplasmosis: systematic review of evidence of efficacy of treatment in pregnancy. BMI. 1999;318:1511–1514.
Watts DH. Management of Human Immunodeficiency Virus Infection in Pregnancy. N engl J Med. 2002; 346:1879–1891.

Weidner W, Schiefer HG. Urethro-Adnexitis des Mannes und sexuell übertragbare Erreger. Urologe. 1988; A 27:123–131.

Werner H. Anaerobier-Infektionen. 2nd ed. Stuttgart: Thieme; 1985.

Werner H. Anaerobe gramnegative Stäbchen. DGHM-Verfahrensrichtlinien. Stuttgart: Fischer; 1991.

Weström L. The risk of pelvic inflammatory disease in women using intrauterine contraceptive devices as compared to non-users. Lancet. 1976;II:221.

Weström L. Chlamydieninfektionen des weiblichen Genitalbereichs. FAC 6–2. 1987:277–290.

Weström LV. Sexually transmitted diseases and infertility. Sex transmitt Dis. 1994;21:32–37.

Weyers W, Diaz C, Petersen EE. Indikation zur Vulvabiopsie. Gyne. 2002;1.

Whitley RJ, Nahmias AJ, Visintine AM, Fleming CL, Alford CA. The natural history of herpes simplex virus infection of mother and newborn. Pediatrics. 1980;66:489–494.

Wölbling RH, Fuchs J, Milbradt R. Systemische Antimykotika. Arzneimitteltherapie. 1985;3:200–208.

Wright R, Johnson D, Neumann M et al. Congenital lymphocytic choriomeningitis virus syndrome: a disease that mimics congenital toxoplasmosis or cytomegalovirus infection. Pediatrics.1997;100:1–6.

Wutzler P et al. Ist eine Elimination der Varizellen durch eine allgemeine Impfung möglich? Dtsch Ärzteblatt. 2002;99 B:850–856.

Yeager AS. Genital herpes simplex infections: Effect of asymptomatic shedding and latency on management of infections in pregnant women and neonates. J Invest Dermatol. 1984;83:53–56.

Zur Hausen H. Papillomavirus in human cancer. Cancer. 1987;59:1692–1696.

Zur Hausen H. Papillomvirusinfektionen als Ursache des Gebärmutterhalskrebses. Dtsch Ärztebl. 1994;91 B: 1488–1450.

Index

Page references in **bold type** refer to illustrations.

U

V

W

Y

Z